Barbara Steck

Adoption as a Lifelong Process

A Psychiatric Analysis

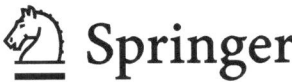 Springer

Barbara Steck
Department of Psychiatry
University of Basel
Basel, Switzerland

ISBN 978-3-031-33040-7   ISBN 978-3-031-33038-4   (eBook)
https://doi.org/10.1007/978-3-031-33038-4

This Springer imprint is published by the registered company Springer Nature Switzerland AG
The registered company address is: Gewerbestrasse 11, 6330 Cham, Switzerland

Preface

Adoption is a significant, socially recognized and legally regulated form of family foundation. It represents an encounter of several life stories: the story of a family unable to raise their child, the story of a child who has lost his parents, and the story of a couple who desires to welcome a child; finally, an institution is responsible for the protection of the child. Adoption is not just a one-time act of accepting a child, but a long-term process that shapes the entire life of adoptive parents and adopted children, as well as biological parents.

Adoption or the fate of children without parents has always aroused lively interest and has been and still is the subject of myths, fairy tales, and novels. The history of adoption is as old as humanity itself. Adoption processes were and remain very different, depending on the location, era, context, and adoption goals. There are great changes today due to the evolution of the family, the society, scientific knowledge, and social protection measures. In the past, adoption was primarily intended to solve inheritance issues. Today, the best interests of the child are of utmost importance. The United Nations Convention defines the needs and rights of a child.

Adoption provides a family and an upbringing for a child who is not directly related to the adopter. Those involved in the adoption situation, a triangle consisting of adoptive parents, adopted child, and biological parents, usually experienced critical life events or personal losses. For the child, it is the loss of his biological family, and very often his cultural, ethnic, and linguistic roots; for the biological parents, it is the loss of their child; for the adoptive parents, it is in most cases the loss of their reproductive capacity. Adoption may represent an opportunity for personal and family development for those affected in this lifelong process, but is a highly complex, unpredictable experience that can be associated with a variety of challenges. Coping with and ultimately working through critical life events is an individual task and depends on multiple intrapsychic and external factors. The subjective experience of difficulties associated with the adoption situation is unique for each subject involved. The individual attribution of meaning and significance to the adoption event helps those concerned creating a sense of continuity in their personal life story, as well as building connections between past, present, and future. The parent-child relationship in adoptive families thus gains a very special quality.

Adoption, a child protection measure, is considered the best solution for the development of a child without a family, compared to the alternatives of placement in a foster family or institution. It guarantees the child a maximum of attachment- and relationship-continuity and legal affiliation.

Adoption is a universal and worldwide tradition, yet the practice has evolved differently according to historical, legal, cultural, and environmental contexts. Adoptive parenting requires specific learning and understanding of the prospective child's preadoption experiences, of his racial, ethnic, linguistic, or cultural origin, and of his need for contact with birth parents or -relatives.

Adoption is a process with continuously changing needs and aspirations of the evolving family members throughout the various life phases. It requires a sincere dialogue between all parties involved and the acceptance of differences between adoptive parents and biological parents, as well as between adopted child and biological child. These prerequisites ensure the creation of a shared history of adoptive parents and adopted children.

The adoption situation presents with multiple risks, such as psychic traumatization and complicated identity formation. On the other hand, adoption has a particularly protective quality, offering opportunities for developmental processes. Research results demonstrate that most adoptees do neither suffer from long-term psychosocial disorders nor need psychiatric treatment. Nevertheless, adopted children are often using child and adolescent psychiatric or psychological services. This fact will hardly change, as older and partly disabled children with personal experiences of neglect, mistreatment, or multiple placements are increasingly accepted for adoption.

For the child, adoption always means breaking off the relationship with biological parents and establishing a new relationship with adoptive parents, a lifelong challenge for all persons involved. For most adoptive parents and adopted children, adoption is a highly gratifying experience. Adoptive parents, however, are confronted with specific problems on the way to realizing their wish for a child and on the common life path with their adopted child. The personal life story of the adopted child, adolescent and young adult is shaped by the adoption situation, raising questions and concerns, expressed in different forms at each stage of development or during developmental transitions. Adoption—like other existential events—brings something unforeseen and unpredictable, as it is linked to many, partly unconscious, personal, and family variables, carrying almost fateful features.

In this book, the historical development of adoption is reviewed. Adoption is regarded as the most comprehensive way, ubiquitously used by society, of ensuring family continuity. Attention is given on self-development and parenthood, new forms of parenthood by reproductive medicine and by surrogacy as alternatives to adoption are mentioned, as well as parenthood of foster children, adoption by sexual and gender minorities and of older children.

Adoption-related stress is an important issue. In young children, regardless of the actual stressors, different types of stress reactions are distinguished, based on their potential to cause lasting physiological disorders. Prenatal stress, stress in infancy

Adoption as a Lifelong Process

and in separation situations, as well as the pain-related aspects of stress and its neuro- and psychobiological effects are discussed.

The scientific literature on adoption is vast and includes studies of interactions of genetic, family, and environmental influences on adopted children's development. Numerous variables such as age, gender, protective, and risk factors are explored, as well as potential vulnerable situations that contribute to the psychosocial adjustment or lead to psychosocial disorders of adopted children. Other works seek to identify key differences in early versus late adopted children, and in national versus international adoptions.

For the child, adoption always represents a filiation breakup with the biological parents as well as a filiation creation with the adoptive parents. Adoption is a life-long process for the biological parents, the adoptive parents, and the child. Their specific challenges are described.

The filiation breakup with biological parents, a potential psychic trauma, early childhood adversities, developmental trauma disorders and its posttraumatic consequences are reviewed. Critical life events are expressed in coping- and grieving processes but may lead to the formation of secrets and be intergenerationally transmitted.

The filiation creation with adoptive parents, revelation of the adoption filiation, loyalty conflicts, identity formation, search of origin and adoptees narratives are discussed; clinical vignettes of adoptees of different age are presented and illustrated by drawings.

The integration of an adoptive child into his new family is a difficult and often turbulent process that requires substantial time, strength, emotional availability, and commitment from adoptive parents. Psychotherapeutic interventions with the adoptive family and adoptive parents are addressed. For the adopted child or adolescent, a psychoanalytical psychotherapy offers a meaningful dialogue and a sustainable relationship within a safe and reliable framework and helps the child to unfold his fantasies and to express his pain and suffering. Psychic processing of traumata attempts to reduce the high intensity of emotional distress, to elaborate meaning and sense of the lived experiences, and to understand its impact on the adoptee's development. The task of the placement agencies is to offer an interdisciplinary team, available for the adopted child, his parents, and the adoptive family, ensuring continuous care and support before adoption, during the care relationship and after the legal adoption.

Basel, Switzerland   Barbara Steck

Acknowledgments

I am very thankful to Gregory Sutorius, senior editor and Melanie Zerah, Editor Clinical Medicine at Springer New York for their personal commitment and support for this project. I express my appreciation to Eric Bernardi for his professional drawing of the figures. Many thanks to the Springer Team, Marie Felina Francois and Rekha Muthusamy, Project Coordinators, for their careful attention to the production of the book.

Many years of work with adoptive families, adopted children, adolescents, and adults led to the desire to present in the framework of a book the challenges faced by all those involved in the adoption process. An earlier book published by Karger in 2007 in German served as a template for this new English book, allowing to review the many societal changes that shape adoption in today's time. Some previously published material of Chaps. 4, 6, 10, 13, 14, and 16 from *Brain and Mind* (2016) is presented.

The multifaceted exchange with professionals, who take care of adoption: child and adolescent psychiatrists, adult psychiatrists, psychologists, psychotherapists, psychoanalysts, educators, schoolteachers, child and adolescent protection- and guardianship authorities, attorneys, placement officials, and adoption commission's members led to a continuous discussion of complex and manifold questions concerning the adoption of a child. The book shows only a subjectively selected excerpt from the much richer experiences in the area of the adoption situation.

My sincere thanks go to all patients: adoptive families, parents, children, adolescents, and adults who enabled me to gain insight into and understanding of their unique situation. Thanks to their trust, openness, and responsiveness, they allowed me to share their personal experiences and emotional burdens, their pain and grief, but also their joy and hope. They gave me insight into their biographical history and their tireless commitment to the adoption relationship, borne of the all-encompassing desire for a successful parent-child encounter.

I am especially grateful to my husband Andreas Steck for his careful lecture of the manuscript and his valuable comments.

For simplification and readability, we use mostly the male form. All names of the clinical vignettes have been changed. Translations are by the author.

Contents

About the Author

Barbara Steck is a lecturer emeritus in Child and Adolescent Psychiatry and Psychotherapy of the University of Basel. She trained in psychoanalysis and family therapy and worked many years in the child and adolescent psychiatric departments of the Universities of Lausanne and Basel and in private practice. Her longtime interest in the fields of adoption, traumatization, grief, and families with ill parents, as well as individual psychotherapy and group psychodrama lead to numerous publications. She is author or co-author of books on adoption, psychosomatics in children and adolescents, indication for psychotherapy for children and adolescents, psychic pain in children and adolescents and with her husband Andreas on brain and mind and on art and creativity. She works as a psychoanalytic therapist and supervisor.

Chapter 1
Introduction: History of Adoption

Aion pais esti paizon. Life is a playing child. Heraclitus of Ephesus, [1] Fragment 52 [1].

This playing child—Heraclitus spoke about more than 2000 years ago—may arouse human beings' desire for parenthood, as it brings existential and essential meaning and significance into their lives.

The word "adoptare" in Latin signifies "to choose" and means to legally name someone as one's own son or daughter. From a historical point of view, adoption can be regarded as the most comprehensive way, ubiquitously used by society, of ensuring family continuity.

Already ancient legends and myths address the needs of adoptees to unveil the mystery of their origins. Let us think of Oedipus, who exclaims: "Break out what will! I at least shall be willing to see my ancestry, though humble." ([2], verses 1232–1233).

The Egyptians and Hebrews tell probably the most famous example of adoption in their legend: Pharaoh's daughter rescues a child, abandoned on the Nile, and calls it her own; his name Moses—in Hebrew Moshe, from "mose" in Ancient Egyptian—means "is born". Finally, Moses, as a grown man, frees his Jewish people from the Egyptian chains and leads it back to its homeland, the promised land.

The adopted child is characterized by a double position, that of an abandoned and at the same time chosen person. In mythology, there are often outstanding people who, due to their double parenthood, were capable of special deeds that fate required. Examples can already be found in Greek and Roman mythology. Heracles, son of Zeus and Alcmene, is called—as his name indicates [2]—to honor, through his heroic deeds, the goddess Hera, jealous wife of Zeus, [3] who sent two serpents to kill

---

[1] Heraclitus (c. 535–c. 475 BC) was a pre-Socratic Greek philosopher.

[2] Ἡρακλῆς in ancient Greek, from Ἥρα-κλέος, Hera-kleos, the glory (kleos) of Hera.

[3] Hera persecuted Herakles for the reason that Zeus was his father, but another woman, Alcmene, was his mother.

© The Author(s), under exclusive license to Springer Nature Switzerland AG 2023
B. Steck, *Adoption as a Lifelong Process*,
https://doi.org/10.1007/978-3-031-33038-4_1

1

the newborn Heracles. Romulus and Remus, children of the god Mars and the Virgin, were abandoned and raised by a mother wolf. According to the legend, Romulus founded Rome; to him the Romans attributed the foundations of the political and military constitution of their city [3].

Right and Law

The Babylonian collection of laws, dating from 2500 BC and carved on a diorite block, is the oldest written and documented law. The restored black diorite block, over two meters high with 44 columns of text, can be admired and "read" today in the Louvre Museum in Paris. The collection of laws contains a section on adoption, which addresses issues still relevant today, such as the traumatic impact on the child following his separation from previous caregivers. Further it outlines that adoptees—who wish to be reunited with their biological parents—may return to them, even if this means hurting their adoptive parents [4].

In ancient Greece, the father had the right, until the fifth day after birth, to decide about life and death of his child, i.e., whether to accept or reject it. In the Athenian Republic, there was the legal possibility of exposing a child, which was contrary to the customs of neighboring countries, where illegitimate children were killed. Sophocles dramatized in his work *Oedipus the King* the birth parents' fear of revenge by the exposed child, expressed in the statement of the Oracle of Delphi: "If you do not kill this child, it will kill you." An "exposure" table near the Agora created the possibility of saving children deposited there thanks to "adoption".

Roman law already knew adoption, called—before Justinian (527-565 AD)— "adoptio plena", i.e., an adoption endowed with all implications of a filiation and consequences of parenthood. In ancient Rome, paternity was always determined by "adoption", as the Roman decided whether to become the father of a child or to abandon the child. A Roman citizen was allowed to adopt the legitimate son of another citizen. These were young men with special qualities and not orphans or abandoned children. Adoptions were carried out by Roman emperors, e.g., Cesar adopted Octavius, Claudius adopted Nero. Legal adoption was a privilege of citizens. The person to be adopted had to be an adult and agree to his adoption; the biological father had to consent to the adoption and lost all rights over his son. The adoptee would take the name of his adoptive father, often keeping the name of his birth father as a byname. The adopted son became heir to his adoptive father but lost all rights over his biological father's goods. Originally, these adoptions were concerned with continuing the cult of the ancestors, an important religious task. Over time, the purpose of adoption was to ensure progeny and thus "bypassing" finitude and death, however, often on the background of political aspirations to preserve power. Women were not allowed to adopt under Roman law. They were used as instruments in the adoption process, which was carried out by men. The prospective adopted son was always informed. He was not separated from his family of origin; on the contrary, he maintained affective relations with his biological family.

Constantine, the first Christian emperor of the Roman Empire, forbade the abandonment of children in the fourth century, claiming that each child is a child of God.

During the Middle Ages, cribs were provided at the entrance of churches or in hospices, serving to accommodate unwanted children. In the Christian Middle Ages, adoption was not promoted because of the belief in indissoluble family ties.

Alfonso X, Spanish King of Castile and Leone, one of the most erudite princes of the Middle Ages, gave in his thirteenth century collection of laws consideration to the welfare of adoptees. For instance, an evaluation of the adoptive parents' suitability was required, if the child to be adopted was under the age of 15 years [5].

In France, adoption was introduced in 1804 by the Civil Code of Napoleon the First. It allowed the adoption of children under the age of 15, but their adoption could only be legalized after the child had reached majority. It was not until 1923 that the adoption of minors became legal in France.

Islam does not recognize adoption but allows to take outcast children into the family, thus fulfilling the duty of mercy.

Until the nineteenth century, adoptions were only realized among the upper classes, i.e., among the population group that enjoyed the highest social prestige; among the lower classes, there were various forms of hiring out children who were remunerated for their labor with board and lodging. Illegitimate children, so-called "bastard" children, were treated as slaves. The abandonment of unwanted children was the most common practice up to the middle of the nineteenth century. Jean Jacques Rousseau tells in his *Confessions*, an autobiographical book, how he relinquished his oldest child by leaving him with a midwife who took the child to the hospice for foundlings ("hospice des enfants trouvés").

Through adoption, rich Egyptians, Chinese and Indians, who had no children, obtained an heir. In India, adopting a male child was a way for Hindus to fulfil religious duties. The last Maharaja in India adopted his grandson (his daughter's son) in 2003, as he had no son of himself.

Adoption procedures depend on countries, epoch, circumstances, conditions, and adoption aims. In the past, adoption was primarily intended to resolve inheritance issues. It was only later that the affective needs of parents and children were considered. Today, finally, the focus is on asserting the needs and rights of the child. Adoption is based on the concern for children's well-being, however sociocultural factors such as race, class, religion, economics, as well as demands and biases of the other parties in the adoption process do have important impacts [6].

In the United States of America, adoption was first legislated and regulated in 1851, by the Adoption of Children Act, in the U.S. state of Massachusetts, with the aim of ensuring the well-being of children; it is considered as the first adoption law in modern times.

Today, in the United States a child can be adopted internationally or through the foster care system, with the help of a local adoption agency or private attorney.

About 135'000 children are adopted in the United States each year, according to the US Adoption Statistics. The impact of the Covid-19 pandemic in the US resulted in an enormous reduction of adoptions.

Across the EU, between 2004 and 2014, there were on average 18' 366 domestic adoptions per year, with 19 adoptions per 100' 000 children.

According to the *United States Children's Bureau*, there are over 440,000 children in the foster care system, over a quarter have been legally "freed" for adoption. International adoption has been declining in recent years. The procedures vary by the individual countries' adoption laws. To adopt an infant domestically can be realized by an adoption agency or independently by a private adoption lawyer. Same sex married couples can adopt children in every state in the United States.

Countries regulate adoption differently: In England adoptions occur without parental consent in almost 50%, while in Sweden adoption without parental consent is an exception. In certain countries grandparents or other relatives are allowed to adopt. In some countries (e.g., Sweden and The Netherlands), adoptions are mostly international. In other countries (e.g., Portugal and the UK) domestic adoptions are predominant. In countries such as Australia, France, Italy, Spain, USA, there are both domestic and intercountry adoption [7]. Within-country relinquishments of a child are often the result of court-ordered terminations of parental rights [8].

Open adoption is characterized by the possibility of various contacts and may take place before, during, and after placement. More and more state courts allow adoptees to have access to their original birth records. The search for finding births parents, as well as establishing contacts differ greatly: there are today many means of contact, and the moments chosen by adoptees vary.

The number of adoptions has been declining, due to child protection laws, a drop in unwanted pregnancies and a better acceptance of and support for single mothers in society. The medically assisted procreation has led to a decrease in adoption requests. However, the number of adoptions might eventually increase because of orphaned or abandoned children due to migration, wars, pandemics, or as a consequence of the growing sterility affecting young men. As few babies are available for adoption at the national level in Europe and North America, the majority of adoptions are international, or from the welfare system. Children with special needs, e.g., older than 5 years, members of a minority or sibling groups, or with physical, emotional, or developmental problems [9] are usually from welfare states. Adoption helps many of these children to grow up in permanent families rather than in foster homes or institutions.

UN Convention on the Rights of the Child

The United Nations Convention on the Rights of the Child is an international human rights treaty which sets out the civil, political, economic, social, health and cultural rights of children. Among the rights of all children is the right to live their childhood, with protection, care, and provision of basic necessities.

In matters of adoption, the UN Convention aims to ensure the best interests of the child and to safeguard fundamental rights in international adoptions. In particular, its goal is to prevent child trafficking by ensuring that professional standards are observed in international adoptions in all signatory/contracting states.

References

1. Heraklit, Fragment 52: Kirk et al. Die vorsakratischen Philosophen im Verlag Metzler 1994.
2. Sophocles. Oedipus the king. The University of Chicago Press; 2010.
3. Knibiehler Y. Formes anciennes d'adoption. Neuropsychiatr Enfance Adolesc. 1995;43(10-11):420–6.
4. Clothier F. Some aspects of the problem of adoption. Am J Orthopsychiatry. 1939;41:863–71.
5. Dreixler M. Der Mensch als Ware. Frankfurt a.M.: Peter Lang, Europäischer Verlag der Wissenschaften 1998.
6. Baden A, Zamostny KP, O'Brien KM, Wiley MO'L. The practice of adoption: history, trends, and social context (Department of Counseling Scholarship and Creative Works. 92. 2003. https://digitalcommons.montclair.edu/counseling-facpubs/92
7. Palacios J, Adroher S, Brodzinsky DM, Grotevant HD, Johnson DE, Juffer F, Martínez-Mora L, Muhamedrahimov RJ, Selwyn J, Simmonds J, Tarren-Sweeney M. Adoption in the service of child protection: an international interdisciplinary perspective. Psychol Public Policy Law. 2019;25(2):57–72.
8. Brinich PM. Varieties of adoptive experience.wpd Paul M. Brinich 2012.
9. Barth RP, Berry M. Adoption and disruption: rats, risks and response. Hawthorne, NY: De Gruyter 1988.

Chapter 2
Self Development and Parenthood

There are two things children should receive from their parents: roots and wings.
Johann Wolfgang Goethe

Self-Development

The development of self and the building of self-representations take place in a continuous process between the infant and his primary caregivers. These processes are based on interpersonal communications with all their asymmetrical needs, desires, and satisfactions. The Latin term infans (from the Greek φημί, phēmí = "I speak", in = not, meaning "one who does not speak") refers to the baby before he acquires speech, however the infant disposes of a great diversity of preverbal communications. It is the mother who holds the role of a "word-bearer" for the infant. She verbalizes the baby's expressions and provides meaning for the infant's manifestations [1].

Numerous authors use for the importance of the primary care of an infant and child the expression "mother-baby" or "mother-infant" or "mother-child relationship or interaction," a role which can of course be assumed by a father, a parent, or another significant caregiver. Most of the available research is centered on mothers as primary caregiver for children, but currently roles and functions are often equally performed by fathers and mothers.

According to Winnicott [2] [1] there is no baby without a mother. The infant's externalized emotions are recorded, retained, and transformed by a "good enough mother" ([3, 4]) [2] and retransmitted to the infant. For the baby to be recognized

---

[1] Donald Woods Winnicott was an English pediatrician and psychoanalyst.

[2] A good enough mother provides a holding environment, which means safeguarding and maintaining the continuity of the infant's or child's experience of being and being alive over time ([3], 1955–1956).

© The Author(s), under exclusive license to Springer Nature Switzerland AG 2023
B. Steck, *Adoption as a Lifelong Process*,
https://doi.org/10.1007/978-3-031-33038-4_2

visually by mother's face and acoustically by mother's voice are the building blocks for intrapsychic representations, self-constitution, and subjective awareness. Learning the language and its meaning takes place in the emotional interaction with primary caregivers. The process of acquiring speech has been called "the emotional history of words" [5]. According to Bollas [6] the voice, with its components such as melody, pitch, timbre, rhythm, tempo, and loudness, underlies verbal communication and is influenced by the different interacting elements of body, emotions, language, music, culture. Bollas [7] considers the infant's earliest experience of his mother as an ongoing process: the mother's psychic attitudes, and physical handling of her baby continuously transform the infant's emotional state and bodily being. When the child has acquired language and thought capacities, a self-narrative process begins in which the child addresses himself as an object in inner discourse: "'I said to myself'" ([8]: p. 348). "From this moment on, the child constructs fantasized self-other scenes based on previous and current experiences and uses language retroactively (nachträglich) to give affective meaning to earlier experiences" ([5]: p. 305).

The fundamental building blocks in the development of the self and self-representation in infancy and early childhood include "affect attunement" [9] and "social referencing" [10]; they represent particularly meaningful communication interactions between infant and primary caregivers. The term affect attunement has its origins in infant research; in the relational interaction between mother and infant, a continuing shared emotional experience is being built up. Primary caregivers assimilate—mainly by imitation—the infant's signals, record them, and behave nearly identically. While the received "information" is then slightly but clearly modulated in frequency, amplitude, or even in the sensory disposition, it is still recognized by the infant and awakes his interest. This kind of playful interactions activates a progressive discovery by the infant of his own capacities. In a social context where the infant is not able to decide on his own behavior, he—by means of social referencing—explores the facial expression of his mother and according to her emotional information (e.g., encouraging or warning) regulates his own behavior. Fear and uncertainty are reduced by social referencing, thereby creating room for curiosity and exploration.

The repeated internalization of the image processed by the mother of the infants' thoughts and feelings provides a "containment", [3] which represents an ongoing dynamic emotional interaction process [12]. The internalization of holding and containing experiences constructs a system of internal relational representations. When primary caregivers lack these holding/containing functions, the infant and young child may present multiple fears and narcissistic rage, [4] which can affect the development of his impulse and affect regulation functions. Since feelings in the mother-child interaction can also be interpreted as physical states, it is difficult for the infant

---

[3] Containment is concerned with the processing of thoughts derived from lived emotional experience [10].

[4] Narcissistic rage [12] is the reactive anger following a narcissistic injury [13], a threat to a person's self-esteem.

or toddler to distinguish physical from psychic reality on the one hand, and reality from fantasy on the other. An emotionally inconsistent availability of a parent often gives rise to multiple anxieties and intense anger. The disruption in the "continuity of being" within a child's development may represent a basic injury [15]. When holding and containing functions of the primary caregiver are missing, infants' and toddlers' learning process to cope with aggressive affects is impaired, as well as other psychological functions associated with aggressiveness such as to separate, to assert autonomy, to achieve a desired state of satisfaction, or to eliminate a source of pain or frustration [16].

In a continuous, secure relationship, the sensitivity and availability of the caregiver ensure the building of a representational system of inner states and the internalization of the containment experience. However, even in good relationships, only one third of the encounters come to a pleasurable contact; however, this is sufficient for normal development [17]. If insufficient meaning is attributed to the infant's communication, if there is no connection to the infant's experience, the infant is unable to acquire a symbolic representation of its mental states [18].

The cognitive integration of emotional experiences of inner and outer reality is an ongoing task from the first day of life and ensures the infant's fundamental experience of the "continuity of being." The continuity of experiences (e.g., the predictability of emotional, cognitive, and relational experiences, as well as the sequence of multiple needs, wishes, and desires and their fulfillment or non-fulfillment) is an essential achievement of the infant to better orient himself.

The more intense, differentiated, and structured the world of internal representations and skills acquired by the infant and the young child is, the greater his autonomy from the caregivers, on both psychic and bodily levels. The development of early object relations takes place through the inferring and attributing of an internal state to the primary caregiver. The intersubjective state allows for the development of perceiving and understanding mental states in oneself and in others (mentalization) [5] and is a prerequisite for the child to perceive the psychic reality of his caregiver [19].The capacity to differentiate but also to link internal and external reality calls for increasing regulation of impulses and emotions. In the dyadic play with a significant person, the child learns—with interpersonal communication—alternative solutions and ideas and broadens his subjective experience. Disturbances of affect attunement and social referencing can result in severe disappointment and withdrawal behavior in the infant as well as in feelings of self-depreciation, shame, and guilt. "…it is the overall quality of the emotional relationship between infant and caregiver, and its internalization as part of the representational world, which is of crucial importance for growth and development" ([20]: p. 105).

---

[5] In cognitive psychology mentalization is called theory of mind.

True and False Self

The term self is a description of subjectivity; it is the sense of feeling real, feeling in touch with others and with one's own body. Only the true self can be creative and only the true self can feel real [15].

The true self is a kind of a hereditary potential or constitutive core and permits—under suitable environmental conditions—the experience of a continuity of being. An average primary caregiver helps the infant—through proper care in the first months of his life—to experience an illusory omnipotence. This allows the true self to become alive. If a mother fails to adapt "good enough" to the infant's needs, he will "comply" with his mother's "handling". "Compliance" by "the infant is the earliest stage of the false self and belongs to the mother's inability to sense her infant's needs" ([15] p: 145).

Gradually the infant is able to acknowledge that he is not omnipotent; he is then ready for disillusionment. Disturbances in the subsequent necessary gentle disillusionment-process, which leads to the recognition of the reality principle, can also give rise to the formation of a false self. A false self means excessive docility toward latent or manifest demands of the outside world. The false self is something like a protective shell around the true self in order to hide it. Any threat to the true self is felt like an assault and causes an all-encompassing vital anxiety in early developmental stages of an infant. The formation of a false self may thus be the best possible defense against such violations of the true self, however, at an extremely high price, namely, the loss of authenticity.

When mothers or parents are not able to empathetically mirror their child's inner experiences, the child will then tend to avoid engagement with his true self. Infants and young children search the face of their primary caretaker; they depend upon the containment and reflected feedback of an emotionally attuned significative adult person to be able to identify themselves with these intersubjective relational experiences and to integrate them as part of their representational world. Accordingly, children develop a sound perception of self as a desiring, thinking, and confident subject. When this existential mirroring-need of every infant is not met, the building up of his own mind, identity, and self are insufficient or inadequate.

There exist in the field of clinical manifestations many variations and severity degrees of a false self. If a primary caregiver impacts his own intentions and desires on the infant instead of supporting the formation of the spontaneous gestures of the baby, then the ability for symbol formation is impaired and the implementation of illusion and omnipotence in play and imagination does not get started. If a child is forced into a false self or seduced into this form, he reacts with symptoms such as irritability and nutritional and functional disorders. In developing a false self, the infant gives up his own creative gestures, imitates his caring environment, and identifies with caregivers who neither understand nor can represent the infant's feelings and intentions, but replace the emotional expressions with their own mostly nonverbal communications.

An infant or young child who internalizes emotionally unresolved representations of the mother into a personal self-image on mental and bodily levels will develop inadequate representations of the intentional self, resulting in distorted body- and self-images. The infant or small child's experience of self and self-awareness—markedly influenced by early perceptions of thoughts and feelings of the mother—has then no connection to present or actual emotions, feelings, and experiences. The developmental task of the process of individuality, independence, and separateness cannot be fulfilled. At the adolescent stage, the subject may be overwhelmed by fears of falling, disintegration, and depersonalization and will search to free the core or true self through self-destructive, even suicidal behavior, or establish mental representations through somatization, a predisposition to eventually harm his body.

Neglected or abused infants or toddlers may not be able to develop object permanence and suffer therefore from separation anxiety and form intense fusional relationships. They remain existentially dependent on the physical presence of a related person. The false self is an early form of defense against impingements of the environment or against a lack of protection by the primary caregivers from outside attacks. According to Winnicott [15], a false self brings the child's own self-development and self-fulfillment to a standstill.

The following vignette demonstrates how free, liberated a patient feels, when she is able to discard her false self—described by her as a shell—and discovers her true self.

Vignette
Sophia is a young woman adopted from a South American country. In a session towards the end of her psychoanalytical therapy, she tells her therapist with pride: "I would like to discard the Sophia who no longer fits into the shell; I have - thanks to the psychotherapy - come to terms with the death of my adoptive mother and the rejection of my adoptive father. I have searched and found my birth mother. I was able to separate from my partner - all this is an amazing development.

Now I can finally accept my face in the mirror, I am a beautiful woman. I feel like a new human being having turned my inner self outside. To sense myself, to know who I am, to accept me as I am and to be my one master are incredible feelings! I am confident and know what I want. It is as if floating building blocks settled into a path on which I can now walk; I think that I do deserve it, because I have fought so hard."

Time and Temporality in Childhood and Adolescence [6]

Child development is also marked socially, in the form of birthdays, anniversaries, pre- school and school entries, religious events, and other transitions. Young children try with magical effort to stop or advance time, wishing to prove that they are

---

[6] While time is related to the passing or the flowing of time occurring in the present, temporality is related with the concept of past, present, and future.

not subjected to it. One of the main tasks during adolescence is to renounce infantile omnipotent entitlement, immortality fantasies, perfection ideals, and to recognize gender and generational differences, and the irreversibility of death. Accepting temporality as a human condition is a psychic process where the self on the one hand denies temporality and, on the other, accepts the reality of unilinear time [21].

Adolescence

Puberty is closely associated with amplification of intensive drive impulses, needs, and feelings, as well as with the reactivation of infantile conflicts. This process may lead to confrontation with narcissistic, libidinal, and aggressive impulses. Adopted adolescents may be overwhelmed by strong emotions of anger, sadness, and pain experienced in critical life events in their early childhood. These past experiences cannot be remembered by conscious awareness and therefore cannot be expressed by words. The genital sexual maturation at the beginning of adolescence changes the relationship of the young person with his own body. This process may be associated with numerous conflicts, sometimes leading to irresponsible behavior of adolescents with respect to their own body, such as auto-aggressive behavior manifested by repetitive accidents, by substance abuse (alcohol, nicotine, drugs), by neglecting bodily care, or by promiscuity.

> Encourage and support your kids because children are apt to live up to what you believe of them. Lady Bird Johnson

> We cannot always build the future for our youth, but we can build our youth for the future. Franklin D. Roosevelt

Parenthood

Parenthood is based on the notion of kinship in its dual biological and social dimensions. According to Lebovici [22] parenthood is the fruit of an encounter between the biography of both parents and their baby and made up of parents' mental representations, affects, desires, and behaviors in the relationship with their child. The future child may only be a project of his future parents, is expected during pregnancy, or may be already born. What constitutes the parents' intrapsychic reality will unfold in fantasied and emotional interactions with the baby, then with the child, by intersubjective exchanges and interpersonal relationships and thus contribute to the attachment-modalities of the young child to his parents and family. According to Manzano et al. [23], it is mandatory that identificatory changes take place in parents during the pregnancy period.

Psychic elaboration of each future parent's past includes processing their own internalized parental images. This process represents a period of psychic growth; if this elaboration does not take place, parents will not be apt to recognize and accept their child's "otherness". The child will then be the receiver of parental projective identifications. [7]

Transgenerational inheritance consists of psychic experiences—emotions, fantasies, images, and identifications—and is organized into a mythical narrative from which each individual takes up essential elements for the formation of his personal family history. The child inscribes himself in his dual maternal and paternal filiations, thus joining and belonging to his family. At the same time, he will be part of the unfolding history of his family.

Transmission of parents' unconscious desires and fantasies to their children takes place through nonverbal communication, the variants being of sensorimotor nature, tactile, visual, and auditory modalities. During breast- or bottle-feeding, for example, multiple modes of communication are used: the gaze; the respective postures of the mother and her baby and their mutual adjustment; the prosody and tonality of the dialogue; the holding, the contact, and the touch; the speech and the vocalizations; as well as gustatory and olfactory experiences [8] of the baby. The child will react to the messages expressed by the communicative behavior of his parents according to his own motivations, in particular his desire for communication and his need for relationship and holding, deriving from his own impulses and defenses. The newborn disposes of an important number of skills he brings into play for the "parentalisation" of his parents. A baby already has the ability to establish triadic exchanges [25].

The parents' biographical history cannot be dissociated from the child's personal history. Under certain conditions, the impact of critical events or psychic trauma can be transmitted from one generation to another. What happened in the parents' past is transmitted to the child and becomes his present reality. Unconscious conflictual patterns of the child's primary caregivers may be internalized by a child, through his identification with the parental lived emotional experiences.

Early Parent–Child Relationship

The family is the place where a child's genealogy and filiation are inscribed. This integration is required for the formation of his identity; but the family is also a place of confrontation with differences between self and others, gender, and generations. Infant research demonstrates a major influence of family relationships on child development processes. The observation of parent–child interactions in their

---

[7] Projective identification is a process, in which in a close relationship, such as between mother and child, an unconscious fantasy of aspects of the self or of an internal relation representation is attributed to an external person.

[8] The olfactory system appears to outperform other senses such as vision or audition, since it can discriminate more than 1 trillion different odors [23]. By comparison, the discriminating power for color is in the order of 2–7 million, for tones about 350,000.

behavioral, emotional, and phantasmatic aspects marked an important step in understanding the infant and child's self-formation and-maturation and associated disorders [22, 25–27].

A subject is not able to construct his personal history alone; he is always anchored in a family history containing significant events prior to his life. As part of a mental transmission process, a person receives elements of cultural heritage from preceding generations. A baby inscribes himself in the longitudinal history of his mother and father. Infants need for the construction of their mental life not only a biological or genetic makeup but also a relationship history. A baby's lived experience consists of his desire for interpersonal emotional exchanges, which he can only express through nonverbal communication. The satisfaction of his vital needs is almost always linked to communicative exchange activities. Positive and negative interaction experiences are stored as corresponding relationship representations and are further elaborated by fantasy activities of the infant. The representations contain the desire and longing to continue the relationship and lustful and pleasurable emotional exchanges with the caring person. With the help of these intrapsychic representations and fantasy activities, the baby tries to bridge the separation anxiety situation with his mother.

Early Relationship Disorders

The parent's intrapsychic representations of their child will contribute to the child's self-development. Transgenerational adverse inheritance consists of raw elements—not elaborated by previous generations, marked e.g., by traumatic experiences, bereavements—and are left unspoken. The burden of the parental personal history permeates the mental development and psychic maturation of the baby. The infant builds up his inner world out of his desire for his mother or primary caregiver and out of his motivation to attribute and understand meaning in the feelings and behaviors of others. The child identifies himself totally or partially with the parental representations projected onto him, which may considerably reduce his degree of freedom and sometimes alienate him [28]. His mental development may be affected, leading to symptoms. These manifestations often reflect strong invested narcissistic [9] parent-child or family ties and can be considered as an indicator of transgenerational transmission of something unnamed, not-thought, revealing an unconscious alliance.

Multiple parental representations of their baby blend and alternate with the "real" baby, creating an imaginary and phantasmatic dimension of early interactions between the baby and his parents. This parent-child interaction is a complex sequence of bidirectional processes which do not develop in a closed circle, but rather in a spiral. It includes the expression of unconscious conflicts of the parents

---

[9] The child serves as an essential source of the parental self-esteem.

and is sometimes the source of disharmony in their relationship with the baby, who then becomes the container for projections of these conflicts.

Parenting—created by the arrival of a child—leads mother and father to identify with their own parents' parenting functions. This reidentification reactivates experiences and conflicts with internalized parental figures and can then be projected onto the child. Aspects of unresolved parental conflicts may be expressed by the child through symptomatic manifestations such as sleep-, respiratory-, or eating disorders.

Unconscious communications occur in the mother or parent–child relationship by nonverbal interactions; a mother, father or parents may unconsciously attempt to mourn certain losses, or some critical events experienced in their own childhood by projecting their unresolved grief onto the child. The child—with his extreme sensitivity and responsiveness—reacts to the expressed emotions and signs of his mother or parent. For parents with severe emotional disturbances, parenthood can be seriously compromised.

When there is a combination of several destabilizing factors (social precarity, unemployment, transculturation, break-up with the extended family, bereavement, illness, breakdown of the family environment), the time, space, safety, availability, and necessary motivation are missing to promote and support a child's development.

Parents can be so overwhelmed by their problems that they hardly perceive the child's signals or ignore them, neglect his needs, and avoid playful contacts. They may react unpredictably or overstimulate their child until he withdraws himself. A fundamental refusal by the child may also occur in the case of a mother who is unable to identify with her maternal role. Two extreme forms of parental insensitivity are intrusion and deprivation. In the case of intrusion, for example, an infant or small child is compelled to fulfill his mother's narcissistic needs. In physical or affective deprivation, the infant or small child's sense of continuity of being is interrupted, affecting his development process and personal life experience.

A mother or parent may have given the baby an exceptionally good start, but cannot handle the next developmental phase, the first separation–individuation process, which a mother often experiences as being rejected by her child. She is then no longer able to fulfill the baby's needs. Thanks to the initial overinvestment at the baby stage—which represents a "primary maternal preoccupation" [29, 30]—the child is sometimes able to draw enough strength to organize and defend himself with respect to his mother. However, later in his development, the child may relive these extremely chaotic and unpredictable circumstances. Psychoanalysts like Bion [12, 31], Winnicott [32], and Ogden [33] describe the consequences of a disruption of the mother-infant bond, which leaves the infant or young child in a state of primitive agony with feelings of "endless falling," "nameless dread", a threat of nonexistence. An infantile event of "primitive agony", [10] of an original break-down, remains actual, unrepresented, and can only be inscribed into the past if taken up by the ego in present experiences and having been worked

---

[10] "Primitive agonies" are characterized by the "return to an unintegrated state," the sensation of "falling forever," "the failure of indwelling," the "loss of the sense of the real," and the "loss of the capacity to relate to objects" ([30]: p 104).

through, integrated, and remembered. Experiences from the time of early child-hood may only later—as memories—have a traumatic impact [34]. At a very young age, a child cannot react adequately to an event that will only later be understandable [35]. A "repressed" memory can thus subsequently lead to trauma-tization. Likewise, threats endured in childhood can have pathogenic effects after-ward [36].

The intense or constant desire of the mother to protect her child usually reflects her own traumatic separation experiences or her non-elaborated or reactivated mourning. A revival of the mother's past traumatic events during pregnancy and birth can lead to a serious failure in her primary maternal capacities. Respiratory difficulties or allergic skin manifestations, for example, may represent maternal anxieties, overprotection, and/or excessive arousal of the child. In a child with sleep disorders, one often finds an anxious mother waking up her child, in an attempt to reassure herself. Other disorders such as anorexia and vomiting may result from the child's opposition to the mother's intrusive behavior. Symptoms vary and change during child development.

Mothers may select and reinforce certain of the child's expressions, which then become part of a specific mother-child communication system. For example, when a baby is expected to replace a deceased person, such as a brother, sister, or grand-parent, whose mourning has not been elaborated, he runs the risk of being a substi-tute. The mother's or father's need to cling to such a substitute child, who also represents their lost love, is above all expressed by their gaze, voice, attitude, and gestures, and less by their words.

Parental psychopathology may deprive a child of his childhood; a child may take over a function of "therapist" for his parents, presenting with a pathological hyper-maturity, which is psychologically extremely costly and significantly reduces the degree of his developmental freedom. These signs of hyper-maturation, which con-sists mainly of an over-adaptation, lead to the formation of a false self, and reveal extreme identification mechanisms, indicative of the child's suffering. The too mature and precocious child manifests a serious and grave adult-like behavior and presents himself as an autonomous and hyper-controlled personality. These so-called model-children, concerned with the care and surveillance of their sick mother or parent, show high vigilance toward a parent who is physically present, but emo-tionally absent, as it is the case in depressed or alcoholic parents.

Studies of interactions between psychotic mothers and their babies have shown the mother's scarcity or avoidance of eye contact. In such a situation, the child directs his gaze to a stranger. At the corporal level, one may observe scenes of rap-prochement and distancing, in which holding and maintaining the baby are chaotic and followed by hyper- or hypotonic reactions. At a vocal level, interactions are poor, and the mother rarely evokes and answers the baby's vocalizations. The play-fulness in interactions is almost absent. The baby then lives to the rhythm of the mother's intensely unpredictable and unconscious emotional fluctuations.

Chronically depressed mothers may be physically present, but emotionally absent for her young child, who is terrified and confused. This interaction has been observed by Stern [9] who states: "Compared to the infant's expectations and wishes, the depressed mother's face is flat and expressionless. She breaks eye contact and does not seek to reestablish it" (p. 12). "After the infant's attempts to invite and solicit the mother to come to life, to be there emotionally, to play, have failed, the infant, it appears, tries to be with her by way of identification and imitation" (p. 12–13).

> The little prince went to see the roses again. … my rose … is more important than all of you… since she's the one I've watered. Since she's the one I put under glass. Since she's the one I sheltered behind a screen…Since she's the one I listened to when she complained, or when she boasted, or even sometimes when she said nothing at all. Since she is my rose.
> *The Little Prince*, Antoine de Saint-Exupéry [37].

Childless Couples with a Desire for Children

Introduction

Adoption and reproductive medicine are today available options for couples with involuntary childlessness as a possibility to realize their desire to have a child. In both situations, the future parents need to grieve their imaginary child, who could not be conceived without the intervention of a third party: adoption agency or reproductive medicine [38].

According to Erikson [39], the desire for children or procreation is a significant psychological developmental task of adulthood, and its realization leads to an additional maturation of the personality. The desire of both parents for a child contains the image of a usually idealized imaginary child; it represents the result of their own relational experience with their parents, as well as the wish for procreative ability and an existential desire from their current relationship [40]. It involves rational and conscious ideas of the future parents but has always an unconscious origin as well. The reasons consciously assumed by the future parents for their desire to have children often do not correspond to the unconscious motivations.

The desire for children usually arises in a significant relationship of a couple and is accompanied by the wish for parenthood. It means for every future mother or father a confrontation with their personal identity, an integration process of their identification with their own parents. For every child's personal development and fulfilment, there is an essential need to be wanted and loved by his parents. Whether legitimate, illegitimate, adopted or conceived with the help of reproductive techniques, it is of unique significance for the child to be the offspring of his parents' desire.

Disappointed Longing

The unfulfilled desire to have children has for every couple, future mother and father, both common and individual conscious and unconscious meanings. It may disappoint the longing to be reproduced in one's own child, to continue one's own life in the child, or to transmit own inner richness to a child. The need to express love and affection in an intimate relationship with the child or the hope to revive own personality traits in the child cannot be realized [41]. The joy of creating a new beginning, a new start in one's own life with a child is spoiled. Women and men experience their own infertility differently, which influences the spouses' psychological processing and mutual support, as well as their ability to decide together on their choice of future parenthood [42].

Grief

The unfulfilled desire to have children represents the loss of parenthood. The inability to realize pregnancy and childbirth—among the most important life events—causes a severe narcissistic injury and self-depreciation. The necessary mourning work is a conscious and unconscious process of dealing with this loss. The grieving process involves the loss of the ability to create a new generation and of transgenerational continuity. The biological incapacity to produce a child interrupts the generational line. The resulting renunciation affects both the individual and the couple as well as the extended family.

Adoption or Reproductive Medicine

In the situation of adoption or reproductive medicine, the understanding and meaning of the specificity of parenthood, of the parent-child bond and of the future child's identity development are of highest significance [43]. In addition, there is the central issue of informing the child about his special filiation.

The following differences can be made:

− The biological child and biological parenthood, whose references are procreation, pregnancy, and birth.
− The imaginary child or imaginary parenthood, which are shaped by emotions, expectations, hopes and projections.
− The social or symbolic parenthood, which allows the transfer of names and inheritances, and which also defines the rights and obligations of the parent-child relationship and affiliation.

Adoption and reproduction are established forms of family formation and established parent-child relationships. They have the same goal, namely, to enable a couple to become parents, when a physical or mental condition has led to infertility.

In both situations, prior grief work of the imagined child is required. The original child will change in the couple's imaginations during their mourning process. Only then the future child does not risk being a "substitute child".

The child must not represent a "means", designated to "cure" the suffering over his parents' loss of fertility, in the sense of a "remedy". No child will ever have the required resources to care for or heal the wounds of his parents, wounds that arose from self-esteem loss or psychic loneliness or impoverishment. The child must not be used to maintain the partnership, to bridge the void in the partnership or to serve as proof of personal or social success of his parents.

Parenthood by Medically Assisted Reproduction

Assisted reproductive technology includes in vitro fertilization, intracytoplasmic sperm injection, cryopreservation of gametes or embryos, and/or the use of fertility medication. According to the Centers for Disease Control and Prevention in the US, assisted reproductive technology is defined as including "all fertility treatments in which either eggs or embryos are handled. In general, assisted reproductive technology procedures involve surgically removing eggs from a woman's ovaries, combining them with sperm in the laboratory, and returning them to the woman's body or donating them to another woman. ...treatments in which only sperm are handled (i.e., intrauterine—or artificial—insemination) or procedures in which a woman takes medicine only to stimulate egg production without the intention of having eggs retrieved" are not included [44].

The World Health Organization also defines assisted reproductive technology [45].

Parents who rear children—created with donated gametes and gestated by a third party—are social but not biological parents. Modern reproductive medicine raises new hopes among unintentionally childless couples. The instrumentalization of sexuality, the disturbed intimacy caused by the medical interventions and the necessary involvement of an external third party [46] represents a strain on the partners' relationship and can lead to emotional distancing. Reproductive medicine also carries the danger of transforming a couple's desire for a child into an entitlement to a child.

The story in the judgment of Solomon [11] shows how the vehemence of the desire for a child is converted into an absolute right to the child, even at the cost of its death. Solomon has judged the woman's statement that the child should be 'neither hers, nor mine', 'share it!' as too murderous to come from the mother. The true (real) mother is ready to renounce her child, as she is inscribing him in a life process, while the other woman wants to possess the child, even at the prize of his death. This example illustrates how the narcissistic mortification caused by one's own childlessness leads to envy, resentment, and ruthlessness, up to murderous rage, which is finally directed against the object of desire.

Advances in reproductive medicine and technology contribute to reinforcing the omnipotent fantasies of having the right to a child because it can be "produced". The

---

[11] The biblical tale from 1 Kings 3:16–28 tells the story of two women who claimed that the child was their own. Solomon orders his soldier to cut the baby in two: the true mother cried out 'Please Lord, give her the living child. Do not kill him!' Solomon thus knows to which mother the newborn belongs.

desire for a child may even lead to the demand for a child or for biological parenthood at any cost. The fact that one of the greatest functions of life, reproduction, can be controlled, gives rise to all-powerful ideas of a perfect product, notions that are no longer in harmony with unpredictable circumstances. The so much desired and expected child, however, risks to be different and not to correspond to the fantasized perfect dream child.

For the parents, there is the additional central question of information to the child. If parents decide to keep the special circumstances secret, namely the fulfilment of their wish for a child through medical help, the necessary processing of the associated feelings with these measures will not take place. The secret in this regard risks becoming a family secret and may later negatively influence the child's identity development and growth.

In adoption as well as in reproduction through medical measures and especially in artificial insemination through donors, the child has a right to information. The question of one's own origin is of central importance to every human being. The legislation also provides the possibility of informing the child about his origin.

From a biological point of view, the child of a heterologous donor (fertilization by sperm cells from a third party) creates an asymmetry between the parents. The father's self-assurance in his role and function may be affected, the couple's communication about the spender avoided, his existence denied [47]. The discussions in this regard raise the question of whether the child of such a donor should be adopted by his social father. The signification of child and parenthood as symbolic creations are always of central importance, regardless of whether it is a biological child, a child conceived by means of reproduction or an adopted child.

Reproductive Medicine and Adoption

Frequently infertility is not only a failure of the body but may also represent an unconscious psychic "no" to the desire for a child. In situations where married couples simultaneously undergo medical interventions and apply for an adoptive child, the desire for a child often results from the unbearable experience of an existential deficiency, which is warded off with painful feelings of annihilation. The impossibility of realizing the biological desire for a child is experienced like a shock and is denied, i.e., can neither be admitted nor accepted. The couple tries to avoid the intrapsychic confrontation with the loss and "takes refuge" in the available options to remedy the deficiency as quickly as possible, "how" seems less essential. The significance of fertility loss remains repressed, and a grieving process does not occur. In vitro fertilization and adoption are sought simultaneously by most childless couples, with women being more favorable for adoption than their husbands [48].

In a consultation with the couple, representations of a future child can hardly be elicited, because the couple's awareness is dominated by the fear of not having a child. This anxiety is presented as a fear related to a somatic disability. However, it is evident that the fear of the couple's inability to accommodate the child on a phantasmatic and mental level is transferred to the body. Infertility anxiety then may be a symptom, either masking another fear, or reflecting the desire that a physical incapacity allows not to face confrontation and processing of a psychic impairment [49].

In such situations the future child is expected with intense fear, which inhibits a phantasmatic representation or allows only unreal and idealistic imaginations. In consultations with future parents, it is essential helping them to listen to their own infantile self, their own inner child, and thereby enabling them to perceive in turn the needs of their future real child [50].

A child at any price represents a treasured jewel and simultaneously a savior or healer child with the implicit expectation that he will restore the narcissistic injury of his parents and reestablish their sexual and social integrity.

When couples are ready to engage in psychotherapeutic work, multiple phantasms, partly conscious but mostly unconscious, arise in both parents, and need to be understood and processed. These are phantasms concerning their bodily integrity, respectively the impairment of the body or the reproductive organs (e.g., the female body or male sperms are fantasized as destructive). The inability to procreate may be lived as an affront on gender identity or as a punishment of sexual desires. A close connection exists between procreativity and male or female sense of self-esteem.

If couples wish to adopt a child after medical measures have been unsuccessful, they lived through episodes of hope and disappointment. The repeated failures of medically assisted reproduction place a great burden on spouses and are accompanied by feelings of anger, hate and envy, as well as by depression, sadness, and pain. The loss of a meaningful way of life, by the bringing up of a child, was sometimes sought in vain over many years. The knowledge of final childlessness often represents the loss of a life perspective; adoption of a child becomes the last resort when the fertility medicine fails [51]. Consequently, it is often particularly difficult for married couples to be confronted with the adoption situation on the one hand and the adoption proceedings on the other. The adoption evaluation extends over months, sometimes over more than a year, and includes the possibility of being rejected as incompetent parents.

Since many couples do not receive a definitive diagnosis of their sterility, they continue to hope for a child of their own. Therefore, identification with adoptive parenthood is demanding and the process of changing identity—from biological parenthood to adoptive parenthood—is ambivalent and long-lasting.

In the couple's phantasms, there may be a conflict between two representations of the child: The couple's imaginary child, affectively highly invested, seems to deny the imaginary adopted child the right to exist. Only grieving over the loss of fertility enables parents to shift their desire for a biological child to the desire for an adoptive child.

Couples with a desire for children have to be informed at the outset by appropriate specialists about the various possibilities of reproductive medicine and adoption. In addition, it seems essential to try to better understand the background of their desire to have children and their essential motivations, based on the basis of an

empathically guided conversation with the couple. Both biological and psychological factors should be included in the evaluation so that adequate therapeutic measures can be proposed accordingly.

Psychotherapeutic processing of, for example, repressed losses and/or unconscious conflicts represents a preventive measure for the future child, whether it is a
child by medically assisted reproduction or an adopted child, since losses can neither be replaced by receiving a child nor can they be bridged by being a parent to a
child. The adopted child is often a traumatized child. Children frequently reveal the
experienced, unprocessed traumas and/or losses of their parents.

Each child will always be somehow unpredictable; parents may remain unaware
of his unconscious phantasms, wishes or dreams. The greatest gift of parents to their
child is providing a loving and protected personal free space and freedom, thus
allowing him to unfold his unique abilities.

Parenthood by Surrogacy

Surrogacy is a form of assisted reproductive technology, where a woman consents
to carry a pregnancy—either altruistically or for financial gains—for another person
or a couple, the child's future adoptive parent(s) after his birth. A surrogate mother
is required to renounce her biological parental rights. In the United States 47 of
50 U.S. states permit commercial surrogacy, which is prohibited in most European
countries. In the European Union altruistic surrogacy is usually the only accepted
method. [12]

Already in the bible (Genesis, 16), the servant Agar bears a child of Abraham at
the request of his wife Sara, who knows that she is sterile. Agar gives birth to Ismail.

The Romans practiced womb rental (ventrem locare). A man whose wife was
fertile and whose children were flourishing could lend or temporarily rent his wife
at the request of a man who had no children. Plutarch, Greek philosopher, and biog-
rapher reported that Cato the younger, after having three children of his wife Marcia,
lent her to his friend Hortensius, whose wife had died, and Marcia bore him an
heir [52].

Parenthood by Adoption

Adoption is a universal and worldwide tradition, yet the practice has evolved differently according to historical, legal, cultural, and environmental contexts [53].

In the last decades research results of adoption and adoptive parenting show the
importance of

---

[12] Gestational Surrogacy: A European Overview. https://www.ejtn.eu

– acknowledging adopted children's birth roots, their cultural, ethnic, racial heritage.
– contact with the child's birth family and/or preadoption significant care persons.
– the adoption situation for same sexual and gender minorities

Adoptive parenting requires specific learning and understanding of the prospective child's preadoption experiences, such as traumatization and/or placements and of his racial, ethnic, linguistic, or cultural origin, as well as of his wishes of contact with birth parents or -relatives. For each child it is essential to be attuned to his specific developmental stage and his needs.

Intrapsychic concerns among adoptive parents are summarized by Schechter [54] as follows:

> The discovery of one's infertility inflicts a narcissistic wound, which requires painful mourning and leads to changes of each parent's self-representation. The associated feelings of anger and the envy of others fertility may be expressed in the relationship with their adopted child or in their phantasms regarding the child's biological parents. These emotions and the resulting intrapsychic conflicts are particularly intense at the puberty of the adopted adolescent and may lead to conflictual problems for the adopted adolescent concerning his sexuality.

Parenthood by Sexual and Gender Minorities

Around two million LGBT people in the United States wish to adopt a child. An extensive review from 2010–2020 on sexual and gender minority (SGM) including lesbian, gay, bisexual, transgender, and queer (LGBTQ) [13] families [55] shows the following results concerning adoptive parenthood. About one in five same-sex couples bring up adopted children, while 3% of same-sex couples raise foster children. Three percent of heterosexual couples bring up adopted children and 4% of heterosexual parents take care of foster children [56]. Some religious related adoption agencies do not permit adoption by sexual and gender minorities [57]. Sexual minority parents may encounter social stigmatization and suffer from lack of acceptance and support [58].

In the United States adoption law and policy are regulated at the state level, in Europe adoption by same-sex couples was for the first time realizable in 2001 in the Netherlands.

An investigation in 28 European countries about the social acceptance of adoption by lesbian women or gay men, found that the adoption by same-sex couples was approved in countries where the legislation allowed these adoption practices [59].

---

[13] In the United States, LGBTQ families may lack financial resources and their children live in poverty; their situation has been aggravated by the COVID-19 pandemic. With adequate living conditions and a supportive environment these parents are competent, and their children show positive adjustment and development.

Lesbian, gay, and heterosexual adoptive parents were investigated with regard to their adopted young children's socialization [60]. When children reach a certain level of cognitive and verbal development, they are able to show interest in and ask questions of their adoptive filiation and awareness of their family structure, thus enabling parents to respond and also to be engaged in preparing them for possible discrimination, which children encounter more often with older age [42, 61, 62]. Parents with own experiences of discrimination are predisposed to prepare their children for racism [63]. Boys tend to be less curious or communicative about adoption than girls [61, 64]. Girls and older children seem to be more willing to speak about racial stigmatization due to their family structure. Parents of color tend to prepare their children for racism more often than white parents. Direct contact with birth parents increases transparency in various issues. With regard to the psychosocial adjustment and behavioral problems of adopted children in lesbian, gay, and heterosexual parented families no significant differences were found [65].

Studies in the past 10 years on comparing children's outcomes adopted by same-sex and heterosexual adoptive parents were reviewed [66]. Knowledge about same-sex adoptive family's functioning, same-sex families with older adopted children, families with gay fathers and those with lower socioeconomic status is still insufficient and results of studies are controversial. Long-term consequences on the transition period in adolescence and on young adult adoptees need to be investigated. Therefore, conclusions relating the influence of parents' sexual orientations on the psychosocial adjustment and development of their adopted children seem to be premature. Further research is needed for the evaluation of long-term effects on psychosocial developments; some authors emphasize the importance of the child having the opportunity to identify with a mother and a father and to interact with their different expressions and behaviors.

Berger [67] argues that the foundation of adoption is "a family for a child and not the other way around", referring to the Article 21 of the 6th International Convention on the Rights of the Child, where adoption is described as a form of child protection. He insists on the following arguments:

– A child has the right and the need to be able to identify with all the dimensions of humanity, both male and female, and to do so during frequent contact, which does not mean equal time with father and mother. Numerous studies show that father and mother offer the baby different and complementary styles of exchange.

– Mothers offer a so-called tonic, emotional dialogue. It is through her voice, her smile, physical support, and search for a comfortable position that the mother expresses her solicitude to her child and contributes to his feelings of confidence and security, thus regulating his states of unease and well-being. Furthermore, at a distance, mothers favor exchanges through the visual channel. The average duration of glances that the baby directs towards adults is systematically to mother's advantage, whereas the relative duration of playing between adults and children is in favor of father. Fathers are more willing for an exchange called phasic dialogue: more physical, more stimulating, discontinuous in nature, with more intense moments, taking place from the end of the first month (such as lifting the baby in the air), and with more body-to-body plays that help the child to control his aggressiveness. Fathers have more expansive motor skills with their child, while mothers awaken emotions more through facial expressions.

– The mother-child dialogue is therefore more related to the expression of emotions, more concerned with care, tenderness, comfort, and protection, whereas the father-child dialogue appears to be more adapted to openness to the environment, even if fathers can be protective. Fathers are more directive, demand more tasks, tease the child, are more "destabilizing", offer the child more "problems" to solve, challenge a child more, and are "catalysts for risk-taking". So, in addition, the father, by the very fact that he has his masculine characteristics, represents an important third party between the child and his mother. The lack of a father, in reality or in the mother's mind, can be the cause of great suffering in children who do not feel they are the "son of", a suffering that can last a lifetime. Conversely, how can a little girl come to understand that two men who do not want to have a wife, wish at the same time to have a daughter? How will she construct her identity?

– Any child who stumbles upon the mystery of his conception, experiences a disturbing excitement in the face of this enigma, as all children are curious about their origin. Whenever filiation is dissociated from birth, the child is confronted with almost insoluble questions. The child of a heterosexual couple can think that he was born of a double desire, the desire of each parent for the other, and the common desire to have a child. The heterosexual couple is therefore the best way to ensure that sexuality, conception, and parental tenderness are inseparably linked.

– Every child needs to be able to imagine a credible origin, a founding scene of his existence. Children who cannot represent themselves as the result of a union between a man and a woman are likely to present significant psychic suffering, usually kept hidden. A child needs to have the notion of a foundational desire for his life.

– Finally, we know that the construction of filiation by adopted children is a complex and laborious process that fails in a number of situations. Adopted children often wonder endlessly about the reasons for their abandonment. They cannot bear the idea of a fault of their biological parents and wonder if they were stolen? Children are constructors of stories, of their personal history, and for them to be able to experience a feeling of psychic filiation, they must have been able to build in thought a phantasmatic filiation.

Parenthood of Foster Children

The Academy of American Pediatrics (AAP) classify children in foster care as a population of children with special health care needs.

Children and adolescents living in foster care, have often experienced adversity and trauma in infancy and childhood and present with multiple health problems (physical, developmental, psychological). [14] They need special care, but the providing of intensive pediatric, developmental, educational, and mental health services are rendered difficult for this population of children who are exposed to relationship breakups, losses, traumatization, lacking future prospects and confidence. Foster care is thought to be transitory, with the goal to realize either the reentry of the child in his original home/family or in a permanent setting such as adoption, guardianship, or placement with relatives [69]. Unaccompanied refugee minors, a small but growing group of adolescents in foster care, represent specific challenges to the welfare system.

In 2020 over 100,000 children and adolescents in foster care have been waiting to be adopted in the US (The Administration for Children and Families ACF), division of the United States Department of Health and Human Services (HHS). Over half are older children, children of racial or ethnic minority groups, children with sibling groups, or children with emotional, behavioral, and developmental disorders. Only about one fifth of foster children may be adopted, mostly by a nonrelative foster parent [70].

For a child in foster care, the project of adoption may represent a highly stressful situation, for which he needs preparation and emotional support. He may have to face the painful loss of his family of origin, siblings, care persons and peers of the institution and simultaneously cope with his integration in the adoptive family and new surroundings, later even with the changing of his name. During this transition period, not only for the child, but also for birth-, foster-, and adoptive families, psychological and social assistance is mandatory. In situations where a child has lived prior to his adoption most of his time with foster parents, who provided a stable and safe relationship, it is indispensable to maintain the child-foster carer relationship over a longer period of time [71].

> Life is not what happened, but what we remember and how we remember it.
> Gabriel Garcia Márquez

Adoption of Older Children

Families adopting an older (5 years old or older) child share often similar experiences, encounter comparable problems, ask the same questions, and have common concerns. Older children who are integrated into their prospective adoptive family face—despite their respective personal histories—adoption-specific adjustment difficulties and go through characteristic stages in their future adoptive family. Building a new attachment and relationship with adoptive parents is more arduous for older children as they have little time to go through earlier developmental phases—in a regression movement—and to grieve their multiple losses with the help of their

---

[14] See also: Callaghan, Fellin, Alexander [61].

adoptive parents before they are already confronted with their pubertal developmental process and the associated tasks [72].

A supportive group program [73] [15] for adoptive families with recently placed school-age (8–13 years) children provided a unique opportunity for parents to deal with their own adjustments, to express and understand common postplacement concerns, to work toward resolution of problems experienced with the adoption of an older child.

The following postplacement issues were raised: adjustment dynamics, symptomatic behavior of the child, loyalty versus disloyalty struggles between new and old families or caregivers, questioning the new affective ties, the shift of family balance, parental adjustments, and the stresses on the marital relationship. Groups consisted of five adoptive couples and met for eleven sessions. The content of the discussion in the group meetings was fully determined by the parents, and the conversations consisted mainly of shared experiences, through which parents could prepare for future possibilities by rehearsing behavior [16] that had been successful for other parents: "…knowing what problems to expect and dealing with them in a supportive atmosphere enabled the families to handle difficult situations successfully" ([73]: p. 273).

Adjustment Dynamics

Three stages are distinguished in which the process of adaptation, the emergence of new affective bonds and the integration of the adopted child into his new family takes place. The initial stage, a kind of honeymoon, during which the child has a great desire to please is very short or hardly noticed. The second, longest and most troublesome stage, during which the child is questioning his parents and acts out his unbearable feelings, breaks out quickly and puts the family in dismay. In the last phase, when the child integrates his adoptive family, he has progressed in building attachments and relationships with his family members; however, there are often relapses.

Regression to earlier phases of development allows the child to receive parental affective concern and attention and to be cherished and cared for—all that he was missing in past years. Often it is hard for adoptive parents to meet their child's intense need for regression, for example when an 11-year-old boy would like to drink at his adoptive mother's breast. An adoptive mother reported that she had "breastfed" her two adopted children for years. Adopted children wish to be wrapped like infants, carried in arms, and rocked like babies. These behaviors are the expression of phantasms, such as wishing to return inside the mother's womb or to have a shared skin with the mother [74].

---

[15] At Lutheran Child and Family Services, River Forest, Illinois, US, only five disruptions in close to 900 placements were experienced over the past ten years.

[16] Behavioral rehearsal is a therapy technique in which behaviors, responses, and social skills are imagined and practiced for being used in real situations.

Even older adopted children may communicate in an infant language, want to be perceived as such and satisfied in their infantile needs. These various manifestations represent a phantasmatic illusion of having been born by the adoptive parents, a necessary illusion for the establishment of primary attachments. Adopted children expect of their adoptive parents to calm their fears, fulfil their desires, understand their needs, and resolve their conflicts. Regressions are often complex and not easy to understand; they can be considered as a kind of replaying past experienced states. Adoptive parents, thanks to their intuitive sensitivity and emotional availability, can help their child, to better reveal and regulate his mental state. Adopted children often express their feelings through the body e.g., they complain of physical pain when overwhelmed by intense emotions. These symptoms provide the opportunity for adoptive parents to contain the child's feelings, distinguish the different emotional qualities, and try to understand the underlying fantasies. The re-experiences of developmental phases help the child integrating into his new family.

The dynamics of each stage are important to understand. At the beginning, the child denies his far too overwhelming fears of being rejected again by his new family. When the child begins to be more aware of his unbearable fears, he starts acting them out with provocative behaviors. Emotionally, the child relives experiences of earlier separation situations, perceived as a rejection of his seemingly worthless person. To protect himself from further hurt, the child tries—in testing the family— to find out which behavior will lead to his abandonment. The child's poor self-esteem is associated with anxieties that the new family will discover his worthlessness, and his trust is too low for believing the reassuring words of the adoptive parents that he will belong to their family forever, since such promises may have been made and broken in the past.

Often the child misjudges ordinary unsatisfactory situations as rejection; a frustration or a simple interdiction already means disapproval. The constant, unconditional emotional engagement of the future adoptive parents for their child leads to his gradually trusting the new relationships and with time to integrate into the new family. Protecting himself from feared rejections, the child may in turn reject the parents, for example by threatening to leave, packing his bags, telling parents that he does not love them and comparing them unfavorably to his former family or care persons. The child reenacts the past endured experience in taking an active role, thus avoiding suffering again a new rejection as a passive victim. In parallel—during the three stages described—the child is obliged to grief the loss of significant persons due to his placement in the new family. Shock and denial are the first reaction, followed by anger and rage, and accompanied by feelings of helplessness and loneliness. Many children remain blocked in their state of anger, unable to accomplish any mourning, as they often suffered recurring separations. Only with help of an emotionally disponible and continuously available adult, will a child be able to engage in a grieving process.

Symptomatic Behavior

At the beginning, the child seems to be very active but has poor attention and concentration skills, which may be a hypomanic defense against his anxiety. When playing, the child has difficulties finishing a game, respecting its rules, or tolerating to lose. Behavioral disorders and school performance problems are frequent. The child's aggressive behavior appears in fights with other children and in destructive activities. A child may hurt himself or suffer accidents. Psychosomatic symptoms such as abdominal pain and headaches are common. A trivial infection may last for a very long time. Parents discover that their child lies and steals and thus expresses his intensive need for attention and care. The child has a hard time attracting attention through positive behavior. He presents symptoms such as nightmares, agitated sleep, night wetting and tends to masturbate and may show particular interest in sexual issues. Certain children suffer from phobias, others behave cruelly towards animals. In general, children prefer to play with younger companions they can dominate. They are frustrated when parents hug each other, feeling left out or they cling to one parent and exclude the other. The child shows no perception of parental needs but arouses their guilt feelings. Outside the family, the child tends to win over other people with charming behavior, and refuses receiving love and tenderness from his parents. Certain children consider only the buying of a gift by their parents as proof of their love. The child's provocative behavior leads to the impression that he seeks to be punished for his bad behavior. The family painfully realizes that the child does not trust them. Parents need to prove again and again that they are different from those their child has known before.

Loyalty Versus Disloyalty

The first task the child faces is to resolve his inner conflict of loyalty. Working out his past affective ties in such a way that creating new affective ties does not mean disloyalty. The loyalty conflict experienced by the child often manifests itself by his naming the new parents. A child may only speak of his former family and not name his new parents. Later, he will try to recognize reaction and attitude of his parents by naming the former mom and dad. Once the child realizes that his new parents can accept that he calls his former parents mom and dad, i.e. that he does not have to renounce his past, he will in time call his present parents mom and dad, what, however, does not mean that the child has completed his intrapsychic processing of loyalty conflicts.

A child may re-experience the loss of previous important attachment figures. He is confronted with an extremely complex task to reconcile the inner relational representations of significant persons of the past with the building up relationship-representations of his present parents, a long-lasting intrapsychic process, which will be re-actualized in adolescence. How painful the associated emotions of this elaboration can be is demonstrated by the example of an adopted teenager, shouting desperately to her adoptive mother: "I don't have a mom!" She felt that a part of her being, the one connected to her birth parents, had been dismissed or denied by her adoption. She lamented the loss of this absent, however present part inside herself and said, that she would never be able to recover this part of her being.

At the beginning, the adoptive child usually does not speak about his memories in his new family, since the feelings associated with these experiences are emotionally far too overwhelming. Later, when he feels at ease in his new family, he starts recounting good memories, generally idealizing his stories. Compared to his previous caregivers, the present parents appear in an unfavorable light. Thanks to positive experiences in his new family and increasing trust the child gains a sense of belonging and begins to narrate in a more adequate way.

Children may test their family by suggesting that their first name be changed, for what they give "valuable" reasons. However, the child's desire is quite different, namely that his parents keep his first name, symbol of his unique personality with his individual history and past. Often children cling to their family or first name during a certain period, then suddenly refuse to pronounce their family name and destroy objects carrying their name. These behaviors show how hard children struggle with their conflictual identity. The child's wish and expectation are that his parents recognize his past identity and help him to preserve it.

Questioning the New Affective Ties

When children show their affection in the relationships with their adoptive parents, they begin to integrate into their new family. The creation of affective ties may be threatening and is questioned again and again, as the child needs to protect himself from future hurts. Gradually, the child also perceives feelings and needs of his parents, which at the beginning he ignored. Future projects can now be discussed, and events—experienced and shared with the new family—can be remembered. The anniversary of the child's placement into his new family is celebrated together, and the affective bonds deepen. Finally, the child dares to talk about his birth parents and/or his previous suffered rejections. This is the time when behavioral symptoms diminish, and the child begins to become an authentic member of his adoptive family.

The Family System

Parents immediately feel the changes in the family balance after the placement of an older child. The family has been compared to a decorative mobile, to which a new element is added. Each family member is affected until the establishment of a new balance. Even if the adoptive parents are prepared and informed about possible troubles, they usually find the adjustment more difficult than they imagined. They have to recognize that there is no spontaneous love between child and parents and the child is felt as a stranger in their family. Often a reevaluation of their adoption motivation takes place. Very frequently other children in the family are upset about the arrival of an additional child, which further complicates the situation. Negative fantasies may arise, such as the family or one of its member could be hurt by a "dangerous" child.

Parental Adjustment

At a certain point, parents begin to doubt their competence to raise and educate another child. Negative emotions may be overwhelming and leading to parental guilt feelings, which are exacerbated when people outside the family express their appreciation for the parents' readiness to accept an older child for adoption. The repeated reenactment of the child's previous conflictual relationships is getting increasingly unbearable for the adoptive parents. Their impression is that the child takes revenge on them for his past suffered relational injuries. The child's unconscious hope is that his adoptive parents will help him to cope, understand and coming to term with his past traumatic experiences. Adoptive parents may also feel threatened when their child demands his birth parents back. Only the working through and the shared emotions of sorrow, pain, and sadness of the child's lived traumatic events and losses will lead to greater intimacy, closeness, and a sense of belonging between parent and child.

Marital Relationship

Spouses feel a great need to communicate and support each other. Conflicts between spouses may arise when the child plays one parent off against the other. The relationship with the child varies and each parent may have different and distinct feelings regarding the child. Jealousy or incompetence may arise in a parent when the child splits his feelings and assigns the "bad" role to one parent. Re-evaluation of personal rules, of disciplinary measures in the family, of the way parents have processed their own losses and related feelings of pain and sadness, as well as re-evaluation of the couple's relationship and intimacy are considered the most important factors helping the family to integrate the older child—with his already marked personality—as a new member into their family.

Suggestions for New Parents Adopting an Older Child

Too high parental expectations to integrate their adoptive child within a determined period of time lead to disappointment of both parents and child. For the first phase of adjustment, it seems important to maintain a daily routine, helping the child to learn a sense of regularity, familiarity, and security. New rules and values should be introduced slowly and carefully, and disciplinary measures used sensitively and explained. When addressing behavioral disorders, a priority needs to be chosen for the most disturbing behavior, while other problems have first to be ignored. Changes are taken place step by step and at times there may be the impression of no progress at all.

Compared with biological or previously adopted children, the newly placed child has spent very little time in the family. Recognizing and empathically receiving the child's emotions, associated with his symptomatic behavior, is a challenging but rewarding task for adoptive parents. It is crucial to realize that the child's behavior, despite its disruptive character, has a significant meaning. Adoptive parents need to be aware that their child's rejecting behavior only seemingly is directed at them; in fact, they are standing in for former caregivers and are being tested by the child for their reliability. Parents ought not to feel threatened by their child's past. Showing the child physical affection and tenderness, even in critical situations or difficult times is essential. Opportunities such as the child's illness or injury allow parents to touch and hold their child. In the process of building a sustainable and supportive relationship, parents need to seize every occasion to strengthen their child's self-esteem. When the child succeeds talking to his parents about his abandonment, in expressing fears and feelings associated with his past traumatic experiences, he achieves a better emotional balance and creates new significant bonds with his parents. Open communication about meaningful persons of the past helps to prevent re-experiencing intense unbearable feelings. Humor is a vital resource and creates space and emotional distance in certain emotionally blocked moments.

References

1. Castoriadis-Aulagnier P. The violence of interpretation: from pictogram to statement. Hove, U.K. and Philadelphia: Brunner/Routledge; 2001. Translated by Alan Sheridan
2. Winnicott DW. Playing and reality. Routledge. London. Basic Books. New York 1971.
3. Winnicott DW. Transitional objects and transitional phenomena. Int J Psychoanal. 1953;34:89–97.
4. Winnicott DW (1955–1966) : Clinical varieties of transference. In: Collected papers. Through pediatrics to psychoanalysis. London: Tavistock; 1958.
5. Rizzuto AM. Psychoanalysis: the transformation of the subject by the spoken word. Psychoanalytic Quarterly, LXXII. 2003.
6. Bollas C. The shadow of the object: psychoanalysis of the unthought known. London: Free Association; 1987.
7. Bollas C. The transformational object. Int J Psychoanal. 1979;60:97–107.
8. Bollas C. On the relation to the self as an object. Int J Psychoanal. 1982;63:347–59.
9. Stern DN. Affect attunement. In: Call JD, Galenson E, Tyson RL, editors. Frontiers of infant psychiatry, vol. 2. New York: Basic Books; 1984. p. 3–14.
10. Klinnert MD, Campos JJ, Sorce JF, Emde RN, Svejda M. Emotions as behavior regulations: social referencing in infancy. In: Plutchhick R, Kellermann H, editors. Emotion: theory, research, and experience. New York: Academic; 1983.
11. Ogden TH. On holding and containing, being and dreaming. Int J Psychoanal. 2004;85(Pt 6):1349–64.
12. Bion WR. Learning from experience. London: Heinemann; 1962.

13. Kohut H. Thoughts on narcissism and narcissistic rage. Psychoanal Study Child. 1972;27:360–400.
14. Freud S. Beyond the pleasure principle. In: Complete psychological works, standard ed, vol. 18. London: Hogarth Press: 1920, p. 7–64. Reprinted in 1955.
15. Winnicott DW. The maturational processes and the facilitating environment. New York: International Universities Press; 1965.
16. Kernberg OF. Barrier to falling and remaining in love. J Am Psychoanal Assoc. 1974;4:743–68.
17. Tronick EZ. The neurobehavioral and social-emotional development of infants and children. New York: Norton; 2007.
18. Tronick ED, Beeghly M. Infants' meaning-making and the development of mental health problems. Am Psychol. 2011;66(2):107–19. https://doi.org/10.1037/a0021631.
19. Fonagy P, Gergely G, Jurist EL, Target M. Affect regulation, mentalization, and the development of the self. New York: Other Press; 2002.
20. Bürgin D. From outside to inside to outside: comments on intrapsychic representations and interpersonal interactions. Infant Ment Health J. 2011;32(1):95–114. https://doi.org/10.1002/imhj.20285.
21. Ladame F. Einschreibung in die Zeitlichkeit: ein Hauptthema der Adoleszenz. EPF-Bulletin. 2007;61:103–8.
22. Solis-Ponton L. La parentalité. Paris: Un hommage international à Serge Lebovici. Le fi l rouge. PUF; 2002.
23. Manzano J, Palacio Espasa F, Zilkha N. Les scenarios narcissiques de la parentalite, clinique de la consultation therapeutique. Paris: PUF. Le Fil Rouge; 1999.
24. Bushdid C, Magnasco MO, Vosshall LB, Keller A. Humans can discriminate more than 1 trillion olfactory stimuli. Science. 2014;343(6177):1370–2. https://doi.org/10.1126/science.1249168.
25. Fivaz-Depeursinge E, Corboz-Warnery A. The primary triangle. New York: Basic Behavioral Science; 1999.
26. Manzano J. Les relations précoces parents-enfants et leurs troubles. Suisse: Médecine et Hygiène. Chêne-Bourg; 1996.
27. Stern DN. The interpersonal world of the infant. New York: Basic Books; 1985. ISBN 978-0-465-09589-6
28. Knauer D, Palacio-Espasa F. Interventions précoces parents-enfants: Avantages et limites. Psychiatr Enfant. 2002;XLV:103–32.
29. Winnicott DW. Primary maternal preoccupation. 1956. In: Winnicott DW. Through pediatrics to psychoanalysis. London: Tavistock; 1958, p. 300–5.
30. Winnicott DW. The theory of the parent-infant relationship. Int J Psychoanal. 1960;41:585–95.
31. Bion WR. Attention and interpretation. London: Karnac; 1970.
32. Winnicott DW. Fear of breakdown. Int R Psychoanal. 1974;1974(1):103–7.
33. Ogden TH. Fear of breakdown and the unlived life. Int J Psychoanal. 2014;95:205–23.
34. Freud S. Studies on hysteria, vol. II. SE Hogarth Press. London; 1893–1895.
35. Freud S. An infantile neurosis and other works, vol. XVII. London: SE Hogarth Press; 1917–1919.
36. Freud, S. Analysis of a Phobia in a Five-Year-Old Boy. SE 10: 1-150. Hogarth Press. London; (1909).
37. Saint-Exupéry A. The little Prince Richard Howard (Translator) 1943.
38. Casonato M, Habersaat S. Parenting without being genetically connected. Enfance. 2015;3(3):289 à 306. ISSN 0013-7545. https://doi.org/10.3917/enf1.153.0289.
39. Erikson EH. Life history and the historical moment. New York: W.W. Norton; 1975.
40. Bürgin D. Triangulierung; der Übergang zur Elternschaft. Stuttgart: Schattauer Verlag; 1998.
41. Küchenhoff J, Könnecke R, Schilling S. Wenn der Übergang zur Vaterschaft misslingt – zur Psychodynamik des unerfüllten Kinderwunsches beim Mann. In: Bürgin D, editor. Triangulierung; der Übergang zur Elternschaft. Stuttgart: Schattauer Verlag; 1998.
42. Freeark K, Rosenberg EB, Bornstein J, Jozefowicz-Simbeni D, Linkevich M, Lohnes K. Gender differences and dynamics shaping the adoption life cycle: review of the literature and recommendations. Am J Orthopsychiatry. 2005;75(1):86–101.

43. Golombok S, Cook R, Bish A, Murray C. Families created by the new reproductive technologies: quality of parenting and social and emotional development of the children. Child Dev. 1995;66:285–98.
44. CDC. What is assisted reproductive technology? Reproductive Health; 2019.
45. Zegers-Hochschild F. International Committee for Monitoring Assisted Reproductive Technology (ICMART) and the World Health Organization (WHO) revised glossary of ART terminology, 2009 (PDF). Fertil Steril. 2009;92(5):1520–4. https://doi.org/10.1016/j.fertnstert.2009.09.009. Archived (PDF) from the original on 2016-11-29
46. Hoksbergen R, Textor MR. Adoption. Grundlagen, Vermittlung Nachbetreuung, Beratung. Freiburg i. Br.: Lambertus 1993.
47. Wyverkens E, Veerle Provoost V, Ravelingien A, Pennings G, De Sutter P, Buysse A. The meaning of the sperm donor for heterosexual couples: confirming the position of the father. Fam Process. 2017;56(1):203–16. https://doi.org/10.1111/famp.12156. Epub 2015 Apr 23
48. Williams LS. Adoption actions and attitudes of couples seeking in vitro fertilization. An exploratory study. J Fam Issues. 1992;13(1):99–113.
49. Stoléru S. Neuropsychiatrie de l'enfant. 1995;43(4/5):164–70.
50. Sabatello U, Natali P, Giannotti A. Pre-adoptive diagnosis: the meaning of a crisis. Br J Psychotherapy. 1989;6(2):160–9.
51. Dreixler M. Der Mensch als Ware. Frankfurt a.M.: Peter Lang, Europäischer Verlag der Wissenschaften 1998.
52. Means T, Dickison SK. Plutarch and the family of Cato minor. Class J. 1974;69:210–5. The Johns Hopkins University Press
53. Grotevant HD, Lo AYH. Adoptive parenting. Curr Opin Psychol. 2017;15:71–5.
54. Schechter MD. About adoptive parents. In: Anthony EJ, Benedek T, editors. Parenthood: its psychology and psychopathology. Boston: Little, Brown; 1970. p. 353–71.
55. Reczek C. Sexual- and gender-minority families: a 2010 to 2020 decade in review. J Marriage Fam. 2020;82(1):300–25. https://doi.org/10.1111/jomf.12607.
56. Goldberg SK, Conron KJ. How many same-sex couples in the U.S. are raising children? The Williams Institute; 2018. https://williamsinstitute.law.ucla.edu/wpcontent/uploads/Parenting-Among-Same-Sex-Couples
57. Farr RH, Ravvina Y, Grotevant HD. Birth family contact experiences among lesbian, gay, and heterosexual adoptive parents with school-age children. Fam Relat. 2018;67(1):132–46.
58. Carone N, Bos HMW, Shenkman G, Tasker F. Editorial: LGBTQ parents and their children during the family life cycle. Front Psychol. 2021;12:643647. https://doi.org/10.3389/fpsyg.2021.643647.
59. Takacs J, Szalma I, Bartus T. Social attitudes toward adoption by same-sex couples in Europe. Arch Sex Behav. 2016;45:1787–98. https://doi.org/10.1007/s10508-016-0691-9.
60. Goldberg AE, Smith JZ. Predictors of race, adoption, and sexual orientation related socialization of adoptive parents of young children. J Fam Psychol. 2015; https://doi.org/10.1037/fam0000149.
61. Freeark K, Rosenblum KL, Hus V, Root BL. Fathers, mothers and marriages: what shapes adoption conversations in families with young adopted children? Adopt Q. 2008;11:1–23. https://doi.org/10.1080/10926750802291393.
62. Wrobel GM, Kohler JK, Grotevant HD, McRoy RG. The family adoption communication (FAC) model: identifying pathways of adoption-related communication. Adopt Q. 2003;7:53–84. https://doi.org/10.1300/j145v07n02_04.
63. Hughes D, Rodriguez J, Smith EP, Johnson DJ, Stevenson HC, Spicer P. Parents' ethnic-racial socialization practices: a review of research and directions for future study. Dev Psychol. 2006;42:747–70. https://doi.org/10.1037/0012-1649.42.5.747.
64. Brodzinsky D. Children's understanding of adoption: developmental and clinical implications. Prof Psychol Res Pract. 2011;42:200–7. https://doi.org/10.1037/a0022415.

65. Costa PA, Tasker F, Leal IP. Different placement practices for different families? Children's adjustment in LGH adoptive families. Front Psychol. 2021;12:649853. https://doi.org/10.3389/fpsyg.2021.649853.

66. Schumm WRA. Review and critique of research on same-sex parenting and adoption. Psychol Rep. 2016;119(3):641–760.

67. Berger M. Homoparentalité et développement affectif de l'enfant. Gallimard « Le Débat ». 2014/3 n° 180 | pages 139 à 146. 2014 ISSN 0246–2346.

68. Callaghan JEM, Fellin LC, Alexander JH. Mental health of looked-after children: embodiment and use of space. In: Evans B, Horton J, Skelton T, editors. Play, recreation, health, and well being. Geographies of children and young people, vol. 9. Singapore: Springer; 2015. https://doi.org/10.1007/978-981-4585-96-5_22-1.

69. Szilagyi MA, Rosen DS, Rubin D, Zlotnik S. Health care issues for children and adolescents in foster care and kinship care. Pediatrics. 2015;136:4.

70. Barth R, Green R, Guo S. Kinship care and foster care. Arch Pediatr Adolesc Med. 2008;162(6):586–7.

71. Boswell S, Cudmore L. Understanding the 'blind spot' when children move from foster care into adoption. J Child Psychother. 2017;43(2):243–57. https://doi.org/10.1080/0075417X.2017.1323946.

72. Ozoux-Teffaine O. Enjeux de l'adoption tardive. Nouveau fondementspour la clinique. La vie de l'enfant. Ramonville Saint-Agne : Edition eres 2004.

73. Gill MM. Adoption of older children: the problems faced. Soc Casework. 1978;59:272–8.

74. Anzieu D. Le Moi-peau. Paris: Dunod; 1985.

Chapter 3
Stress and Pain

"Turmoil
   Happiness is often accompanied by suffering.
   It hurts, I want to scream my pain.
   The suffering of a child rises to the surface, overflows,
   a river coming out of its bed, submerging the earth.
   This suffering knows no limits, it invades me, destroys me,
   it destabilizes my structure, it makes me doubt about myself,
   it is anchored in my flesh, my guts.
   This pain is not due to any hazard, its origin is called abandonment,
   the abandonment of a father and a mother, the weakness of two beings.
   I wish so much being able finally to turn the page, not to be tormented anymore."
   Adopted youth

Stress

Every crisis has both its dangers and its opportunities—Martin Luther King

Introduction

The "stress model"—stress reaction or stress response system—consists of two different levels, the soma, and the mind. While on the somatic level, basic functions are postnatally established, mental structures are substantially built up after birth. Harmful stress impairs the organization of these mental structures. External stress has very different impacts, corresponding to specific times of exposure during the development process. The stress response is considered an innate, mind and body encompassing function; stress reactions are mainly characterized by the infant's

B. Steck, *Adoption as a Lifelong Process*,
https://doi.org/10.1007/978-3-031-33038-4_3

genetic predispositions, environmental influences, and the associated exchange processes.

From a biological perspective, the brain is the central organ for adaptive processes not only for our living in the physical environment as part of a homeostatic regulation, but also for our life in the social environment. Our lived experiences modulate brain structures and functions, they induce changes, termed adaptive plasticity. In response to critical life events, so-called stressors, there is a coordinated and energizing response, which maintains our physical integrity and psychic well-being. Mind—and by association the brain—facing threats and potentially stressful situations initiate physiological, emotional, and behavioral responses. These reactions can either be adaptive or detrimental to health. Stress is always based—by means of the autonomic nervous system and endocrine mechanisms—on a bidirectional communication between different systems (e.g., brain, heart, circulation, immune and metabolic networks). The complex interactions of these different systems lead to positive or negative changes in brain, mind, and body. The hormones associated with stress exposure protect the body in the short term and promote adaptation. In the long term, however, exposure to chronic stress causes changes in brain and body with subsequent illnesses.

Neurobiological Responses to Stress

The central components of the stress system are located in the hypothalamus and the brain stem. They form parts of a neuroendocrine control system, the hypothalamic-pituitary-adrenal axis, and of the autonomic nervous system, namely the sympathetic-adreno-medullary system. The activation of these systems results in increased secretion of stress hormones (corticotropin-releasing hormone, cortisol, noradrenaline, and adrenaline). At the same time increased inflammation-related cytokines, [1] responsible for the coordination of the immune system, are released, followed by the activation of the parasympathetic nervous system, the other part of the involuntary nervous system, which begins to rebalance both the sympathetic activation and the inflammatory reactions [1].

The stress system has two main operational modes of functioning. The immediate mode is the fight or flight response, [2] which is triggered by a rapid activation of the sympathetic nervous system as a result of the release of adrenaline. In parallel, the hypothalamic-pituitary-adrenal axis (HPA axis) is stimulated. Two important hormones from the hypothalamus and the pituitary gland are released, the corticotropin-releasing hormone (CRH) and adrenocorticotropic hormone (ACTH). They serve the coordination of rapid metabolic and behavioral responses. The

---

[1] Cytokines are peptides that regulate growth and differentiation of cells, mostly in the immune system.

[2] The fight or flight response was first described by Walter Cannon (1871–1945) as a reaction in animals to a threatening event. It can also give rise to a freezing of mental functions.

ACTH effect on the adrenal cortex leads to the release of glucocorticoids; they are responsible for the multiple physical reactions and behaviors that occur during an acute stress reaction.

The other mode consists of a long-lasting influence on social behavior and plays probably a key role in dealing with everyday social stress. This mode involves many circuits in the limbic system. The CRH has an important function in the regulation of behaviors associated with chronic stress [2].

Stressful experiences in early childhood negatively affect an individual's ability to cope with stressful events later in life [3]. The failure of coping mechanisms is accompanied by several changes, namely abnormal activity of the HPA axis and altered limbic functions. The neurobiological consequences of molecular and cellular changes occur not only in the limbic system, especially the amygdala and hippocampus, but also in the prefrontal cortex. While the exact molecular mechanisms responsible for stress-induced cognitive impairment are not yet known, there is evidence that changes in the anchoring properties of synapses by cell adhesion molecules are involved. Dysregulation of synaptic adhesion molecules by stress leads to synaptic changes and memory deficits [4].

Stress-related learning deficits may be caused by suppressed neurogenesis in the hippocampus. These changes are reversible. Individual differences in vulnerability to stress can be explained by a greater or lesser regeneration capacity in brain circuits and functions after stress-induced changes. Stressful events in early childhood, such as the death of a parent, impair hippocampal integrity, resulting in subsequent reduced cognitive performance. In children with severe deprivations, an increased amygdala volume and a lower total brain volume were found [5].

Psychobiological Effects of Stressful Experiences

Adverse experiences during critical developmental periods in early childhood greatly influence brain development and can have long-lasting effects. However, brain development retains its plasticity into adulthood [6, 7]. Stressful events in early childhood that give rise to epigenetic modifications altering gene expression play an important role in the development of stress-related mental disorders and other health problems later in life. These changes are often ongoing but need not be permanent [7, 8].

In humans, the development of the brain, especially the cortex, takes place largely postnatally. Epigenetic changes are associated with changes in both gene expression and synaptic development [9]. However, mental illnesses cannot be reduced to a simple genetic or molecular level but must be understood as a large-scale dysfunction. Not only the genetic and biological factors of the brain need to be considered, but also the complex environmental factors and personal life experiences, which may be associated with acute or chronic emotional stress [10].

Both the psychic and biological confrontation-, conflict-, and coping processes as reactions to stress, as well as the nature of recovery from stress are fundamental to understand the extent of psycho-physical consequences in situations of chronic stress. A direct effect of chronic stress is seen in the impaired ability to cope effectively with stress. An exaggerated or reduced stress response may indicate a dysregulation of those systems responsible for maintaining homeostasis and good health. Adverse early childhood experiences are associated with decreased stress reactivity and increased impulsive behavior. Young adults who experienced a high level of adverse experiences before the age of 16, showed reduced cortisol and heart rate reactivity, decreased cognitive performance and unstable affect control, often associated with impulsive behavior and antisocial tendencies [11].

The reduced stress reactivity (reduced cortisol release), resulting from early childhood stressful experiences, causes decreased dopamine activity and provides a basis for the development of risky behaviors, because it alters cortisol feedback responses in critical brain systems.

Certain areas of the brain need to be sufficiently stimulated at crucial stages of development to function optimally later on. Critical stressful experiences in early childhood not only affect the development of the cerebral cortex and the limbic system, but also lead to multiple long-term changes in several neurotransmitter systems. The specific connectivity of dendritic branches and neuronal synapses is shaped according to the frequency of their use. Thalamus, amygdala, hippocampus, and prefrontal cortex are all involved in the gradual integration and interpretation of incoming sensory information [12]. This integration process can be disrupted by high arousal.

Although genetic variability in stress reactivity is undoubtedly significant, early life experiences and environmental influences convey considerable effects. The mere exposure of a fetus to maternal stress can later influence its readiness to react, i.e., its response to stress. While temporary increases in stress hormones are protective and even necessary for survival, excessively high levels or prolonged exposure can be harmful or downright "toxic". Dysregulation of this network of physiological mediators (i.e., too much or too little cortisol, for example) can give rise to a chronic "wear and tear" effect of multiple organ systems, including the brain [1]. Cumulative, stress-inducing strains ultimately make it impossible to cope with stress and return to a homeostatic balance. Certain neurobiological changes are reversible through treatment measures. Various studies show that the negative consequences of early environmental stress, i.e., the corresponding psychopathological disorders, can be alleviated by preventive interventions [13].

Three Different Types of Stress Reactions in Young Children

In young children, regardless of the actual stressors, three different types of stress reactions are distinguished, based on their potential to cause lasting physiological disorders: a positive, a tolerable, and a toxic stress [1].

Positive Stress The concept of positive stress relates to a short and easily to regulate physiologic state, whereby the availability of caring and responsive adults is essential to help the child reduce the stress, in providing a protective effect, which enables the stress response system to quickly return to its initial state. Positive stress responses can be a growth-promoting element in a child's normal development. The quality of the relationship translates directly into the physiological and functional processes of the brain, the autonomic nervous, and the endocrine systems.

Tolerable Stress It is—in contrast to the positive stress—linked to an exposure to non-normative experiences that contain a higher degree of strain or threat. The triggering factors can be, for example, a serious illness, an injury, or a conflictual divorce. However, even in these cases, if there is sufficient protection from supportive adults, the risk that these circumstances produce excessive activation of the stress response systems, leading to psycho-physiological damage and long-term consequences for health and learning processes, is greatly reduced.

Toxic Stress This is caused by too strong, too frequent, or too long-lasting activation of the physical stress reaction systems. In most cases, no protective and supportive adult relationship has been available. All forms of emotional unavailability of primary care persons in early childhood, for example neglect, substance abuse or depression, are likely to induce a toxic response to stress. In addition to the more short-term changes in observable behavior, toxic stress in young children can result in little outwardly visible signs but permanent changes in brain structures and functions. The plasticity of the fetal, infant, and early childhood brain makes it particularly sensitive to hormonal influences. Prolonged elevated levels of stress hormones interrupt and alter the size of glucocorticoid receptors in the amygdala and modify the development of brain architecture in the cortex. At the same time, chronic stress can lead to the loss of neurons and neuronal connections in the hippocampus and medial prefrontal cortex.

Although the hippocampus can turn off elevated cortisol, chronic stress reduces its ability to do so and may lead to impaired memory and mood. Exposure to chronic stress and high cortisol levels inhibits neurogenesis in the hippocampus, which plays an important role in encoding memories and other functions [1]. Toxic stress limits the ability of the hippocampus to promote contextual learning, which is associated with difficulties in distinguishing potentially dangerous from safe circumstances, as is the case in post-traumatic stress disorders.

Stressful experiences in early childhood can impair the development of adaptive and coping skills needed to deal with later challenges. Unhealthy lifestyles, lack of coping strategies and environmental disruption are often responsible for children's physiological, psychic, and behavioral responses to significant adversity in early childhood. The long-term adverse consequences can best be avoided by having available, stable, and responsive caregivers who help children develop a reliable sense of security that promotes the return and restoration of their stress response systems to baseline. Stressful events alone do not lead to adverse outcomes; it is rather the absence or inadequacy of protective relationships, which hinder the healthy adaptation to stress. In the presence of severe adversity, there is a toxic stress response, associated with disturbing physiological responses, which may generate "biological memories" and increase the risk of negative health outcomes. Toxic exposure in childhood is associated with the development of unhealthy lifestyles (e.g., substance abuse, poor eating and exercise habits), as well as persistent social impairment such as school failure and poor health (e.g., diabetes and cardiovascular disease) [13].

The toxic stress response affects the neuroendocrine immune network and causes a persistent and abnormal cortisol response. The resulting immune dysregulation, including a persistent inflammatory state, increases the risk and frequency of infections in children. The toxic response to stress plays a role in the pathophysiology of depressive and psychotic disorders, as well as in behavioral and post-traumatic stress disorders. Adults who had to endure adverse early childhood circumstances, are more likely to suffer physical illnesses and to show unfavorable health issues (alcoholism, chronic obstructive pulmonary disease, depression, malignant tumors, obesity, more frequent suicide attempts, ischemic heart disease, and others) [14]. Excessive stressful early childhood life experiences seem to cause lifelong immune dysregulations [15]. In toxic stress, there is an interaction of environmental influences with psychic, cerebral, and whole-body processing, resulting in mental and/or somatic disorders.

Stress at Different Ages

Prenatal Stress

When a mother suffers major stress during pregnancy, there are profound influences on the endocrine functions of the fetus, which may extend throughout his life. These effects appear to a large extent dependent on the timing of the maternal stress, as specific stages of brain development are likely to be more sensitive to the impact of intrauterine exposure to glucocorticoids. Moreover, these effects appear to be strongly sex-dependent [16]. Diseases occurring during pregnancy can also be transmitted to the fetus and thus passed on to future generations [17]. Maternal stress resulting from critical life events during pregnancy is linked to impaired attention and spatial working memory in offspring's early childhood [18]. These associations vary depending on the sex of the child and the intensity of maternal anxiety during pregnancy, as well as on the maternal care after pregnancy.

Stress in Infancy

It is well known from child psychiatry clinics that maternal depressive symptomatology is associated with reduced sensitivity to infants and young children and with behaviors of non-engagement and withdrawal [19].

The development of the child's amygdala takes place from the first year until late childhood. The amygdala seems to have a particularly high sensitivity to the quality of maternal care [19]. Infants with depressed mothers showed larger volumes of the amygdala and higher glucocorticoid levels. Similarly, children who have grown up in orphanages also show an increased amygdala volume, which suggests that the amygdala is particularly sensitive to severely disturbed (i.e., discontinuous, or neglectful) care in early childhood. The volume of the hippocampus remained the same in children of mothers who had suffered from depression since birth than in a control group of children with non-affected mothers. Stressful experiences during gestation may have an influence on neurodevelopment, especially the connectivity between the amygdala and the medial prefrontal cortex, a circuitry important for emotion regulation in later development [20].

Stress in Separation Situations

Extensive studies in animal research show that opiates, endorphins, oxytocin, and prolactin are released in the central nervous system as regulators during separation anxiety [21]. In addition, the reactivity of the sympathetic nervous system is increased [22].

According to Panksepp [23], there are six emotional systems [3] helping the organism to feel affectively balanced or unbalanced. The panic system is responsible for the psychic pain of separation distress. It involves a panic protest, immediately following social losses, triggering intense sadness and pain.

In the case of social loss or prolonged separation of an infant from his mother, a transition from feelings of panic to despair takes place, a reaction, which—without sufficient relational help by adequate substitute persons—may give rise to the so-called "anaclitic" depression in the young child. [4]

Long-lasting neurobiological changes (especially of neurotransmitters such as serotonin and catecholamines) can be the consequences, with disturbances of cardiac rhythm, body temperature and sleep disturbances as well as changes of neurohormones, e.g., oxytocin, which promotes empathy and attachment development.

Children, who have experienced stressful separations, remain vulnerable because disturbances in the neurotransmitter and neuroendocrine systems are long-lasting and can be reactivated later in other stressful situations, such as the loss of affective relationships. They are also more susceptible to physical disorders and especially to infectious diseases.

---

[3] The primary emotional systems in mammals are seeking, anger, fear, desire, caring, panic, and play.

[4] Anaclitic depression is a short-term life-sustaining shutdown mechanism (Robertson and Robertson [24]: Young Children in Brief Separation. In: Psychoanal. Study Child, 26: 264–315); it was first described by Spitz RA (1946): Anaclitic depression; an inquiry into the genesis of psychiatric conditions in early childhood. Psychoanal Study Child. 2:313–42.

Pain

> When deprived of something, children react with such a great intensity, either of protest or
> sadness, that it seems as though the experience they are living at the moment completely
> invades all aspects of their life… ([25]: p. 239)

Neurobiological Aspects of Pain

There is a wide spectrum of pain sensations. Nociceptive pain arises from mechanical, thermal, chemical, or electrical stimulation of pain receptors, the nociceptors, which map to the sensory cortex via afferent pain fibers. In medical examination, pain is measured with clinical scales, while neuroscience attempts to visualize it through brain imaging techniques [26].

Darwin [27] showed the evolutionary origin of pain expression in his book *The Expression of Emotions in Man and Animals*. Facial expression and vocalization of pain are behaviors representing calls for help and trigger prosocial responses. The function of pain in all living beings is to protect the body from harm, ultimately pain serves to prolong life.

Very large neural networks are mobilized during emotional pain, and their interactions during varying pain states remain to be understood in more detail. However, extensive imaging studies demonstrate a network of brain structures, which process pain-related information. This includes the thalamic nuclei, which play a key role in receiving and processing sensory information, and the somatosensory, insular, and anterior cingulate cortex. The latter two are important for the affective and behavioral aspects of pain [28]. Prefrontal cortical as well as subcortical areas such as the amygdala contribute to the awareness and cognitive appraisal of pain [29]. The amygdala is a key element in the affective components of pain and, together with the prefrontal cortex, forms part of the multimodal fields of the pain processing network. Through its connection with the reward-aversion system, the amygdala also plays an important role in the modulation of pain.

The same neurotransmitters (opiates, endorphins, oxytocin, and prolactin) that regulate physical pain also control the feelings of pain e.g., in separation situations. The complex nature of pain leads to the activation of extensive neuronal networks that influence the emotional state of a subject. The affective and sensory components of pain are closely linked. In humans who respond empathically to the pain of another person, the same brain regions are activated which are also involved in physical pain [30]. Psychic pain in humans (e.g., in mourning processes) activates the same neuronal pathways as physical pain (namely the anterior cingulate gyrus, the dorsomedial thalamus, and the periaqueductal grey [31].

With increasing encephalization of the pain system, neural mechanisms evolved, which enabled the transition from pain as a purely physical phenomenon to the experience of psychological pain. Thus, the pain system, with all its complex sensory and affective components, is an important self-regulating network of visceral and somatic functions. It controls bodily integrity and plays an important role in the formation of attachment [5] and empathy [34].

Pain and Stress Processing

Infants and toddlers have not yet acquired the ability to reflectively perceive and express their feelings in a stressful situation. An emotionally too violent or painful experience may be expressed by the body in behavioral manifestations, psychosomatic disorders, or developmental dysfunctions [35, 36].

Psychic pain is caused by a real or imagined loss of a loved person. The significant person is irretrievably lost, but the deprived subject nevertheless holds on to the loved one by emotionally investing his internal representation [37]. Where there is pain, the absent, lost person is still present.

Pain perception is modulated by the influence of emotional and cognitive components. Negative emotions of intense and short duration, such as those associated with physical injury, diminish pain perception. They lead to stress-induced hypoalgesia. Long-lasting influences of psychosocial stress, overwhelming an individual, are associated with negative emotions of anxiety and depression and result in constant distress. The pain threshold is lowered, pain perception is increased, and hyperalgesia develops [38]. The central stress processing system includes various areas of the prefrontal cortex, the rostral and dorsal anterior cingulate gyrus, the anterior insula, the amygdala, and the hippocampus. Pain and stress are processed in the same brain regions.

Infancy, childhood, and adolescence are particularly vulnerable periods with increased susceptibility to stress [39]. If a child's basic needs are not met by continuous, loving, and reliable caregivers, the development of his personality and health is persistently at risk. Aversive childhood experiences can be linked to sustained modification of pain processing, leading to increased pain sensitivity, heightened pain significance with associated negative feelings, and a greater risk of pain disorders in adulthood.

Cumulative stress experiences lead to modified cellular and neuroendocrine expression at different levels of pain processing. Chronic stress experiences result in pain amplification mechanisms and cerebral sensitization to pain. Central features in pain disorders are hyperalgesia, an increased pain sensation, which is also accompanied by sensitivity to touch and hypersensitivity, due to a lowered pain threshold, as well as by affective symptoms, such as increased anxiety reactions or more

---

[5]According to the attachment theory, somatization is the failure to build up a secure attachment in infancy; in early development, the integration of sensory, visceral, and motor excitations with images and words does not take place. "A fundamental aspect of this learning is dependent on the parents' ability to mirror and regulate the infant's emotional states and in this way help the infant to convert emotional arousal into psychic elements that can then be thought about, named and communicated" (Fonagy et al. [32], cited in [33]: p. 122).

frequent depressive states. Victims of aversive childhood experiences show an elevated sensitivity and a chronicity of pain and anxiety.

An emotional evaluation of the pain stimulus occurs primarily in the anterior cingulate gyrus. The affective state of anxiety or depression influences the experience of pain. Social rejection or exclusion are associated with increased pain perception via activation in the region of the dorsal anterior cingulate gyrus [40], while the cognitive evaluation takes place in the prefrontal cortex. When a stressful situation is emotionally assessed as a catastrophe, no cognitive evaluation takes place and a heightened perception of pain results [41]. If a significant person providing emotional security is present, activation of the ventromedial prefrontal cortex occurs, and pain sensation is attenuated [42].

Early childhood painful, stressful experiences can interfere with the development of adaptive and coping skills, necessary to deal with later challenges. Stable and responsive relationship persons, helping children cope with emotional pain and providing a reliable sense of safety, support a return and restoration of children's stress response systems to baseline. The absence, or inadequacy of protective relationships impedes healthy adaptation to stress and psychic pain.

Pain and Attachment

> . . .for a person to know that an attachment figure is available and responsive gives him a strong and pervasive feeling of security. . . ([43] : p. 27).

Oxytocin—in addition to its importance during pregnancy—is involved in secure attachment in early childhood and provides a basis for the development of good-quality social relationships in adulthood [44].

Parental relationship models affect their child's attachment security, with each parent transferring their own internalized relationship pattern to the child, independent of the other parent. The child will eventually seek to integrate the two internalized relationship models of his primary caregivers. A secure internal relationship model is thought to be a sufficiently protective factor and contributes to the child's resilience in a deprivation situation [45].

Appropriately behaving caregivers activate a safety-signal-related neural area and reduce pain experiences. They provide a child with a sense of security in threatening situations. Underlying attachment-induced safety is based on the activation of neural regions signaling safety and reducing distress or threat. Visual contact with a caregiver during the experience of physical pain causes increased activity in the ventromedial prefrontal cortex, which is associated with decreased pain appraisal and reduced activity in neural pain regions [42].

Experiences of social rejection, exclusion or loss are among the most painful. Individual efforts to avoid such situations can be considerable. The question arises as to why these negative social experiences have such a profound impact on emotional well-being. New findings suggest that the experiences associated with social pain—such as painful feelings during social separation experiences—have the same underlying neurobiological substrates as physical pain experiences. Certain basic neural systems (involved in pain and reward) may have been co-opted to support more complex social experiences. The relevance of the overlap between physical and social pain helps to understand surprising findings: "In children, factors that increase the experience of physical pain (such as injury or sickness), also increase the child's sensitivity to the whereabouts of their caregiver, leading to more frequent experiences of distress upon separation "([40]: p. 428); there is "the reduction in physical pain that occurs in the presence of social support and the increase in feelings of social disconnection that accompanies physical pain" (idem: p. 431).

Parents and meaningful caregivers, by virtue of their behavior, play a significant role in their child's pain. Their own and the family's handling of pain (whether they overemphasize it, do not take it seriously enough, or react inadequately to it) forms the first resonance element with which an infant identifies. Their confidence in their child's ability to overcome pain is shown by their commitment to protect and monitor the child [46].

The Lancet Child and Adolescent Health Commission [47] highlights the fact that the experience of pain affects all children, from infants to adult age; pain is multifaceted, ranging from acute to chronic, arising from illness and physical interventions, but also in multiple other situations. Pain is omnipresent and poses a great challenge to the affected children and their families, as well as to the treating professionals and to society. The personal, psychic experience of pain often goes unnoticed, is not verbalized, or even ignored. Untreated, unrecognized, or poorly treated pain in childhood leads to serious and long-lasting negative consequences that persist into adulthood and include chronic pain, disability, and suffering. The authors point to the urgent need to ensure that pain is neither silenced nor its treatment ignored. Better ways to assess and identify pain must be made available, easier access to treatments for pain must be provided, and more affordable models of treatment must be developed.

References

1. Shonkoff JP, Garner AS. The committee on psychosocial aspects of child and family health, committee on early childhood, adoption and dependent care, and section on developmental and behavioral pediatrics. Technical report. The lifelong effects of early childhood adversity and toxic stress 2012.
2. Hostetler CM, Ryabinin AE. The CRF system and social behavior: a review. Front Neurosci. 2013;7(92):1–15.
3. De Kloet ER, Joëls M, Holsboer F. Stress and the brain: from adaptation to disease. Nat Rev Neurosci. 2005;6(6):463–75.
4. Wang XD, Su YA, Wagner KV, Avrabos C, Scharf SH, Hartmann J, et al. Nectin-3 links CRHR1 signaling to stress induced memory deficits and spine loss. Nat Neurosci. 2013;16(6):706–13.
5. Mehta MA, Golembo NI, Nosarti C, Colvert E, Mota A, Williams SCR, et al. Amygdala, hippocampal and corpus callosum size following severe early institutional deprivation: the English and Romanian adoptees study pilot. J Child Psychol Psychiatry. 2009;50(8):943–51.

6. Weder N, Kaufman J. Critical periods revisited: implications for intervention with traumatized children. J Am Acad Child Adolesc Psychiatry. 2011;50(11):1087–9.
7. Weder N, Zhang H, Jense K, Simen A, Jackowski A, Lipschitz D, et al. Child abuse, depression, and methylation in genes involved with stress, neural plasticity, and brain circuitry. J Am Acad Child Adolesc Psychiatry. 2014;53(4):417–24.
8. Nemeroff CB, Binder E. The preeminent role of childhood abuse and neglect in vulnerability to major psychiatric disorders: toward elucidating the underlying neurobiological mechanisms. J Am Acad Child Adolesc Psychiatry. 2014;53(4):395–7.
9. Gabel HW, Greenberg ME. Genetics. The maturing brain methylome. Science. 2013;341(6146):626–7. https://doi.org/10.1126/science.1242671.
10. Solms M. Freud returns. Sci Am. 2004;290(5):82–8.
11. Lovallo WR. Early life adversity reduces stress reactivity and enhances impulsive behavior: implications for health behaviors. Int J Psychophysiol. 2013;90(1):8–16.
12. Van der Kolk BA, Alexander C, McFarlane AC, Weisaeth L. Traumatic stress: the effects of overwhelming experience on mind, body, and society. New York: Guilford Press; 2007.
13. Garner AS, Shonkoff JP. Early childhood adversity, toxic stress, and the role of the pediatrician: translating developmental science into lifelong health. Pediatrics. 2012;129:e224–31.
14. Franke HA. Review: toxic stress: effects, prevention and treatment. Children. 2014;1:390–402.
15. Fagundes CP, Kiecolt-Glaser JK. Stressful early life experiences and immune dysregulation across the lifespan. Brain Behav Immun. 2013;27C:8–12.
16. Kapoor A, Dunn E, Kostaki A, Andrews M.H, Matthews SG. Symposium report fetal programming of hypothalamo-pituitaryadrenal function: Prenatal stress and glucocorticoids. The Journal of Physiology. 2006;572(1):31–44.
17. Cheong JN, Wlodek ME, Moritz KM, Cuffe JSM. Topical review: programming of maternal and offspring disease: impact of growth restriction, fetal sex and transmission across generations. J Physiol. 2016;594(17):4727–40.
18. Plamondon A, Akbari E, Atkinson L, Steiner M, Meaney M, Fleming AS. Spatial working memory and attention skills are predicted by maternal stress during pregnancy. Early Hum Dev. 2015;91:23–9.
19. Lupiena SJ, Parent S, Evanse AC, Tremblayc RE, Zelazoi PD, Corboj V, et al. Larger amygdala but no change in hippocampal volume in 10-year-old children exposed to maternal depressive symptomatology since birth. Proc Natl Acad Sci U S A. 2011;108(34):14324–9.
20. Humphreys KL, Camacho MC, Roth MC, Estes EC. Prenatal stress exposure and multimodal assessment of amygdala–medial prefrontal cortex connectivity in infants. Dev Cogn Neurosci. 2020;46:100877.
21. Panksepp J. Neuroscience. Feeling the pain of social loss. Science. 2003;302(5643):237–9.
22. Kossowsky J, Monique PHD, Pfaltz C, Schneider S, Taeymans J, Locher C, Gaab J. The separation anxiety hypothesis of panic disorder revisited: a meta-analysis. Am J Psychiatry. 2012;AiA:1–14.
23. Panksepp J. The psycho-neurology of cross-species affective/social neuroscience: understanding animal affective states as a guide to development of novel psychiatric treatments. Curr Top Behav Neurosci. 2017;30:109–25.
24. Robertson J, Robertson J. Young children in brief separation. Psychoanal Study Child. 1971;26:264–315.
25. Matte-Blanco I. The unconscious as infinite sets. An essay in bi-logic. London: Karnac; 1975.
26. Steck A, Steck B. Brain and mind. New York: Springer; 2016.
27. Darwin CR. The expression of the emotions in man and animals. 1st ed. London: John Murray; 1872.
28. Price DD. Psychological and neural mechanisms of the affective dimension of pain. Science. 2000;288(5472):1769–72. Review
29. Neugebauer V, Galhardo V, Maione S, Mackey SC. Forebrain pain mechanisms. Brain Res Rev. 2009;60(1):226–42. https://doi.org/10.1016/j.brainresrev.2008.12.014.

30. Bernhardt BC, Singer T. The neural basis of empathy. Annu Rev Neurosci. 2012;35:1–23. https://doi.org/10.1146/annurev-neuro-062111-150536. Review

31. Eisenberger NI, Lieberman MD, Williams KD. Does rejection hurt? An FMRI study of social exclusion. Science. 2003;302(5643):290–2.

32. Fonagy P, Gergely G, Jurist E, Target M. Affect Regulation, Mentalization and the Development of the Self. London. Karnac. (2002).

33. Gubb K. Psychosomatics today: a review of contemporary theory and practice. Psychoanal Rev. 2013;100(1):103–42. https://doi.org/10.1521/prev.2013.100.1.103.

34. Tucker DM, Luu P, Derryberry D. Love hurts: the evolution of empathic concern through the encephalization of nociceptive capacity. Dev Psychopathol. 2005;17(3):699–713.

35. Bürgin D, Steck B. Seelische Schmerzen als übergreifendes Element. In: Bründl P, Scheidt CE, editors. Psychosomatik-Sadomasochismus-Trauma. Klinische und entwicklungstheoretische Perspektiven. Frankfurt: Brandes & Apsel; 2020. p. S.18-37.

36. Bürgin D, Steck B. Seelischer Schmerz bei Kindern und Jugendlichen. Psychoanalytisch-psychotherapeutische Perspektiven. Frankfurt am Main, Deutschland: Brandes & Apsel (Verlag); 2021. 978-3-95558-317-0 (ISBN)

37. Pontalis JB. Entre le rêve et la douleur. Paris: Editions Gallimard; 1977.

38. Egle UT, Egloff N, von Känel R. Stressinduzierte Hyperalgesie (SIH) als Folge von emotionaler Deprivation und psychischer Traumatisierung in der Kindheit. Schmerz. 2016;30:526–36.

39. Charmandari E, Achermann JC, Carel JC, Soder O, Chrousos GP. Stress response and child health. Sci Signal. 2012;5(248):mr1.

40. Eisenberger N. The pain of social disconnection: examining the shared neural underpinnings of physical and social pain. Nat Rev Neurosci. 2012;13:421–34.

41. Bushnell MC, Ceko M, Low LA. Cognitive and emotional control of pain and its disruption in chronic pain. Nat Rev Neurosci. 2013;14:5012–5011.

42. Eisenberger NI, Master SL, Inagaki TK, Taylor SE, Shirinyan D, Lieberman MD, Naliboff BD. Attachment figures activate a safety signal-related neural region and reduce pain experience. Proc Natl Acad Sci USA. 2011;108:11721–6.

43. Bowlby J. A secure base: parent-child attachment and healthy human development. Basic Books, USA; 1988. p. 27.

44. Heinrichs M, Baumgartner T, Kirschbaum C, Ehlert U. Social support and oxy-tocin interact to suppress cortisol and subjective responses to psychosocial stress. Biol Psychiatry. 2003;54(12):1389–98.

45. Fonagy P, Steele M, Steele H, Higgitt A, Target M. The Emanuel miller memo-rial lecture 1992. The theory and practice of resilience. Review. J Child Psychol Psychiatry. 1994;35(2):231–57.

46. Jaaniste T, Jia N, Lang T, Goodison-Farnsworth EM, McCormick M, Anderson D. The relationship between parental attitudes and behaviours in the context of paediatric chronic pain. Child Care Health Dev. 2016;42(3):433–8.

47. Eccleston C, Fisher E, Howard RF, Slater R, Forgeron P, Palermo TM et al. Delivering transformative action in paediatric pain: a Lancet Child & Adolescent Health Commission. Published online 2020. https://doi.org/10.1016/S2352-4642(20)30277-7

Chapter 4
Adoption Studies

Research in the field of adoption has been ongoing for decades and deals with manifold and highly complex issues. Investigations include studies of interactions of genetic, family, and environmental influences on the psychosocial development of adopted children. Numerous variables such as age, gender, protective and risk factors are explored, as well as potential vulnerable situations that contribute to the psychosocial adjustment of adopted children or lead to psychosocial disorders. Other works seek to identify key differences in early versus late adopted children, and in national versus international adoptions. Adoption research includes also epidemiological studies. The following is an attempt to draw some conclusions from the abundance of results and to point out controversial findings. Adoption research allows a unique insight into the malleability of child's development, also demonstrating children's ability to recovery from adversities in infancy.

Adoption is uniformly described in the literature as the best solution for the development of a child without a family, compared to institutional or foster care placement [1–3]. Adoption guarantees the child maximum attachment- and relationship continuity and legal affiliation [4]. Adoption should not be considered as a cause of future psychopathology; however, it must be taken seriously as a *risk* situation, because all participants share the experience of loss: for the adopted child it is the loss of his biological parents, for the latter the loss of their biological child, and for the adoptive parents usually the loss of their biological parenthood [5, 6].

The human being is not a prisoner of its genome. François Jacob [7]

© The Author(s), under exclusive license to Springer Nature
Switzerland AG 2023
B. Steck, *Adoption as a Lifelong Process*,
https://doi.org/10.1007/978-3-031-33038-4_4

Genetic and Environmental Factors

The contribution of genetic factors on the family environment and the relationship between the family environment and developmental processes has been investigated in complex projects [8–10]. Developmental research allows us to understand environmental factors and their influence on child development, and to know the processes by which genetic predispositions emerge, i.e., genotypes develop into phenotypes [9, 11–13]. Numerous studies deal with the gene-environmental interaction in the origin of mental illnesses [14, 15]. Research results indicate that identical twins inherit the same genetic characteristic in only 45% [16]. Offspring of parents with severe mental illness (schizophrenia, bipolar disorder, major depressive disorder) are at a higher risk to develop psychiatric disorders; a third may eventually suffer from a severe mental illness at the time of young adulthood [17, 18]. Schizophrenia has a heritability of 60–80%, much of which is attributable to common risk alleles. A large genome-wide association study analyzed the gene variants that contribute to the pathogenesis of this disorder [19]. This study points to genes involved in functions related to synaptic organization, differentiation, and transmission as the most important site of pathology in schizophrenia.

Bipolar disorders and schizophrenia have shared genetic risk factors [20]. Large studies of heritability in twins have shown that the risk is higher for schizophrenia than bipolar disorders [21, 22]. Major depression, often coexisting with anxiety, represents a disease which is etiologically heterogeneous with regard to genetic and environmental factors. Offspring of mothers with major depression and antisocial life history are exposed to multiple adverse experiences and have a greater risk for early onset psychopathology, compared to children of mothers with depression without antisocial history [23, 24]. Offspring of other parental psychopathology (such as severe personality disorders, parental substance abuse, parental imprisonment, or the consequences of familial disruption) are at risk for developmental and psychosocial disorders [25, 26]. In a complex interplay parental and offspring factors determine ultimately a child's psychosocial development.

Vignette

Ten years old, adopted Lucas shouts in a psychotherapeutic session: "She (the birth mother) lied! if she puts me into the world, she should take care of me". Lucas suffers from nightmares, in which he hears voices—of his birth mother: "I don't want to know you, I don't want to hear about you" and can no longer fall asleep. He continues: "I hope the dream is not true; if she wants to see me once, I ask her for a photo of her and for a cell phone so I can contact her. I will tell her about me, but I don't dare to ask her: Can I visit you for a weekend? Especially I will never ask her, if she could not take care of me because she has been taking drugs."

Comment

Information by the adoptive parents revealed that the biological mother was a drug abuser.

Environmental influences do not have the same effects on individuals, a reason why children in the same family are different. "So often we have assumed that the key influences on children's development are shared: their parents' personality and childhood experiences, the quality of their parents' marriage relationships, children's educational background, the neighborhood in which they grow up, and their parents' attitude to school or to discipline. Yet to the extent that these influences are shared, they cannot account for the differences we observe in children's outcome" ([11]: p. 23).

The behavior of the child influences the behavior of parents and family environment—and vice versa. The family process is thus a double-directed one [27]. The problems of fit between adoptive parents and adopted children intensify as children grow older [28]. Hereditary influences become more apparent with age. Over the years, children can more easily choose a social context that suits their dispositions, i.e., with greater independence children increasingly shape their environment themselves [11, 29]. Certain genetic factors therefore will be apparent only at a specific developmental age [30].

The parent—child relationship was examined in over 9′000 twin pairs by parents' rating of their children's prosocial behavior (at ages 3, 4, 7, and by teachers at age 7), by describing their feelings (positive or negative) towards their children and their discipline practices (positive, noncoercive or coercive, punitive). Results indicate that the children of parents with positive feelings and exercising positive, noncoercive discipline showed relatively more prosocial behavior than the children of parents with negative feelings and a coercive punitive discipline [31].

Over 200 adopted children and their biological and adoptive parents, as well as over 200 nonadoptive control parents and their offspring were investigated from infancy through adolescence about their cognitive abilities. Conclusions are that adopted children resemble their adoptive parents slightly in early childhood but not at all in middle childhood or adolescence, a time period, where their cognitive abilities are similar to their biological parents, a result, which is equally true for children and parents in control families. Genetic factors play an important role in the development of offspring's cognitive abilities [32].

Risk and Protective Factors

Risk factors are variables increasing the likelihood that a child will develop a mental disorder or that his development will be unfavorable [33]. They usually have a cumulative effect [34]. Protective factors, on the other hand, have a favorable influence on psychic development. Risk, protective or vulnerability factors [35] have independent influences. Therefore, more relevant than the identification of such variables or factors is to explore the processes underlying these factors. Only the respective social or cultural context decides whether a feature, situation or circumstance is protective or associated with risks [36].

Adoptive families have a protective effect on their adoptive child, often at high risk resulting from negative early childhood experiences [37].

Longitudinal studies among adopted children, their birth parents, adoptive parents, and siblings compared to nonadopted children, and their parents, and siblings have been conducted in the United States since 1975 [11]. The examined children in these studies were followed from birth into adulthood. Results show that disorders are multifactorial determined: several genes are partly responsible for a genetic predisposition, and combinations of different environmental risk factors are involved [30]. Most reviews from behavioral genetics ascertain that the occurrence of behavioral problems follows a genotype—environment—interaction model [28, 38] For example, a temperamentally predisposed child may have a stimulating effect on his adoptive parents.

Even if there is agreement in the literature that certain behavioral characteristics are inherited, there is less certainty about the heredity of specific behaviors. Most adopted children show good psychosocial adjustment despite a potentially pathologic biological family background [39]. Behavioral genetics convey the best available evidence for the importance of nongenetic factors in behavioral development. Children play an active role in the creation and interpretation of their experiences [40].

Adoption research thus allows a unique insight into how hereditary and environmental factors influence the mental development of children. Studies examining this interaction on psychosocial disorders in adoptees reveal that genetic predispositions are expressed when activated by environmental factors. Children of biological parents with established mental illnesses such as schizophrenia have a higher risk of mental illness when they grow up in psychopathological adoptive families [28, 33, 41–47].

Prospective longitudinal studies ([46, 48–53]; Wynne et al. 2006), show that genetic risk factors in the child and severe communication disorders of the adoptive parents interact and together have a negative impact on the adopted child. 200 children of schizophrenic mothers adopted at birth or before the age of 5 years were compared with adopted children of non-schizophrenic mothers. The children's genetic risk to develop schizophrenia was reduced by a protective family environment: Children who grew up in healthy adoptive families did not show severe mental disorders, while children growing up in dysfunctional adoptive families with severe communication disorders of the adoptive parents developed schizophrenic disorders.

A confirmation of gene-environment interactions in the development of psychiatric disorders shows the following results [54]: Adoptees, living in dysfunctional families with maladaptive conflict solving, disturbed emotional expressions, unclear boundaries, or unstable family patterns, have an increased probability to develop psychiatric disorders, especially those with a genetic vulnerability to schizophrenia.

There is less genetic influence in depression [55–57]. Estimates of heredity in childhood depression from twin and adoption studies vary widely, and no definitive conclusions regarding a genetic etiology of depressive symptoms in childhood can be drawn. Thus, there is no correlation between depression in the adopted child and depression in the history of the biological family. Adoption may protect against the onset of depressive development through the caring and supportive relation with the child by the adoptive family.

In a study of adoptive families from the general Swedish population, genetic and rearing effects on the parent-offspring transmission for major depression were investigated. The findings suggest that the risk for major depression is the consequence of genetic factors and rearing experiences to an approximately equal degree, i.e., transmission for major depression seems to result equally from genes and rearing. If biological and adoptive parents are affected, the risk for major depression for adoptees offspring was additive [58, 59].

An evaluation of studies assessing early life stress (sexual-, physical-, and emotional abuse, poverty, physical illness/injury, death of a family member, domestic violence, natural disaster) and the presence or absence of major depressive disorder before age 18 years found that children and adolescents with a history of early life stress experiences have a higher risk for developing major depressive disorders before age 18 than youth without such a history [60].

The onset of depression is associated with serious environmental factors that occur before the age of 18, such as the death or psychiatric illness of an adoptive parent [28]. The death of an adoptive parent in early childhood may represent for the child a loss of part of his self since the separateness between parent and child is not yet well established in the child's inner representations. The parental loss causes a severe narcissistic injury to the child and may be associated with confusing and contradictory images, memories, and emotions.

Other studies show significant relationships between affective disorders in adopted adults (e.g., depression)—who were older at the time of their placement (e.g., after institutionalization)—and their ill birth parents (e.g., alcoholism, antisocial personality structure). Similarly, adverse psychosocial experiences prior to adoption and disruption of the adoptive relationship led to affective illness or disorders in adoptees in adulthood. Correlations were found between the socioeconomic situation of the adoptive family, an alcohol problem in one of the adoptive parents and antisocial behavior in adopted adolescents who were born of birth parents with a personal history of delinquency or criminality [61, 62]. Children of delinquent parents thus run the risk of antisocial development themselves, if there are financial difficulties or alcoholism in the adoptive family.

Early Versus Late Adoption

Children who are adopted as infants enjoy continuous care from their adoptive parents, while children adopted at a later age have experienced at least one significant change in caregivers when they are integrated into the adoptive family. Very often, older placed children have suffered in their pre-adoptive history adversities such as abuse, neglect, or rejection [63]. It is well known that the attachment histories, established in relationships with primary caregivers and internalized as representations, are reactivated in the interaction with new caregivers. Likewise, there is a correlation between the child's age at the time of adoption and his psychosocial development. Results suggest that children adopted as infants have few developmental risks associated with adoption [64] and as adults show good psychosocial adjustment, with slightly increased vulnerability in adopted males compared to adopted females [65]. In some studies findings conclude that physical and cognitive developments of adopted infants fare as well as those of non-adopted children in comparable families of similar socioeconomic status [44, 66, 67]. Other results show—for children adopted as infants—a slightly increased risk for developing problems in social behavior, as evidenced, for example, by poorer peer relationships, difficulties with their adoptive parents and increased referrals to child and adolescent psychology and psychiatry services [44, 68–71].

The results of a longitudinal study demonstrate that in the area of cognitive development, adopted children with similar birth circumstances as non-adopted children performed even better in cognitive domains such as reading, mathematics and general intellectual skills and maintained these qualifications at school graduation and later as adults [72]. The main variables responsible for these results were the socioeconomic status, the educational and vocational training of the adoptive family members, and parental interest in their children's education. Infants or toddlers placed after 12 months of age or—according to some researchers—after 6 months of age, are at increased risk for developmental impairments, especially in the areas of emotional, social, and behavioral development [66, 67, 69, 71, 73].

Long-term studies of severely deprived children in Romanian institutions, who were adopted by well-functioning British families, did not show persistent effects of deprivation if adopted before the age of 6 months; however, children who were adopted at 6–12 months showed multiple impairments, which persisted for many children up to age 11. Some children were able to improve their cognitive functions between the ages 6 and 11. The findings show great heterogeneity in outcomes [74]. The quality of the adoptive mother–child relationship plays an essential role [75].

Studies on the development of specific executive functions demonstrate their contribution to adaptive and maladaptive socio-emotional outcomes among children having experienced early psychosocial deprivation [76]. Data are still inconclusive with regard to the moderating factors that promote resilience in children who have experienced extraordinarily severe deprivation. Research on deprivation-specific psychological patterns demonstrates their persisting influence up to the age of 15 years [77, 78].

However, the risk appears not to be simply due to age at the time of placement; older placed children may have suffered pre-adoptive experiences of deprivation, neglect, rejection, and abuse. They have acquired problem behavior and adaptation and coping strategies prior to their adoption, which they express in their relationship with their adoptive parents [71, 73, 79].

A prospective study investigated the mental health of children, adopted from the public care system in the United Kingdom, over 4 years after their placement. The consequences of pre-adoptive risk factors (adverse childhood experiences, number of moves, days spent with birth parents and days spent in care) on children's internalizing and externalizing problems [1] were explored. Results show the negative impact of adverse childhood experiences on adopted children's internalizing and externalizing problems and confirm the necessity to identify and inform caregivers of children's experienced adversity, with the aim to provide early intervention measures and support for adoptive families [80].

Older placed children who lived with their biological parents prior to adoption are likely to be even at a higher risk of having been victims of maltreatment (physical and/or sexual abuse), rejection, and/or neglect than children who were placed in institutions [37]. The development of children having experienced extremely negative relationships with their biological parents in early childhood may differ from institutionalized children who—because of their emotional deprivation—were not able to form selective attachments [81]. Adoptees with pre-placement experiences of parental mistreatment are at higher risk of presenting attachment disorganization, adjustment- and dissociative disorders [44, 69, 71, 73, 82–85]. The question arises if older adopted children with personal adverse experiences of abuse, neglect, and rejection can catch up developmental milestones if they are placed in a well-qualified, caring environment. The results are encouraging. Although early deprivations and disadvantages are associated with an increased risk of developmental impairment, behavioral problems and relational difficulties, many cases show good psychosocial outcome [57, 86–88].

A study of adult adoptees revealed that those placed early were more likely to rate their adoption experience positively, while those placed after age two were twice as likely to testify that they had not been loved by their adoptive mother [63].

Investigations on Adopted Romanian Orphans

After the Romanian Adoption Law came into force in August 1990, thousands of Romanian children were adopted who had suffered severe neglect in their early childhood. This presented an opportunity to document, through numerous research studies, developmental changes following their placement in adoptive families [30, 45, 57, 87–89].

Rutter et al. [45] noted that 165 children, who had been placed in Romanian orphanages for at least 2 years before their adoption in England, presented with specific and different outcomes in response to the severe deprivations suffered in institutions, compared with nondeprived children, born in England, and adopted as infants. The children were assessed in seven different areas at the ages of four and six. Results show attachment problems, attention deficit disorder and hyperactivity, as well as autistic-like characteristics and cognitive impairment associated with severe institutional deprivation, while emotional difficulties, poor peer relationships and behavioral

---

[1] Internalizing problems are characterized by anxious and depressive symptoms, social withdrawal, and somatic complaints. Externalizing problems are defined as aggressive, oppositional, and delinquent behavior.

problems were not associated with severe institutional deprivation. One fifth of children presented normal functioning despite having spent the longest time in institutions.

Attachment Disorders [2]

> ... for the child, the physical realities of his conception and birth are not the direct cause of his emotional attachment. This emotional attachment results from the daily care of his needs for physical nurturance, nutrition, well-being, love, and stimulation [90].

The lack of a consistent caregiver for the infant is considered to be a decisive factor for the occurrence of severe attachment disorders. "To say of a child that he ... has an attachment to someone means that he is strongly disposed to seek proximity to and contact with a specific figure and to do so in certain situations, notably when he is frightened, tired, or ill" ([91]: p. 371).

Studies that examine attachment disorders and their consequences come to different results [57, 87, 92–94]. The findings of Rutter and collaborators demonstrate that attachment disorders were associated with the duration of the child's experience of severe deprivation, i.e., the longer the deprivation lasted, the higher the risk of developing attachment disorders [95]. However, not all children, who experienced severe deprivation, developed attachment disorder. Thus, deprivation is not the only cause of severe attachment disorders; for example, 70 out of 100 children adopted from a Romanian orphanage before the age of two did not show severe attachment disorders [87].

Because infants with insecure attachment behaviors may overburden prospective adoptive parents [95], preventive measures through early interventions in adoptive families have been proposed [96], such as support for the adoptive mother during the interaction with her infant. The mother-infant attachment, the maternal response to the infant's behavior, and the infant's competence need to be promoted.

Autistic Disorders

Autistic-like behavioral patterns were found in 6% of 111 children adopted from Romania with severe early childhood deprivation; isolated autistic features were detected in another 6% [97]. In contrast to autism spectrum disorders, the considerable improvement of autistic symptoms at the age of 4 and 6 years, as well as the great social interest of these children are to be emphasized. Also, the gender distribution between girls and boys was almost balanced and the head circumference was not increased, as is often the case in autism [98].

---

[2] Attachment Disorders are psychiatric illnesses that can develop in young children who have problems in emotional attachments to others (American Academy of Child Adolescent Psychiatry)

These autistic-like behavioral patterns appear to be related to a prolonged state of sensory and experiential deprivation, with cognitive impairment and an inability to develop attachment relationships. Autism may develop based on non-genetic brain damage [99, 100], or severe sensory deprivation may impair normal brain development. A severe developmental delay and a head circumference below the third percentile are indicative of organic brain dysfunction.

The changes in various brain regions detected in these children by magnetic resonance imaging (MRI) may represent consequences of the ongoing stress associated with early global deprivation and lead to long-term cognitive and behavioral deficits [88, 101–103]. In their studies, Rutter et al. [57] demonstrate that children adopted prior to 6 months made up all their cognitive deficits, while those adopted before 2 years improved but did not normalize their cognitive functioning. At age 11, profound institutional deprivation is associated with autistic-like patterns and disinhibited attachment, to a lesser degree also with cognitive impairment and inattention/overactivity [88, 104].

The age at entry into the adoptive family was the most important predictor of cognitive functioning at age four. The level of cognitive development of the children adopted after 6 months varied greatly when tested at age 11: some improved their cognitive functioning, for many the cognitive impairments persisted [74]. The remaining cognitive deficit is probably a consequence of massive early deprivation, with emotional deprivation playing a more important role than nutritional deprivation. Long-term studies revealed the most pronounced positive changes in the quality of the parent-child relationship among those children who caught up in their cognitive development between examinations [105].

Hoksbergen [106] refers to the children originating from Romania as survivors. Their survivor behavior is shown by the fact that they are completely focused on their own interests, on the "here and now"—without any future perspectives—, undifferentiated in emotional relationships but with a great need for attention. Despite the often-serious psycho-social problems while raising their Romanian adopted child, adoptive parents face the challenges to deal competently with their task. Their resilience is much higher than the one of other parents. Adopted children are desired children for whom the adoptive parents are extraordinary committed for their best possible upbringing. The behavioral characteristics of Romanian adopted children require from adoptive parents great educational knowledge, dedication, engagement, and empathy. Adoptive parents have a clear need for support.

The Mental Health Long-Term Outcomes of Young Adopted Adults

Research on adults, who were internationally adopted around 2 years of age, showed that early severe or multiple adverse experiences increased their risk of psychiatric disorders in adulthood. However, children having suffered from less severe early adversity seemed to be resilient [107].

A longitudinal investigation of children having lived up to 43 months in Romanian institutions, suffering from severe deprivation, were followed up in young adulthood (22–26 years). The adverse neurodevelopmental and mental health disorders may have long-term damaging and harmful effects in "three symptom domains: inattention and overactivity, disinhibited social engagement, and autism spectrum disorder, despite the positive influence of well resourced, caring, and supportive adoptive families. By contrast, early problems in cognitive impairment were rarely carried into young adulthood. There was an emergence of emotional problems among the young adults who experienced extended deprivation. A substantial minority who appeared resilient, showing no core problem at any age" ([108]: p. 2). The profound impact may lead to low educational achievement, unemployment, and the need of mental health service. 20% of the adoptees were without problems.

Summary

Children adopted from institutions having experienced global deprivation present—with increasing age at the time of adoption—social and behavior problems, particularly in adolescence and enduring into adulthood. In the first 2 years of life a child is highly vulnerable to adversity, and early stress experiences lead later among others to emotion regulation-, attention-, and executive dysfunctions. Resilient and genetic factors, epigenetic changes, insufficient environmental- and inadequate relationship stimulation are some main factors contributing to the outcome [109].

Epidemiological Studies

Epidemiological studies reveal that adopted children use more often child and adolescent psychiatric institutions compared to their proportion in the general population than non-adopted children. Adoptive parents seem to refer their adopted children more frequently for evaluation. The confrontation-, coping skills and strategies of adoptive parents play an extremely important role in the psychosocial development of the adopted child [37].

Various studies demonstrate that adoptive families seem to have greater social and psychological resources than families with biological children [1, 42]; adopted children thus benefit from positive childhood experiences, better socio-economic conditions, greater family stability and better mother-child interactions during their childhood in the adoptive family [6, 44, 110].

Nevertheless, adopted children are overrepresented in child and adolescent psychological and psychiatric assessments and treatment [111–113]. They present a significantly higher rate of behavioral disorders than children growing up in biological families [44]. Mostly aggressive and antisocial problems, as well as learning difficulties are reported [113–118].

An analysis of 62 studies (of over 17,000 adopted children) compared the intelligence quotient and school performance of adopted and non-adopted children: there was no difference of the intelligence quotient between adopted and non-adopted children, but school performance and language skills of adopted children were poorer and learning difficulties more frequent. The study concludes that adoption has positive effects on the cognitive development of adopted children, however, adopted children present delayed school performance. Psychosocial problems associated with their adoption situation may inhibit their ability to concentrate on schoolwork [119].

Behavioral problems seem to occur more frequently than average in adoptions of older, neglected and/or abused children [47, 69, 120–125] as well as of children with prenatal drug exposure and multiple institutional placements [105, 126]. The burden is higher for adoptive parents with children who were victims of sexual or physical abuse, prior to their integration into the adoptive family, than for adoptive parents whose children had previously suffered neglect [105].

A greater risk and/or vulnerability for mental disorders has been postulated for adoptees [114, 127, 128], but they are probably referred for assessment more frequently [39, 129, 130]. The threshold of tolerance for the manifestation of symptoms seems to be lower for adoptees than for non-adoptees [118].

Comparative long-term studies speak for an interactive protective effect through adoption; it reduces children's psychiatric risk, resulting from the lack of care by their biological parents [37]. In the USA, a survey comparing adopted and non-adopted adolescents concludes that adopted adolescents do not experience themselves differently from other adolescents; in 90–98% they consider their adoption positive [131]. These results do not correspond to clinical experience; do they reflect adopted adolescents' wishes or their adjustment efforts? Adopted youths' perceptions of positive family relationships proved to be the best predictor for their identity development and their social adjustment. According to adolescents' assessments, factors such as school success and self-confidence correlated with the openness of their family's communication about adoption issues. For their part, adoptive parents consider the adoption successful in 85% of all cases. However, these results are hardly representative since it is likely that adoptive parents of conflict-affected or failed adoptions do not participate in such surveys due to their feelings of shame and guilt.

90% of 42 interviewed Swiss adoptees were positive towards their adoption. However, one third experienced their adoption as a burden. Psychosocial adjustment was found to be poor in 10% [132].

Other studies show no significant differences in various adjustment variables between adopted and nonadopted children [133], i.e., most adopted children present with similar patterns of behavioral problems as non-adopted children [41]. A distinct group of dissocial adopted youth [134] may indicate the existence of an adoption-specific psychiatric risk, especially during adolescence [135, 136], what is confirmed by an elevated prevalence of dissocial disorders in adopted girls [117, 137].

Differences in psychosocial adjustment were found in nationally adopted adolescents compared to non-adopted adolescents, which were related to their developmental phase and gender [138]. There was no correlation between the increase of externalizing disorders (such as aggressive behavior) in adolescence and adverse influences before the adoption [124]. Longitudinal studies with control groups found differences between adoptees and non-adoptees at a certain age and no differences at other ages, indicating that adjustment problems in adopted children may be temporary [129].

A comparative study—using standardized psychiatric interviews—in the Netherlands of nationally adopted and non-adopted young adults found a higher risk for mental health problems among adoptees compared to non-adoptees of the same age. Adopted males were more likely to be affected than adopted females. Male adoptees - one assumes - have a higher vulnerability to early childhood negative experiences or to the adoption situation than female adoptees. However, most of the international adoptees did not present serious psychic problems [139].

Studies investigating mental health problems in over 17'000 internationally adopted adolescents and over one million non-adopted peers were analyzed. The results obtained are that the 12–19 years old adopted adolescents experience more mental health problems than their non-adopted peers [140]. The reports of parents showed even higher rates than the self-reports of the adolescents, maybe due to parents' sensitive responsiveness to their children's emotional disorders.

A Dutch review of research results over the past 10 years concludes the following: adoption is associated with developmental opportunities and risks. Many adoptees show surprisingly good psychosocial adjustment, but some subgroups present difficulties. Infant-, international and transethnic adoptions may complicate adoptees' identity development. Post-infant adoptees may present with developmental delays, attachment-, and post-traumatic disorders. Useful interventions include preventive counselling, post-adoption support, group services for adoptive parents and adopted children. Both adoptive parents and adopted children need to be assisted by child and adolescent psychiatrists [64].

Reviews of adopted children's attachment studies display that children, adopted in their first year of life, have the same values of secure attachment as non-adopted children; this is not the case for children adopted later than 12 months. Children with pre-adoptive adverse experiences are at risk for building an insecure attachment style to their adoptive parents compared to non-adopted children. Even if adoption improves attachment security for deprived children, adversity in early childhood has long-lasting effects on adopted children's attachment representations and attachment styles may be transgenerational transmitted in adoptive families [141, 142].

Early attachment experiences have critical effects on later attachment behavior in adolescence, both with peers, in school with teachers, and in intimate relationships. The development of pathological attachment patterns should be recognized and treated in early childhood, since—when chronic in adolescence—treatment may be demanding. Yet experiencing new secure attachments may change inner attachment models, even in adolescence, a period, in which adolescents search for other and new secure attachment figures outside the family; adults or intimate peers, who are sensitive to the adolescent's need for emotional security, may thus contribute to the teenager's better attachment behavior [143].

The partly contradictory results of the research studies can tentatively be explained as follows: In some studies, the results were collected from a clinical population, i.e., children and adolescents with mental health problems (children in outpatient consultations or hospitalized adolescents), while other studies were conducted in a non-clinical population. Some studies concerned infants and toddlers, while others included older children with specific needs. Different comparison groups and methodological analyses are cited as additional factors for the inconsistent results [123, 129]. In bivariate analyses, for example, adopted boys had a greater incidence of psychiatric disorders than nonadopted boys and there was a greater prevalence of substance dependence among adopted girls than nonadopted girls. In contrast, multivariate analysis showed that adoption status was not related to psychiatric disorders, substance abuse, or school failure [144].

Summary

Risk or higher vulnerability are registered among children with adverse pre- adoptive experiences such as neglect, maltreatment, or multiple placements [28, 33, 41–47]. Most adoptees do not suffer from mental or somatic illnesses and show little or no influence of adoption on their personal development.

Factors and interactions leading to positive development and good psychosocial adjustment in most adoptees need to be investigated [28, 127, 145].

Domestic, International, Transracial [3] or Transcultural Adoptions

International adoptions between 2003 and 2013 totaled more than 300,000 worldwide; most of these placements were transracial. In the United States transracial placements account for 85% of all intercountry adoptions [146], involving White parents and Black, Asian, Latino, or Multiracial children.

Intercountry, foreign, transnational adoptions are often criticized and there are increasing calls for more help for families and children in their country of origin. For UNICEF a placement outside the country is to be considered only when all other care options in the child's home country have been exhausted. Placement with local adoptive or foster families is always preferable to adoption abroad. Intercountry

---

[3] Transracial adoption, placing a child of one racial or ethnic group with adoptive parents of another racial or ethnic group.

adoption, according to UNICEF, is only justifiable under the following conditions: the child has been abandoned, there are no alternative options in the home country, the placement does not represent a commercial interest, the adoption applicants are prepared by reputable placement agencies and are accompanied during and after the adoption. International adoption is advocated when children are rejected in their country of origin because of their ethnicity, their birth out of wedlock, their infirmity or disability. Intercountry adoptees are believed to experience more complicated adoption processes than those adopted domestically and are therefore at greater risk for mental health problems [135, 136, 147]. Studies in this regard vary widely in design and are inconsistent in their findings.

In a prospective longitudinal study, 160 infants (up to 6 months old), adopted internationally, were followed from infancy to 14 years to examine their social development and to determine the influence of adoption on early and middle childhood, as well as current factors on their social development in adolescence. Outcomes reveal that both, early childhood, and current experiences, play an important role in social development. Adoptive parents do influence the social development of their adopted child. Child temperament, as well as maternal empathy contribute to the adolescent's social development. Early adoptive parent—adoptive child relationships do not directly determine social development in adolescence; yet the influences of adoptive parents on their adoptive child's social development during his childhood creates an essential basis [148].

Review articles summarizing studies of the parent-child relationship in domestic [149, 150] or intercountry adoptions [151, 152] suggest that close bonds exist between most adopted children and their parents. The parent-child relationship is predominantly viewed positively by both parties [153]. In two thirds to three quarters of cases, both adoptive parents and adopted children evaluate their intercountry adoption as positive. They report being satisfied with the adoption or consider their adoption successful. 80% of children and adoptive parents view their family relationship as positive [122, 132, 152]. If the adoption cannot be concealed, due to the child's appearance, adoptive parents recognize the otherness of their child, and his integration usually succeeds within the first year after the child's arrival.

A review of over a hundred studies (including over 25,000 adoptees of all ages and a control group of over 80,000 non-adoptees) concludes that most international adoptees manifest favorable psychosocial adjustment, although they use mental health services more often than non-adoptees. International adoptees present fewer behavioral problems and are less likely to be referred to psychiatric services than national adoptees [154].

Yet a study of seven-year-old children, adopted internationally and across ethnic groups as infants, found that they were at higher risk for manifesting behavioral disorder at home and, according to their parents, occurring more often in boys. However, these children showed a favorable psychosocial adjustment at school, their school performance was within the normal range, in some cases even above the mean value. Since various research findings conclude that adopted youth show an increased risk of behavioral problems in adolescence, the question arises whether the difficulties at home, identified at a younger age, are not temporary disturbances, which are manifested outside the family during adolescence [71]. Of over 1500 internationally adopted adolescents 22% of males and 18% of females presented with psychosocial disorders, compared to 10% of an adolescent control group from the general population [125].

A comparative study of domestically adopted children in the United States and children adopted from Romania reveals that behavioral disorders in both groups were associated with negative pre-adoption experiences of abuse and institutionalization. In both groups, the children suffered in the past stressful situations or traumatic experiences of different causes, which eventually led to similar behavioral disorders [121]. The adoptive parents rated the parent-child relationship in both groups as satisfactory.

In a 17 years longitudinal investigation of 224 transethnic or same-race adult adoptees, their psychosocial adjustment was examined [155]. The results show correlations between adoptees' psychosocial adjustment and their ethnicity, gender, and the structure of their adoptive family. Age at placement did not play a significant role in psychosocial adjustment outcomes [156, 157]. However, selected examples from the literature indicate that the adoption outcomes of adoptees—who belonged to a different ethnicity than their adoptive parents—were influenced by their older age at adoption and by pre-adoptive experiences of neglect and institutional placements [158]. A review of various studies of placements across color and ethnicity concludes that psychosocial adjustment was satisfactory in 70% [159].

The apparent and immutable racial and ethnic differences between parents and children are considered as the basis of the transracial adoption paradox [4] ([160]: p.8). Four cultural socialization strategies for adoptive families are described: in cultural assimilation parents engage their adopted child into the majority culture; enculturation means that adoptive parents acknowledge racial and ethnic differences and enhance their adopted child's knowledge of his birth culture and heritage. In racial inculcation [5] parents teach their children how to cope with racism and discrimination. In child choice, parents give the adopted child the opportunity to choose his racial and cultural identification. Transracial adoptive families may engage during the development of their child in various strategies. [6]

A detailed review of transracial adoption research (from 1990 to 2003) indicates that domestic and international transracial adoptees "are psychologically well adjusted, exhibit variability in their racial/ethnic identity development, and along with their parents, engage in a variety of cultural socialization strategies to overcome the transracial adoption paradox" ([160]: p.13).

The adopted child in intercountry adoption is a "foreigner" in a double sense: as an recipient for parental unconscious projections (as this is the case for any child, also for biological children) and because of his ethnic strangeness [162]. Feelings of

---

[4] Racially different parents and children in adoptive families

[5] The teaching of coping skills to help children deal effectively with racism and discrimination.

[6] See also: Antares [161].

loneliness and strangeness evolve progressively due to the child's appearance, characterized by his specific ethnicity, as well as his distant origin. Unfamiliar, alien, and foreign affects are intensified by projections of mostly unconscious similar feelings of the adoptive parents and, above all, by the discriminatory attitude of the environment. This double strangeness is sometimes associated with Freud's [163] concept of the uncanny. Freud describes the uncanny as a perplexity that may seize us in front of certain objects or in certain situations and arouse fear or anxiety; he discusses this emotional situation in relation to fears of death and castration.

The impact of racism on children is enormous and they may experience discrimination at the place where they live, where they go to school, economically and by non-respect of their rights. Racism and its presuppositions about faculties, motives, and interests of black children affect their care, support, encouragement, and their health [164]. Children internalize negative racial events and associated emotions. Racial stereotypes consist of distorted images and built-up beliefs, that members of a particular race share the same features or character traits. These racial attitudes and prejudices are still present and influence greatly children's psychosocial development, personal achievements, and mental and somatic health [165]. Internalized negative racial stereotypes have numerous impacts: self-perception and perceptive capacities deteriorate, and subjects may unconsciously search others for confirming negative aspects of their race identity. [7] Yet if adolescents are resilient to build up positive racial identity—an authentic sense of who they are, to which culture and race they belong—they will be able to cope with discrimination, racial negative attitude, and prejudices of others [166], without having the need to demonize other cultures or races.

Not only children and adolescents are suffering from experiences of racism, but also bystanders are significantly affected. Adults, who in their youth witnessed racism and victimization, are overwhelmed by psychic and physiological reactions, when recalling these past events. The abuse may involve an individual's physical injuries and psychic hurt, an experience of power dominance, such as a demonstration of difference in age, stature, status, harming tremendously a person's self-esteem and—with repetitive abuse—increasing stress reactions, leading to chronic stress levels, impairing adequate coping, and finally a subject's fearful anticipations of maltreatment [167]. Victims are highly vulnerable and are prone to further victimization.

> To mediate the effects of institutional and personally mediated racism in the educational setting and prevent internalized racism, studies show that a positive, strong racial or ethnic identity and parental engagement in families is protective against the negative effects of racial discrimination on academic outcomes. ([168], p. 5; [169]).

Adopted children have to cope not only with their special filiation, but often with negative experiences linked to their ethnic and racial status. Transracial adopted children and adolescents face multiple challenges and need specific comprehension

---

[7]Racial identity and ethnic identity are terms that refer broadly to how individuals define themselves with respect to race and/or ethnicity.

with regard to their affiliation to double minority groups. Adoptive parents must be aware of the cultural background of their adopted child and of his preadoption experiences. Their task is to help their child with his cultural socialization and to prepare him how to deal with prejudices, unfairness, bias. Cultural socialization includes exposure to birth culture, supporting ethnic identity and pride in ethnic background, connecting to cultural group with its activities and lessons of language [170].

Preparing children means to teach awareness of stigmata and how to cope with them. "Racial microaggressions are brief, commonplace daily verbal, behavioral or environmental indignities, whether intentional or unintentional that communicate hostile, derogatory or negative slights toward people of color" ([171], p. 271). Microaggressions concerning adoption are messages that convey negative assumptions about adoption, birth parents, adoptees and/or adoptive parents [172]. [8]

International transracial adoptions are frequent in France and microaggressions towards adoptive parents and their adopted adolescents happen repetitively. Adopted children having experienced critical or traumatic events, rendering them particularly vulnerable, are exposed in the country of their adoptive parents to discrimination, prejudice, exclusion, and isolation due to their origin and their physical differences. Their problematic behaviors may be understood as the consequence of their lived past rejections and additional negative responses from the environment, leading to an escalation of their challenging behavior [173].

51 French adoptive parents, who adopted one or more children internationally, were investigated in a semi-structured interview about their parental representations regarding their child's cultural identity. 12 parents considered it essential, that the child adopted their own French culture, thus strengthening his feelings of belonging to the adopted family. 18 parents clearly opted for their child bicultural identities, promoting ethnic and cultural links, and helping their adopted child to learn how to protect himself from discrimination. 21 parents wished to adapt their connections with their child's country of origin and culture according to his interest and own choices [174].

Anderson et al. [175] investigated the impact of adoptive family discussions—concerning racial and ethnic differences—on South Korean adopted adolescents' delinquent behavior. When families acknowledged those differences, their adolescents manifested the fewest delinquent behaviors. Adopted adolescents, whose families were divided in their estimation of the importance of racial and ethnic differences, presented significantly more behavioral problems. Ethnic-racial identity may also be denied by adoptees, because of their negative experiences in social groups [176].

Adoptive parents need to recognize and accept cultural differences, denote the family as multicultural and value the child's exposure to his culture of origin; then

---

[8] Examples of adoption microaggression types include: "Biology is Best," which conveys an assumption that biological or blood ties are superior; "Grateful adoptee," which conveys an assumption that adoptees are lucky to have been adopted and should be grateful; and "Phantom Birth Parents," which conveys an assumption that birth parents are no longer important once they relinquish parental rights ([172]: pp. 13–14).

they are able to provide cultural socialization for their child; their adopted offspring build positive self-esteem and feel connected to their culture and their adopted adolescents take part in family discussion about adoption, manifest fewer externalizing behaviors, and are more interested in activities and enjoy them more [177–181]. Disagreement between adopted offspring and their parents with regard to their values on racial and cultural differences was associated with adolescents' wrongdoing to a greater degree than in families where parents and adopted youth valued these differences equally important or in families where all members denied the importance of racial and ethnic differences [175]. These findings reflect the adolescent's need to live consensus and harmony in his adoptive family.

The results of studies on self-esteem between adoptees and nonadopted youth show no differences in self-esteem. Adoptees from international, domestic, transracial, and same-race adoption show normative levels of self-esteem, suggesting on one hand adoptees' resilience to catch up, on the other hand the adoptive family's great investment [182].

Of particular importance are the comparison of psychosocial outcomes in adolescence and early adulthood between biological children, adopted children, immigrant children and the general population. A study in Sweden of over 11,000 adopted children born abroad (mainly originating from Korea, India, and Colombia) between 1970 and 1979 concludes, that adoptees born abroad have a higher risk in adolescence and early adulthood to be hospitalized for psychiatric illness, depression, alcohol, or drug abuse, to attempt suicide, to dye by suicide or to commit a crime, than this is the case for Swedish-born adolescents [147]. The birth siblings in adoptive families show fewer psychosocial disorders than the adoptees; the results for adoptees and immigrant children are approximately the same. There are no significant differences in the occurrence of schizophrenia or anorexia nervosa; yet there is an increased risk for social maladjustment and mental health problems compared to the general population among male adolescents or young adults, older adoptees, and adolescents who grew up with single parents. Unfortunately, information on events prior to adoption and age at adoption are not obtainable.

A study comparing family interaction composed of one adopted and one biologic adolescent concludes that the parent-adolescent relationship is more conflictual with the adopted adolescent. The authors discuss as reason for their finding the more stressful identity development (differences in appearance, preoccupation regarding biological parents), but also the fact that innate characteristics of the adoptive parents and the adopted adolescent do not fit and become more pronounced during adolescence. Intrafamilial communication is important for preventing negative outcomes [183].

Summary

The risk of internationally adopted children is associated with gender, age at adoption, pre-adoptive and post-adoptive life experiences, and genetic predisposition. However, it must be emphasized that most internationally adopted children differ little from the general population in their psychosocial adjustment, which is positive in over 80% of cases, as studies in Europe and the USA demonstrate. In the follow-up of these children, care should be taken not only to provide anti-discriminatory support but also to promote cultural and ethnic identity. The results of various studies are quite heterogenous and often non-representative [152]. Ethnic–racial socialization in transracial adoptive families is a complex process of multiple interconnecting components and aspects and takes place in the interaction between each adoptive parent (with his personal history), the parental couple, the family, and each individual child, in evolving contexts and various phases of development of all family members during their life course.

Certainly, it is desirable to help unwanted and abandoned children directly in the respective developing country—as Terre des Hommes [184] requires. However, due to population growth and the poor financial situation of developing countries caused by debt and economic problems, as well as the limited possibilities of development aid, it is unlikely that the social care of these children can be ensured in the foreseeable future.

Therefore, intercountry adoptions may still be regarded as meaningful. Accordingly, they were also accepted as a "substitute solution" in the declaration of the United Nations [152]. Nor should one forget, that for a child who cannot be appropriately integrated in their home country because of his ethnic origin, birth out of wedlock, infirmity or any other reason, intercountry adoption is currently often the only real chance to grow up as a "desired and valued family member" [185].

Open Adoption

Open adoption is a collective term for a variety of forms of adoption that differ in the degree and intensity of contact between birth parents and adoptive families ([186]; p. 107). Different stages of open adoption are discussed [187]. The so-called *confidential open* adoption is an exchange of minimal information shared by adoptive and biological parents, which ceases at or shortly after the child's adoption. In *intermediary or limited open* adoption, the adoptive parents regularly send photos and information to the biological parents via the intermediary agency. In *semi-open* adoption, biological parents meet with adoptive parents, but no information permitting mutual identification is exchanged. Only in *fully open* adoption do the child's two sets of parents meet and share identifying information. A continuous open adoption means the maintaining of ongoing contacts by adoptive parents and biological parents throughout the child's development. Initiation of contact may be by adoptive or birth relatives and mediated by a social worker or adoption agency team. The kind of contact may be variable, changing in its frequency and often representing a complex situation: involved family members may vary, forms of communication differ, and relationships change [188].

Different theoretical perspectives and their divergent conclusions for open versus closed adoption are discussed as well as behaviors and experiences of all those

involved in the adoption triad (biological and adoptive parents and adoptees) analyzed [189]. Increasingly, open adoption is proclaimed as the best solution for the
welfare of an adopted child [190, 191]. According to Paulitz [192], incognito adoption represents an injustice to the child, as it does not serve the child's interests, but
rather the supposed well-being of the birth parents and, above all of the adoptive
parents: therefore, this author is unconditionally in favor of open adoption, whereby
he understands the transition from incognito adoption (an adoption in which the
person of the adopter is known but remains unnamed to the birth parents) to open
adoption as a fluent process. In all counselling interviews with biological parents
who release their child for adoption and with adoptive applicants, information
should be provided about the possibilities and conditions of open adoption.

The quality of the parent-child relationship and their communication patterns are
the important elements for the adopted child's adjustment [193]. Directives recom-
mend that the initial contact between biological and adoptive parents serve to
exchange information; both pairs of parents should subsequently be entitled to
maintain information about and contact with the child on an ongoing basis. The
nature and intensity of the relationship should be determined jointly by the adoptive
and biological parents. An advantage of open adoption is that birth certificates no
longer need to be sealed. The frequency and importance of communications between
adoptive parents, biological parents and adopted child vary at different times for the
persons involved, and their individual needs and wishes should be respected and
guided by their empathy for the child [194].

Young, adopted adults usually appreciate their contacts with birth relatives,
on the one hand for receiving information about their background, on the other
as an attestation of their adoptive parents' openness towards their birth family.
167 adoptees (mean age 25 years) were assessed by semi-structured interviews
and self-report questionnaires about their attachment to and communications
with their adoptive family and their contact with birth families. Findings reveal
that a secure attachment relation and positive and open communication with
adoptive parents about the adoption is associated with positive feelings about
birth parents contact; 42% of the adoptees had—within the previous 2 years—
some contact by phone calls, emails, photos, or in-person visits [195]. Adoptive
parents, who favor their adoptee's contacts with biological relatives and discuss
adoption issues in the family, contribute to their child's adoptive identity formation [196].

Controversial Results of Clinical Studies

The evaluation of the advantages of open adoption reveals that adoptive parents in
fully open adoption were more empathetic during the adoption process, spoke more
openly with their children about the adoption and felt less fear that the biological

mother might reclaim their child than adoptive parents in confidential adoption [9] [190]. Adoptive parents succeeded in building a trusting relationship with the biological mother, who assured them that she would never reclaim her child. In the belief to act in the best interests of their child, adoptive parents maintained the relationship with the biological mother.

Open adoption is an ongoing process. For adoptive parents, a transformation of their identity takes place [197, 198]. Adoptive parents need to come to term with their past, deal with the present and face the future. In the present, they feel entitled to be the parents of an adopted child; for the future, they maintain trust in the permanence of the relationship with their child. Such an intrapsychic clarity of identity is reflected in the narratives of adoptive parents [199]. The adoptive mother's contacts with the birth mother positively influence her attitude towards the biological mother and promote a confident attitude of both adoptive parents towards their child.

Neil [200, 201] comes to the following conclusions of her studies: The feelings of the adoptive parents for the personal history and the birth parents of their child, as well as their communication style with their child about his adoption, are important factors influencing the development of the adopted child. In "optimal" communication, adoptive parents are open to discussion and empathetic towards the birth family. Character traits or memories of the child rendering his adoption status clearly evident, influence favorably the adoptive parents' feelings and acknowledging of their child's past.

A key factor is the authenticity of adoptive parents' empathic feelings for their child and his biological relatives. Children in open adoption seem to experience more continuity in their personal history, leading to a reinforcement of their self-esteem [202, 203]. Children in all types of open adoption present with a positive self-esteem and shared their curiosity about their biological parents and their satisfaction with the open adoption situation. Girls were more curious about their biological parents than boys. Information about biological parents do not seem to confuse children's understanding of adoption or diminish their self-esteem but is not associated with a better comprehension of their adoption status, which seems to be linked to their developmental cognitive abilities [204].

In open adoption the biological parents are equally interested in the prosperity of their child and therefore wish to cooperate with the adoptive parents for the child's benefit, an advantage for the child's identity-finding process.

---

[9] The secret, closed, or confidential adoption definition refers to an adoption, in which the prospective birth mother chooses to keep her identity private and exchanges no contact with the adoptive family during or after the adoption process.

Disadvantages and Differences of Open Adoption

The following aspects are claimed to be disadvantages of open adoption, seemingly representing a threat for adoptive parents who do not feel entitled to assume their role as full parents [190, 205]. Open adoption leads to anxiety among adoptive parents that biological parents may interfere in the adoptive family and have a negative influence on the attachment formation between the adopted child and his adoptive parents [206].

Open adoption was satisfactory for future adoptive parents who determined, before the child's placement, the degree of openness either by written consent or by oral contact with the biological mother [207, 208]. Demick and Wagner [187] describe the following advantages and disadvantages of open adoption: on the one hand, adoptive parents felt a sense of meaning and empowerment, on the other hand, adoptive mothers reported lower self-esteem, probably resulting from their greater empathy towards the birth mother. Adoptive mothers—in another study of 190 adoptive families with 4–12 years old adopted children—enjoyed good self-esteem. The specific kind of relationship between adoptive and biological parents is extremely diverse and evolves continuously as do also the members of both families [209]. Openness in adoption may be desired at a particular time by one party, but not by the other, and may change over time. A longitudinal study on open adoption collected information from 190 adoptive families and 169 birth mothers, 4 and 12 years after the child's placement in his adoptive family. There was no evidence of fears that the birth mother would reclaim her child or interfere with the adoptive family. The adoptive parents did not feel that their right to parenthood had been impaired. However, open adoption did not guarantee successful bereavement outcomes for biological mothers [210].

Research with the adoptive kinship network, which includes the adopted child, siblings, his adoptive parents and their extended families, and his birthparents and their extended families concludes that the psychosocial outcome [10] for adopted children is less related to the level of openness than to the dynamics of the adoptive kinship network. Better collaboration in relationships [11] within the adoptive kinship network promotes better adjustment of adopted children [211].

A study in the USA used questionnaires to examine whether contacts between members of the adoptive family and the biological family had an impact on the psychosocial development of adolescents adopted in infancy. The results revealed no differences in the adoptive parents' assessment of the adoptees, while the adopted

---

[10] Child outcomes included their satisfaction with the degree of openness and their curiosity about their birthparents, global self-worth, understanding of adoption and aspects of socio-emotional adjustment.

[11] Characteristics of collaborative relationships: proactive management of the logistics of openness arrangements; management of fears, management of communication flow to the child in a way that is developmentally appropriate; empathy for the child's adoptive situation; empathy for the child's birthmother; maintaining appropriate generational boundaries; and effective management of outside influences, such as agency or extended kin.

adolescents with long-term direct contact with biological parents reported fewer externalizing disorders, such as behavioral problems, than adopted adolescents without contact with birth parents [212].

Open adoption seems to be less frequent in Europe than in the United States, where in domestic infant adoptions contact with birth relatives is maintained in half or even two-thirds of the cases. In international adoption the possibility of contact is dependent on the country of the child's origin; such contacts are rather rare.

The clinical experience points to a highly complex interplay based on the individual child's subjective experience of conflict and loyalty and his personal attachment- and relationship with the dual parental couple, as well as the emotional and cognitive communication between child and adoptive parents on a conscious and unconscious level. To recognize and understand their child's problematic situation and to provide him with the necessary scope for his finding a "solution", requires a self-understanding of parenthood, which offers the child permission and support to co-determine—whenever possible—the relationship with his biological parents. Whether, how, at what moment, where and how often contacts and meetings between the child and his birth parents will take place, needs to be adapted to the individual child and consider all persons involved in the triangle. Above all, the child's stage of development and his psychic well-being are always to be respected.

Adoption Disruption and Dissolution

> Adoption breakdown [12] refers to various situations where children—placed in families with an intent to adopt—exit the family either before or prematurely after the completion of the legal adoption procedures ([213], p 131).

Breakdowns of adoption relationships are less common than those of (long-term) placements in foster care [214]. Approximately 10–16% of adoptions of children with specific needs (generally children adopted after three years) are terminated or dissolved [215, 216]. Children with specific needs include children who were older at the time of placement, disabled, belonging to a minority, or members of a sibling group [92]. According to Terre des Hommes, up to 2% of children are re-placed; they are older or disabled, or have lived adversities in their past, e.g., long stays in institutions [132].

Adopted children being placed in an already existing sibling line, as an intermediate or oldest child in the family, had to be re-placed disproportionately often [217]. Kühl [132] emphasizes the relationship between sibling constellation and adoption success: "The greater the time interval between the arrival of an adopted child and the subsequent admission of another child, the more favorable the mental

---

[12] Disruption: the adoption process ends *before* the adoption is legally finalized. Dissolution: the legal relationship between the adoptive parents and adoptive child is ceased - voluntarily or involuntarily - *after* the adoption is legally finalized. In both situations, the child is placed in foster care or with new adoptive parents.

development of both children seems to be. Adopted children who joined a family with exclusively younger children as the oldest show a less favorable self-concept than adolescents who were adopted as the youngest or as an only child. Socialization outcomes in families with only adopted children appear more favorable than in families where only biological children lived when the adoptive child was received..." (p. 49–50).

In Northern Ireland, interviews with adoptive parents having lived the disruption of their adoption relationship were conducted [218]. The impact of the adopted child's experienced traumatization on his adoptive family might be extreme and parents express exhaustion, stress, grief, despair, shame, anger and finally relief when the child is transferred. In identification with the child, parents assume the child's lived feelings of his traumatization and are finally emotionally so overwhelmed, that they are no more capable to empathically care for their child, suffering from a so-called compassion fatigue. [13]

Relationship Dissolution or Divorce in Adoptive Parents or Same-Sex Parent Couples

190 adoptive couples were investigated during the first 5 years of their adoptive parenthood. 15 (7.9%) couples broke up their relationships: seven of 57 lesbian couples (12.3%), one of 49 gay male couples (2.0%), and seven of 84 heterosexual couples (8.3%) [219]. The likelihood of relationship dissolution was significantly higher for parents adopting not an infant, but an older child, for those who 3 months after the placement of their child described their feelings of being insufficiently prepared for the adoption and finally for parents who told of their preadoption relational maintenance behaviors [14] as being poor or extremely enmeshed.

Failure (terminations and dissolutions of adoption relationships) may only very rarely be attributed to a single cause and is usually due the interaction of several factors [215, 220]. A distinction is made between risk and protective factors, which may impair the adoption relationship or contribute to its good outcome [221].

Risk Factors Child-related risk factors include older age, the number of previous placements and a disability [222]. Nationality and ethnicity are considered by some authors to be a risk factor for the termination of the adoption relationship [223,

---

[13] Compassion fatigue is a condition comprising three elements: burnout, meaning physical and mental exhaustion; secondary trauma stress involving the transfer of trauma symptoms from those who have been traumatized to those who have been hearing the trauma story; and compassion satisfaction which is known to moderate the effects of the other two and is directly related to high quality support from knowledgeable professionals.

[14] Relationship or relational maintenance refers to a variety of behaviors by relational partners in an effort to maintain that relationship; the subjective experience of the relation with the partner may differ with time, the satisfaction within the relationship may increase or decrease.

224], but not in the opinion of others. These results are inconclusive; the same is true for the adoption of a sibling group.

Overall, the adoption relationship with girls, adopted in infancy or latency is found to last longer, but this is not the case for girls in puberty or early adolescence [225]. The adoption relationship fails more frequently with children presenting behavioral or psychic disorders unless special care is provided for the families [226].

Children placed at an older age and having previously experienced severe adverse conditions seem incapable to recover in adoptive families, and—at the time of adolescence—the adoptive relationship breaks up, as the following study demonstrate.

Over 100 children, between 5 and 11 years old with adverse preadoption experiences, placed for adoption from public care (domestic U.K. adoptive placements) were assessed 1 and 6 years later. At the adolescent follow-up, in 23% a placement disruption had taken place, in 49% the adoptive relationship continued positively, and in 28% the adoptive relationship continued despite enormous difficulties. A higher risk for the disruption of the adoptive relationship was found for older children, for children being singled out from siblings and rejected, for children with longer time in foster care and with multiple behavioral problems [227].

Protective Factors Child-related protective factors are primarily considered to be the child's young age, the absence of past adverse experiences (violence or abuse) in the family of origin, and the availability of essential information about the relinquishing family [224].

Pre-adoptive risk factors appear to be less important than the adoptive family's functioning for the outcome of adopted children and adolescents [228]. Specific challenging factors such as loss, adoption communicative openness, and post-adoption contact with birth family relatives influence the adoptive family relationship [229–231].

Adoptive family-related risk or protective factors were identified with regard to the age of the adoptive parents (in families with relatively young or relatively old parents, breakdowns were more frequent), to the quality of their marital relationship and to their parenting skills. According to Barth et al. [220], more flexible parental attitudes prove to be favorable in dealing realistically with problematic behavior of the adopted child; empathetic and loving attention enables the child to gradually build trust and attachment. Other factors such as educational level, financial situation, parental motivation, religious and class affiliation, and social support have been investigated: however, the results of these studies prove to be inconsistent. Nevertheless, it is worth noting that in families who received regular and intensive counseling and support, breakdowns rarely occurred [232].

In the United States breakdowns rates range from 10% to 25%, being higher for older children and depending on the population studied, the duration of the study, geographic and other factors. Rates have decreased slightly since the 1980s and 1990s.

The main factors for breakdowns are the following:

- The adopted child was older, hat endured multiple adverse experiences (abuse, neglect, trauma); placements with resulting behavioral and emotional problems, leading to the breakdown of the adoptive relationship in early adolescence.
- The parental couple's relationship was unstable or characterized by rigidity and the parents' expectations were unreasonable. Parents refused to seek assistance or were inexperienced with children being disabled or having special needs.
- Adoption agencies failures: insufficient preparation of prospective adoptive parents and lack of support for adoptive families [213].

The investigation of failed international adoption cases in Switzerland revealed that children of foreign origin were abandoned after their adoption or never adopted after their arrival [217]; the exact number of those expelled is difficult to estimate. The evaluation of young foreigners, placed for adoption by the private organization "Terre des Hommes", revealed that 14.5% were never adopted [233]. The community has a duty and responsibility to improve the legal status of the foreign child in various respects. It is up to the political authorities to eliminate the uncertainty, in which the foreign child finds himself from the moment he arrives in Switzerland until his adoption, and to integrate him into society - regardless of the future adoptive parents' attitude about their original intention - after the expiration of the period of pre-adoptive foster care prescribed by the civil law.

Outlook

Professionals involved in adoption point out the necessity of scientific research on adoption problems, as well as epidemiological studies on adoptive families [5, 234]. Prospective longitudinal studies on a large scale are required in order to draw comparisons between the different types of placement. Preparedness for future adoptive parents and adoptive child, as well as for their follow-up care and support services need to be assessed. The aim is to gain knowledge about what type of placement leads to the best outcomes for which children and adolescents, what factors are associated with the different outcomes and what consequences arise for all persons involved. Research needs to be multidisciplinary, including psychiatrists, psychologists, social workers, developmental neurologists, and health economists [235].

The evaluation of potential consequences of contacts with the biological family—after the child's placement and adoption—and the well-being of the child and all parties involved is an essential task. Although the importance of the adoption triangle is emphasized, research attention was not equally directed to all sides of the triangle; biological families have been neglected.

Adoption support services aimed at reducing children's problems and addressing parental stress and unreasonable expectations are crucial. Evaluation of such interventions and of the preparation of prospective adoptive parents and children must follow rigorous criteria.

High quality adoption research has significant implications for children who cannot remain with their families of origin. The more adoption practices can be supported by solid, research-based evidence, the lower the risk of adoptive placement terminations will be and the smaller the need for ongoing mental and social health interventions for adoptees and their families [236].

References

1. Johnson DE. Adoption and the effect on children's development. Early Hum Dev. 2002;68:39–54.
2. Van IJzendoorn MH, Juffer F. The Emanuel Miller Memorial Lecture 2006: adoption as intervention. Meta-analytic evidence for massive catch-up and plasticity in physical, socio-emotional, and cognitive development. J Child Psychol Psychiatry. 2006;47:1228–45.
3. Zeanah C. Disturbances of attachment in young children adopted from institutions. J Dev Behav Pediatr. 2000;21:230–6.
4. Duke ML. Groups seeking to eliminate adoption. In: Marshner C, Picroce WL, editors. Adoption factbook III.222. Wahington DC: National Council for Adoption; 1999.
5. Cohen N. Adoption. In: Rutter M, Taylor E, editors. Child and adolescent psychiatry: modern approaches. Oxford: Blackwell; 2002. p. 373–81.
6. Hoksbergen R. The importance of adoption for nurturing and enchancing the emotional and intellectual potential of children. Adoption Q. 1999;3(2):29–41.
7. Jacob F. La logique du vivant. Une histoire de l'hérédité. Paris: Gallimard, coll. « Bibliothèque des sciences humaines » 1970.
8. Plomin R, Scheier M, Bergeman CS, Pedersen NL, Nesselroade JR, McClearn GE. Optimism, pessimism and mental health: a twin/adoption analysis. Personal Individ Differ. 1992;13(8):921–30.
9. Plomin R. Genetics and children's experiences in the family. J Child Psychol Psychiatr. 1995;56(1):33–68.
10. Wadsworth SJ, Corley RP, Hewitt J, Plomin R, DeFries JC. Parent-offspring resemblance for reading performance at 7,12 and 16 years of age in the Colorado adoption project. J Child Psychol Psychiatr. 2002;43(6):769–74.
11. Plomin R, Reiss D, Hetherington EM, Howe G. Nature and nurture: genetic influence on measures of the family environment. Dev Psychol. 1994;30:32–43.
12. Reiss D, Plomin R, Hetherington EM, Howe G, Rovine M, Tryon A, Stanley M. The separate worlds of teenage siblings: an introduction to the study of the nonshared environment and adolescent development. In: Hetherington EM, Reiss D, Plomin R, editors. Separate social worlds of siblings: impact of nonshared environment on development. Hillsdale, NJ: Lawrence Erlbaum Associates; 1994. p. 63–109.
13. Wachs TD. The nature-nurture gap: what we have here is a failure to collaborate. In: Plomin R, McClearn GE, editors. Nature, nurture, and psychology. Washington, DC: AOA Books; 1993. p. 375–91.
14. Rutter M, Kim-Cohen J, Maughan B. Continuities and discontinuities in psychopathology between childhood and adult life. J Child Psychol Psychiatry. 2006a;47(3–4):276–95.
15. Rutter M, Moffitt TE, Caspi A. Gene-environment interplay and psychopathology: multiple varieties but real effects. J Child Psychol Psychiatry. 2006b;47(3–4):226–61.
16. Plomin R. Genetics and developmental psychology. Merrill-Palmer Q. 2004;50(3):341–52.
17. Poletti M, Gebhardt E, Pelizza L, Preti A, Raballo A. Looking at intergenerational risk factors in Schizophrenia spectrum disorders: new frontiers for early vulnerability identification? Front Psychiatry. 2020;11:566683.

18. Rasic D, Hajek T, Alda M, Uher R. Risk of mental illness in offspring of parents with schizophrenia, bipolar disorder, and major depressive disorder: a meta-analysis of family high-risk studies. Schizophr Bull. 2014;40(1):28–38. https://doi.org/10.1093/schbul/sbt114.

19. Trubetskoy V, Panagiotaropoulou G, Awasthi S, et al. Mapping genomic loci implicates genes and synaptic biology in schizophrenia. Nature. 2022;604(7906):502–8. https://doi.org/10.1038/s41586-022-04434-5.

20. Berrettini WH. Are schizophrenic and bipolar disorders related? A review of family and molecular studies. Biol Psychiatry. 2000;48(6):531–8.

21. Giusti-Rodríguez P, Sullivan PF. The genomics of schizophrenia: update and implications. J Clin Invest. 2013;123(11):4557–63. https://doi.org/10.1172/JCI66031.

22. Kendler KS, Gatz M, Gardner CO, Pedersen NL. A Swedish national twin study of lifetime major depression. Am J Psychiatry. 2006;163:109–14.

23. Kim-Cohen J, Caspi A, Taylor A, Williams B, Newcombe R, Craig IW, Moffitt TE. MAOA, maltreatment, and gene environment interaction predicting children's mental health: new evidence and a meta-analysis. Mol Psychiatry. 2006;11(10):903–13.

24. Kozhimannil KB, Kim H. Maternal mental illness. Science. 2014;345(6198):755. https://doi.org/10.1126/science.1259614.

25. Berggink V, Larsen JT, Hillegers MHJ, Dahl SK, Stevens H, Mortensen PB, Petersen L, Munk-Olsen T. Childhood adverse life events and parental psychopathology as risk factors for bipolar disorder. Translational. Psychiatry. 2016;6:e929. https://doi.org/10.1038/tp.2016.201.

26. Bountress K, Chassin L. Risk for behavior problems in children of parents with substance use disorder. Am J Orthopsychiatry. 2015;85(3):275–86. https://doi.org/10.1037/ort0000063.

27. Lollis S, Kuczynski L. Beyond one hand clapping: seeing bidirectionality in parent-child relations. J Soc Pers Relationships. 1997;14:441–61.

28. Peters BR, Atkins MS, McKay M. Adopted children's behavior problems: a review of five explanatory models. Clin Psychol Rev. 1999;19(3):297–328.

29. Rende R, Plomin R. Nature, nature, and the development of psychopathology. In: Cicchetti D, Cohen DJ, editors. Developmental psychopathology, vol. 1 (theory and methods). New York: Wiley; 1995. p. 291–314.

30. Rutter M, Silberg J, O'Connor TG, Simonoff E. Genetics and child psychiatry: I advances in quantitative and molecular genetics. J Child Psychol Psychiatr. 1999a;40(1):3–18.

31. Knafo A, Plomin R. Parental discipline and affection and children's prosocial behavior: genetic and environmental links. J Pers Soc Psychol. 2006;90(1):147–64.

32. Plomin R, Fulker DW, Corley R, DeFries JC. Nature, nurture, and cognitive development from 1 to 16 years: a parent-offspring adoption study. Am Psychol Soc. 1997;8:6.

33. Schleiffer R. Adoption: psychiatrisches Risiko und/oder protektiver Faktor? Prax Kinderpsychol Kinderpsychiat. 1997;46:645–59.

34. Masten AS, Coatswonh JD. Competence, resilience, and psychopathology. In: Cicchetti D, Cohen DJ, editors. Developmental psychopathology, vol. 2 (risk, disorder, and adaptation). New York: Wiley; 1995. p. 715–52.

35. Rutter M. Psychosocial resillience and protective mechanisms. In: Rolf J, editor. Risk and protective factors in the development of psychopathology. Cambridge: Cambridge Univ. Press; 1990. p. 181–214.

36. Cohler BJ, Scott FM, Musick JS. Adversity, vulnerability, and resilience: cultural and development perspectives. In: Cicchetti D, Cohen DJ, editors. Developmental psychopathology, vol. 2 (risk, disorder, and adaptation). New York: Wiley; 1995. p. 753–800.

37. McGuinness TM, Dyer JG. International adoption as a natural experiment. J Pediatr Nurs. 2006;21(4):276–88.

38. Lombroso P, Pauls D, Leckman J. Genetic mechanismen in childhood psychiatric disorders. J Am Acad Child Adolesc Psychiatry. 1994;33:921–38.

39. Wierzbicki M. Psychological adjustment of adoptees: a meta-analysis. J Clin Child Psychol. 1993;22:447–54.

40. Scarr S. Developmental theories for the 1990s: development and individual differences. Child Dev. 1992;63:1–19.
41. Brand AE, Brinich PM. Behavior problems and mental health contacts in adopted, foster, and nonadopted children. J Child Psychol Psychiatr. 1999;40(8):1221–9.
42. Cohen NJ, Coyne J, Duvall J. Adopted and biological children in the clinic: family, parental and child characteristics. J Child Psychol Psychiatr. 1993;34(4):545–62.
43. Dance C, Rushton A, Quinton D. Emotional abuse in early childhood: relationships with progress in subsequent family placement. J Child Psychol Psychiatr. 2002;43(3):395–407.
44. Fergusson DM, Lynskey M, Horwood LJ. The adolescent outcomes of adoption: a 16-year longitudinal study. J Child Psychol Psychiatr. 1995;36(4):597–615.
45. Rutter M, Kreppner JM, O'Connor TG. Specificity and heterogencity in children's responses to profound institutional privation. Br J Psychiatry. 2001;179:97–103.
46. Tienari P, Wynne LC. Adoption studies of schizophrenia. Ann Med. 1994;26:223–37.
47. Verhulst FC, Althaus M, Versluis-den Bieman HJM. Problem behavior in international adoptees: I. an epidemiological study. Am Acad Child Adolesc Psychiatry. 1990;29(1):94–103.
48. Tienari P, Sorri A, Lahti I, Naarala M, Wahlberg KE, Pohjola J, Moring J. Interaction of genetic and psychosocial factors in schizophrenia. Acta Psychiatr Scand., Suppl. No 319. 1985a;71:19–30.
49. Tienari P, Sorri A, Lahti I, Naarala M, Wahlberg KE, Rönkkö T, Pohjola J, Moring J. The Finnsih adoptive family study of schizophrenia. Yale J Biol Med. 1985b;58:227–37.
50. Tienari P. Implications of adoption studies on schizophrenia. Br J Psychiatry. 1992;161(Suppl. 18):52–8.
51. Tienari P, Wynne LC, Sorri A, Lahti I, Läksy K, Moring J. Genotype-environment interaction in schizophrenia-spectrum disorder. Long-term follow-up study of Finnish adoptees. Br J Psychiatry. 2004;184:216–22.
52. Wahlberg KE, Wynne LC, Hakko H, Laksy K, Moring J, Miettunen J, Tienari P. Interaction of genetic risk and adoptive parent communication deviance: longitudinal prediction of adoptee psychiatric disorders. Psychol Med. 2004;34(8):1531–41.
53. Wynne LC, Tienari P, Nieminen P, Sorri A, Lahti I, Moring J, Naarala M, Läksi K, Wahlberg KE, Mittunen J. Genotype-environment interaction in the schizophrenia spectrum: genetic liability and global family ratings in the Finnish Adoption Study. Fam Process. 2006;45(4):419–34.
54. Myllyaho T, Siira V, Wahlberg KE, Hakko H, Laksy K, Roisko R, Niemela M, Rasanen S. Interaction of genetic vulnerability to schizophrenia and family functioning in adopted-away offspring of mothers with schizophrenia. Psychiatry Res. 2019; https://doi.org/10.1016/j.psychres.2019.06.017.
55. Eley TC, Deater-Deckard K, Fombonne E, Fulker DW, Plomin R. An adoption study of depressive symptoms in middle childhood. J Child Psychol Psychiatr. 1998;39(3):337–45.
56. Rice F, Harold G, Thapar A. The genetic aetiology of childhood depression: a review. J Child Psychol Psychiatr. 2002;43(1):65–79.
57. Rutter M, the English, Romanian (ERA) Study Team. Developmental catch-up, and deficit, following adoption after severe early privation. J Child Psychol Psychiatr. 1998;39(4):465–76.
58. Kendler KS, Ohlsson H, Sundquist K, Sundquist J. Sources of parent-offspring resemblance for major depression in a National Swedish Extended Adoption Study. JAMA Psychiatry. 2018;75(2):194–200. https://doi.org/10.1001/jamapsychiatry.2017.3828.
59. Kendler KS, Ohlsson H, Sundquist J, Sundquist K. An extended Swedish National Adoption Study of Bipolar Disorder Illness and cross-Generational Familial Association with schizophrenia and major depression. JAMA Psychiatry. 2020;77(8):814–22. https://doi.org/10.1001/jamapsychiatry.2020.0223.
60. LeMoult J, Humphreys KL, Tracy A, Hoffmeister JA, Ip E, Gotlib IH. Meta-analysis: exposure to early life stress and risk for depression in childhood and adolescence. J Am Acad Child Adolesc Psychiatry. 2020;59(7):842–55.
61. Cadoret RJ, Troughton E, Bagford J, Woodworth G. Genetic and environmental factors in adoptee antisocial personality. Eur Arch Psychiatr Neurol Sci. 1990a;239:231–40.

62. Cadoret RJ, Thoughton E, Moreno-Merchant L, Whitters A. Early life psychosocial events and adult affective symptoms. In: Robins LN, Rutter M, editors. Straight and devious pathways from childhood to adulthood. Cambridge: Cambridge University Press; 1990b. p. 300–13.
63. Howe D. Age at placement, adoption experience and adult adopted people's contact with their adoptive and birth mothers: an attachment perspective. Attach Hum Dev. 2001;3:222–37.
64. Nickman SL, Rosenfeld AA, Fine P, Macintyre JC, Pilowsky DJ, Howe RA, Derdeyn A, Gonzales MB, Forsythe L, Sveda SA. Children in adoptive families: overview and update. J Am Acad Child Adolesc Psychiatry. 2005;44(10):987–95.
65. Collishaw S, Maughan B, Pickles A. Infant adoption: psychosocial outcomes in adulthood. Soc Psychiatry Psychiatr Epidemiol. 1998;33:57–65.
66. Howe D. Adoption outcome research and practical judgement. Adopt Foster. 1998a;22(2):6–15.
67. Howe D. Patterns of adoption: nature, nurture and psychosocial development. Oxford: Blackwell Science; 1998b.
68. Howe D, Hinings D. Adopted children referred to a child and family Centre. Adopt Foster. 1987;11:44–7.
69. Howe D. Parent reported problems in 211 adopted children: some risk and protective factors. J Child Psychol Psychiatr. 1997;38(4):401–12.
70. Humphrey M, Ounsted C. Adoptive families referred for psychiatric advice. Br J Psychiatry. 1963;109:599–608.
71. Stams GJJM, Juffer F, Rispens J, Hoksbergen RAC. The development and adjustment of 7-year-old children adopted in infancy. J Child Psychol Psychiatr. 2000;41(8):1025–38.
72. Maughan B, Collishaw S, Pickles A. School achievement and adult qualifications among adoptees: a longitudinal study. J Child Psychol Psychiatr. 1998;39(5):669–85.
73. Cederblad M, Höök B, Irhammar M, Mercke AM. Mental health in international adoptees as teenagers and young adults: an epidemiological study. J Child Psychol Psychiatr. 1999;40:1239–48.
74. Beckett C, Maughan B, Rutter M, Castle J, Colvert E, Groothues C, Kreppner J, et al. Do the effects of early severe deprivation on cognition persist into early adolescence? Findings from the English and Romanian adoptees study. Child Dev. 2006;77(3):696–711.
75. Stams GJM, Juffer F, van IJzendoorn MH. Maternal sensitivity, infant attachment, and temperament in early childhood predict adjustment in middle childhood: the case of adopted children and their biologically unrelated parents. Dev Psychol. 2002;38(5):806–21. https://doi.org/10.1037/0012-1649.38.5.806.
76. McDermott JM, Troller-Renfree S, Vanderwert R, Nelson CA, Zeanah CH, Fox NA. Psychosocial deprivation, executive functions, and the emergence of socio-emotional behavior problems. Front Hum Neurosci. 2013;77:167.
77. Rutter M, Sonuga-Barke EJX. Conclusions: overview of findings from the era study, inferences, and research implications. Monogr Soc Res Child Dev. 2010;75(1):212–29. https://doi.org/10.1111/j.1540-5834.2010.00557.x.
78. Rutter M, Sonuga-Barke EJ, Castle JI. Investigating the impact of early institutional deprivation on development: background and research strategy of the English and Romanian Adoptees (ERA) study. Monogr Soc Res Child Dev. 2010;75(1):1–20. https://doi.org/10.1111/j.1540-5834.2010.00548.x.
79. Stovall KC, Dozier M. Infants in foster care: an attachment theory perspective. Adopt Q. 1998;2:55–88.
80. Paine AL, Fahey K, Anthony RE, Shelton KH. Early adversity predicts adoptees' enduring emotional and behavioral problems in childhood. Eur Child Adolesc Psychiatry. 2021;30:721–32. https://doi.org/10.1007/s00787-020-01553-0.
81. Zeanah C. Beyond insecurity: a reconceptualization of attachment disorders in infancy. J Consult Clin Psychol. 1996;64:42–52.
82. Jacobsen T, Miller L. Attachment quality in young children of mentally ill mothers: contribution of maternal caregiving abilities. In: Solomon J, George C, editors. Attachment disorganization and foster care context. New York: Guilford Press; 1999. p. 347–78.

83. Liotti G. Disorganization of attachment as a model for understanding dissociative psychopathology. In: Solomon J, George C, editors. Attachment disorganization. New York: Guilford Press; 1999. p. 291–317.

84. Perry BD, Pollard RA. Homcostatis stress, trauma and adaptation: a neurodevelopmental view of childhood trauma. Child Adolesc Psychiatr Clin N Am. 1998;7:33–51.

85. Schore A. Early organization of the nonlinear right brain and development of a predisposition to psychiatric disorders. Dev Psychopathol. 1997;9:595–631.

86. Hodges J, Tizard B. Social and family relationship of ex-institutional children. J Child Psychol Psychiatry. 1989;30:77–98.

87. O'Connor TG, Rutter M, the English and Romanian Adoptees Study Team. Attachment disorder behavior following severe deprivation: extension and longitudinal follow-up. J Am Acad Child Adolesc Psychiatry. 2000a;39(6):703–12.

88. O'Connor TG, Rutter M, Beckett C, Keavency L, Kreppner J, the English and Romanian Adoptees Study Team. The effects of global severe privation on cognitive competence: extension and longitudinal follow-up. Child Dev. 2000b;71:376–90.

89. Castle J, Groothues C, Bredenkamp D, Beckett C, O'Connor TG, Rutter M, the English and Romanian Adoptees Study Team. Effects of qualities of early institutional care on cognitive attainment. Am J Orthopsychiatry. 1999;69:424–37.

90. Goldstein J, Freud A, Solnit A. Beyond the best interests of the child. 2nd ed. New York: Free Press; 1973.

91. Bowlby J. Attachment. 2nd ed. New York: Basic Books; 1982.

92. Groze V, Rosenthal JA. Attachment theory and the adoption of children with special needs. Soc Work Res Abstr. 1993;29(2):5–12.

93. Hughes DA. Adopting children with attachment problems. Cild Welfare. 1999;LXXVIII(5):541560.

94. Solomon J, George C, editors. Attachment disorganization. New York: Guiloford Press; 1999.

95. Chisholm K. A three year follow-up of attachment and indiscriminate friendliness in children adopted from romanian orphanages. Child Dev. 1998;69(4):1092–106.

96. Juffer F, Hoksbergen AC, Riksen-Walraven JM, Kohnstamm GA. Early intervention in adoptive families: supporting maternal sensitive responsiveness, infant-mother attachment, and infant competence. J Child Psychol Psychiatry. 1997;38(8):1039–50.

97. Rutter M, Andersen-Wood L, Bredenkamp D, Castle J, Groothues C, et al. Quasi-autistic patterns following severe early global privation. J Child Psychol Psychiatry. 1999b;40(4):537–49.

98. Woodhouse W, Baily A, Rutter M, Bolton P, Baird G, Le Couteur A. Head circumference and other pervasive developmental disorders. J Child Psychol Psychiatry. 1996;37:665–71.

99. Gillberg C, Coleman M. The biology of the autistic syndromes. 2nd ed. London: Mac Keith Press; 1992.

100. Rutter M, Bailey A, Bolton P, Le Couteur A. Autism and known medical conditions: myth and substance. J Child Psychol Psychiatry. 1994;35:311–22.

101. Chugani HT, Phelps ME. Maturational changes in cerebral function in infants determined by "FDG positron emission tomography". Science. 1986;231:840–3.

102. Chugani HT, Phelps ME, Mazziotta JC. Positron emission tomography study of human brain functional development. Ann Neurol. 1987;22:487–97.

103. Chugani HT, Behen ME, Muzik O, Juhasz C, Nagy F, Chugani DC. Local brain functional activity following early deprivation: a study of postinstitutionalized romanian orphans. Neurolmage. 2001;14:1290–301.

104. Rutter M, Beckett C, Castle J, Colvert E, Kreppner J, Mehta M, Stevens S, Sonuga-Barke E. Effects of profound early institutional deprivation: an overview of findings from a UK longitudinal study of Romanian adoptees. Eur J Dev Psychol. 2007;4(3):332–50. https://doi.org/10.1080/17405620701401846.

105. Erich ST, Leung P. The impact of previous type of abuse and sibling adoption upon adoptive families. Child Abuse Negl. 2002;26:1045–58.

106. Hoksbergen R. Die Folgen von Vernachlässigung. Erfahrungen mit Adoptivkindern aus Rumänien. Idstein: Schulz-Kirchner; 2003.
107. van der Vegt EJ, Tieman W, van der Ende J, Ferdinand RF, Verhulst FC, Tiemeier H. Impact of early childhood adversities on adult psychiatric disorders: a study of international adoptees. Soc Psychiatry Psychiatr Epidemiol. 2009;44:724–31. https://doi.org/10.1007/s00127-009-0494-6.
108. Sonuga-Barke EJS, Kennedy M, Kumsta R, Knights N, Golm D, Rutter M, et al. Child-to-adult neurodevelopmental and mental health trajectories after early life deprivation: the young adult follow-up of the longitudinal English and Romanian Adoptees study. 2017 https://doi.org/10.1016/S0140-6736(17)30045-4.
109. Julian MM. Age at adoption from institutional care as a window into the lasting effects of early experiences. Clin Child Fam Psychol Rev. 2013;16(2):101–45. https://doi.org/10.1007/s10567-013-0130-6.
110. Golombok S, Cook R, Bish A, Murray C. Families created by the new reproductive technologies: quality of parenting and social and emotional development of the children. Child Dev. 1995;66:285–98.
111. Brodzinsky DM. Long-term outcomes in adoption. In: Behrman RE, editor. The future of children: adoption. Los Altos, CA: Center for the Future of Children, the Davis and Lucile Packard Foundation; 1993. p. 153–66.
112. Grotevant HD, McRoy RG. Adopted adolescents in residential treatment: the role of the family. In: Brodzinsky DM, Schechter MD, editors. The psychology of adoption. New York: Oxford University Prerss; 1990.
113. Kotsopoulos S, Cote A, Joseph L, Pentland N, Stavrakaki C, Sheahan P, Oke L. Psychiatric disorders in adopted children. Am J Orthopsychiatry. 1988;58(4):608–12.
114. Hersov L. The seventh annual Jack Tizard memorial lecture, aspects of adoption. J Child Psychol Psychiatry. 1990;34(4):493–510.
115. Jerome L. Overrepresentation of adopted children attending a children's mental health center. Can J Psychiatr. 1986;31:526–31.
116. Kim WJ, Davenport C, Joseph J, Zrull J, Woolford E. Psychiatric disorders and juvenile delinquency in adopted children and adolescents. J Am Acad Child Adolesc Psychiatry. 1988;27:111–5.
117. Rogeness GA, Hoppe SK, Macedo CA, Fischer C, Harris WA. Psychopathology in hospitalised, adopted children. J Amer Acad Child Adolesc Psychiatry. 1988;27:628–31.
118. Warren SB. Lower threshold for referral for psychiatric treatment for adopted adolescents. J Am Acad Child Adolesc Psychiatry. 1992;31:512–7.
119. Van Ijzendoorn MH, Juffer F, Poelhuis CW. Adoption and cognitive development: a meta-analytic comparison of adopted and nonadopted children's IQ and school performance. Psyachol Bull. 2005;131(2):301–16.
120. Bohman M, Sigvardsson S. Outcome in adoption: lessons from longitudinal studies. In: Brozinsky DM, Schechter RMH, editors. The psychology of adoption. New York: Oxford University Press; 1990. p. 93–106.
121. Groza V, Ryan SD. Pre-adoption stress and its association with child behavior in domestic special needs and international adoptions. Psychoneuroendocrinology. 2002;27:181–97.
122. Hoksbergen R, Juffer F, Waardenburg BC, van de Klippe G. Adopted children at home and at school. The integration after eight years of 116 Thai children in the Dutch society. Lisse: Swets & Zeitlinger; 1987.
123. Sharma AR, McGue MK, Benson PL. The psychological adjustment of united adopted adolescents and their nonadopted siblings. Child Dev. 1998;69:791–802.
124. Verhulst FC, Versluis-den Bieman HJM. Developmental course of problem behaviors in adolescent adoptess. J Am Acad Child Adolescent Psychiatry. 1995;34(2):151–9.
125. Versluis-den Bieman HJM, Verhulst FC. Self-reported and parent reported problems in adolescent international adoptees. J Child Psychol Psychiatry. 1995;56(8):1411–28.

126. Simmel BD, Barth RP, Hinshaw SP. Externalizing symptomatology among adoptive youth: prevalence and preadoption risk factors. J Abnorm Child Psychol. 2001;29(1):57–69.
127. Brodzinsky DM. Adjustment to adoption: a psychosocial perspective. Clin Psychol Rev. 1987;7:25–47.
128. Hersov L. Adoption. In: Rutter M, Taylor E, Hersov L, editors. Child and adolescent psychiatry. 3nd ed. Oxford: Blackwell; 1994. p. 267–82.
129. Haugaard JJ. Is adoption a risk factor for the development of adjustment problems ? Clin Psychol Rev. 1998;18(1):47–69.
130. Zill N. Adopted children in the United States: a profile based on a national survey of child health (serial 104–33). Washington, DC: Government Printing Office; 1996. p. 104–19.
131. Stein LM, Hoopes JL. Identity formation in the adopted adolescent. The Delaware Family Study. New York: Child Welfare League of America; 1985.
132. Kühl W. Wenn fremdländische Adoptivkinder erwachsen werden ... Adoptionserfolg und psychosoziale Integration im Jugendalter. Erste Ergebnisse einer Befragung. Osnabrück: Terre des hommes; 1985.
133. Borders LD, Black LK, Pasley BK. Are adopted children and their parents at greater risk for negative outcomes? Familiy Relations. 1998;47:237–41.
134. Schleiffer R. Dissoziale Störungen bei adoptierten Jugendlichen. Eine klinisch-empirische Studie. Z für Kinder- und Jugendpsychiatrie. 1993;21:115–22.
135. Miller BC, Fan X, Christensen M, Grotevant HG, van Dulmen M. Comparison of adopted and nonadopted adolescents in a large. Nationally Representative Sample Child Development. 2000a;71(5):1458–73.
136. Miller BC, Fan X, Grotevant HD, Christensen M, Coyl D, van Dulmen M. Adopted adolescents' overrepresentation in mental health counseling: adoptees problems or parents' lower threshold for referral? J Am Acad Child Adolesc Psychiatry. 2000b;39:1504–11.
137. Goldberg D, Wolkind SN. Patterns of psychiatric disorders in adopted girls: a research note. J Child Psychol Psychiatry. 1992;33:935–40.
138. Burrow AL, Tubman JG, Finley GE. Adolescent adjustment in a nationally collected sample: identifying group differences by adoption status, adoption subtype, developmental stage and gender. J Adolesc. 2004;27(3):267–82.
139. Tieman W, van der Ende J, Verhulst FC. Psychiatric disorders in young adult intercountry adoptees: an epidemiological study. Am J Psychiatry. 2005;162(3):592–8.
140. Askeland KG, Hysing M, La Greca AM, Aarø LE, Tell GS, Sivertsen B. Mental health in internationally adopted adolescents: a meta-analysis. J Am Acad Child Adolesc Psychiatry. 2017;56:203–13. https://doi.org/10.1016/j.jaac.2016.12.009.
141. Raby KL, Dozier M. Attachment across the lifespan: insights from adoptive families. Curr Opin Psychol. 2019;25:81–5. https://doi.org/10.1016/j.copsyc.2018.03.011.
142. Van den Dries L, Juffer F, Van IJzendoorn MH, Bakermans-Kranenburg MJ. Fostering security? A meta-analysis of attachment in adopted children. Child Youth Serv Rev. 2009;31:410–21.
143. Brisch KH, Hellbrügge T, editors. Kinder ohne Bindung. Deprivation, adoption und Psychotherapie. Stuttgart: Klett-Cotta; 2006.
144. Lipman EL, Offord DR, Boyle MH, Racine YA. Follow-up of psychiatric and educational morbidity among adopted children. J Am Acad Child Adolesc Psychiatry. 1993;32:1007–12.
145. Nickman SL, Lewis RG. Adoptive families and professionals: when the experts make things worse. J Am Acad Child Adolesc Psychiatry. 1994;33:753–5.
146. Vandivere S, Malm K, Radel L. Adoption USA: a chartbook based on the 2007 National Survey of Adoptive Parents. Washington, D.C.: The U.S. Department of Health and Human Services, Office of the Assistant Secretary for Planning and Evaluation; 2009.
147. Hjern A, Lindblad F, Vinnerljung B. Suicide, psychiatric illness, and social maladjustment in intercountry adoptees in Sweden: a cohort study. Lancet. 2002;360:443–8.

148. Jaffari-Bimmel N, Juffer F, Ijzendoorn MH, Bakermans-Kranenburg MJ, Mooijaart A. Social development from infancy to adolescence: longitudinal and concurrent factors in an adoption sample. Dev Psychol. 2006;42(6):1143–53.
149. Jungmann J. Forschungsergebnisse zur Entwicklung von Adoptivkindern. Z Kinder Jugendpsychiatr. 1980;8:184–219.
150. Textor MR. Inlandsadoptionen: Herkunft, Familienverhältnisse und Entwicklung der Adoptivkinder. In: Hoksbergen RAC, Textor MR, editors. Adoption: Grundlagen, Vermittlung, Nachbetreuung, Beratung. Freiburg: Lambertus; 1993. p. 41–63.
151. Hoksbergen R. Auslandadoptionen: deutsche, niederländische und andere Forschungsergebnisse. In: Hoksbergen R, Textor MR, editors. Adoption. Grundlagen, Vermittlung Nachbetreuung, Beratung. Freiburg i. Br: Lambertus; 1993. p. 63–90.
152. Textor MR. Auslandsadoptionen. Forschungsstand und Folgerungen Praxis Kinderpsychol. Kinderpsychiat. 1991a;40:42–9.
153. Berry M, Barth RP. Preparation, support and satisfaction of adoptive families in agency and independent adoptions. Child Adolesc Soc Work J. 1996;13:157–83.
154. Juffer F, van Ijzendoorn MH. Behavior problems and mental health referrals of international adoptees: a meta-analysis. JAMA. 2005;293(20):2501–15.
155. Brooks D, Barth RP. Adult transracial and inracial adoptees: effects of race, gender, adoptive family structure, and placement history on adjustment outcomes. Am J Orthopsychiatry. 1999;69:1.
156. Benson PL, Sharma AR, Roehlkepartain EC. Growing up adopted: a portrait of adolescents and their families. Minneapolis, MN: Search Institute; 1994.
157. Lindholm BE, Touliatos J. Psychological adjustment of adopted and nonadopted children. Psychol Rep. 1980;46:307–10.
158. Fensbo C. Mental and behavioural outcome of inter-ethnic adoptees: a review of the literature. Eur Child Adolesc Psychiatry. 2004;13(2):55–63.
159. Rushton A, Minnis H. Annotation: transracial family placements. J Child Psychol Psychiatry. 1997;38(2):147–59.
160. Lee MR. The transracial adoption paradox: history, research, and counseling implications of cultural socialization. Couns Psychol. 2003;31(6):711–44.
161. Antares K. Between two worlds: a phenomenological exploration of experiences and understandings related to race for black transracially adopted emerging adults. 2020. Dissertations. 3658. https://scholarworks.wmich.edu/dissertations/3658
162. Golse B. À propos de l'adoption internationale: la double étrangeté de l'enfant venu d'ailleurs. Arch Pediatr. 2011;18:723–6.
163. Freud S. The uncanny. SE 17. London: Hogarth Press; 1919. p. 217–56.
164. Riera A, Walker DM. The impact of race and ethnicity on care in the pediatric emergency department. Curr Opin Pediatr. 2010;22(3):284–9.
165. Rivas-Drake D, Seaton EK, Markstrom C, et al. Ethnic and racial identity in the 21st Century Study Group. Ethnic and racial identity in adolescence: implications for psychosocial, academic, and health outcomes. Child Dev. 2014;85(1):40–57.
166. Cheng ER, Cohen A, Goodman E. The role of perceived discrimination during childhood and adolescence in understanding racial and socioeconomic influences on depression in young adulthood. J Pediatr. 2015;166(2):370–7.e1.
167. Janson GR, Hazler RJ. Trauma reactions of bystanders and victims to repetitive abuse experiences. Violence Vict. 2004;19(2):239–55.
168. Trent M, Dooley DG, Jacqueline Dougé J. The impact of racism on child and adolescent health. Pediatrics. 2019;144:2. https://doi.org/10.1542/peds.2019-1765.
169. Anderson AT, Jackson A, Jones L, Kennedy DP, Wells K, Chung PJ. Minority parents' perspectives on racial socialization and school readiness in the early childhood. Acad Pediatr. 2015c;15(4):405–11.
170. Pinderhughes EE, Matthews JAK, Zhang X, Scott JC. Unpacking complexities in ethnic–racial socialization in transracial adoptive families: a process-oriented transactional system. Dev Psychopathol. 2021;33:493–505. https://doi.org/10.1017/S0954579420001741.

171. Sue DW, Capodilupo CM, Torino GC, Bucceri JM, Holder AMB, Nadal KL, Esquilin M. Racial microaggressions in everyday life: implications for clinical practice. Am Psychol. 2007;62(4):271–86. https://doi.org/10.1037/0003-066X.62.4.271.

172. Baden A. Do you know your real parents? And other adoption microaggressions. Adopt Q. 2016;19(1):1–25. https://doi.org/10.1080/10926755.2015.1026012.

173. Miller LC, Pérouse de Montclos M-O, Matthews J, Peyre J, Vaugelade J, Baubin O, Chomilier J, de Monleon J-V, de Truchis A, Sorge F, Pinderhughes E. Microaggressions experienced by adoptive families and internationally adopted adolescents in France. Adopt Q. 2020;23(2):135–61. https://doi.org/10.1080/10926755.2020.1719253.

174. Harf A, Skandrani S, Sibeoni J, Pontvert C, Revah-Levy A, Moro MR. Cultural identity and internationally adopted children: qualitative approach to parental representations. PLoS One. 2015;10(3):e0119635. https://doi.org/10.1371/journal.pone.0119635.

175. Anderson KN, Lee RM, Rueter MA, Kim OM. Associations between discussions of racial and ethnic differences in internationally adoptive families and delinquent behavior among Korean adopted adolescents. Child Youth Serv Rev. 2015b;51:66–73. https://doi.org/10.1016/j.childyouth.2015.02.001.

176. Umaña-Taylor AJ, Quintana SM, Lee RM, Cross WE Jr, Rivas-Drake D, Schwartz SJ, Syed M, et al. Ethnic and racial identity in the 21st century study group. Ethnic and racial identity during adolescence and into young adulthood: an integrated conceptualization. Child Dev. 2014;85(1):21–39. https://doi.org/10.1111/cdev.12196. PMID: 24490890; PMCID: PMC6673642

177. Anderson KN, Rueter MA, Lee RM. Discussions about racial and ethnic differences in internationally adoptive families: links with family engagement, warmth, and control. J Fam Commun. 2015a;15:289–308. https://doi.org/10.1080/15267431.2015.1076420.

178. Grotevant HD, Lo AYH. Adoptive parenting. Curr Opin Psychol. 2017;15:71–5.

179. Kim OM, Reichwald R, Lee R. Cultural socialization in families with adopted Korean adolescents: a mixed-method, multiinformant study. J Adolesc Res. 2013;28:69–95. https://doi.org/10.1177/0743558411432636.

180. Pinderhughes EE, Zhang X, Agerbak S. "American" or "multiethnic"? Family ethnic identity among transracial adoptive families ethnic-racial socialization, and children's self-perceptions. New Dir Child Adolesc Dev. 2015;150:5–18.

181. Pinderhughes EE, Matthews JAK, Zhang X. Ethnic identity formation. In: Fong R, McRoy RG, editors. Transracial intercountry adopt. Cult. Guid. Prof. New York: Columbia University Press; 2016. p. 154–92.

182. Juffer F, van IJzendoorn MH. Adoptees do not lack self-esteem: a meta-analysis of studies on self-esteem of transracial, international, and domestic adoptees. Psychol Bull. 2007;133(6):1067–83.

183. Rueter MA, Keyes MA, William G, Iacono WG, McGue M. Family interactions in adoptive compared to nonadoptive families. J Fam Psychol. 2009;23(1):58–66.

184. Terre des Hommes. Massnahmen gegen Privatadoptionen/Kinderhandel. Osnabrück: Selbstverlag; 1989.

185. Zuegg R. Die Vermittlung ausländischer Adoptivkinder als Problem des präventiven Kinderschutzes. Zürich: Verlag Pro Juventute; 1986.

186. Textor MR. Offene Adoptionsformen. In: Nachrichtendienst des Deutschen Vereins für öffentliche und private Fürsorge, Heft 4 1991b.

187. Demick J, Wapner S. Open and closed adoption: a developmental conceptualization. Fam Process. 1988;27:229–49.

188. Grotevant HD. What works in open adoption. In: Curtis PA, Alexander G, editors. What works in child welfare. 2nd ed. Washington, DC: Child Welfare League of America; 2012. p. 309–27.

189. Silverstein DR, Demick K. Towards an organizational-relational model of open adoption. Fam Process. 1994;33:111–24.

190. Grotevant HD, McRoy RG, Elde CL, Lewis Fravel D. Adoptive family system dynamics: variation by level of openness in the adoption. Fam Process. 1994;33(2):125–46.

191. Leon Irving G. Adoption losses: naturally occurring or socially constructed ? Child Dev. 2002;73(2):652–63.
192. Paulitz H. Offene Adoption: ein Plädoyer. Freiburg i.Br: Lamberus Verlag; 1997.
193. Brodzinsky DM. Family structural openness and communication openness as predictors in the adjustment of adopted children. Adopt Q. 2006;9:1–18. https://doi.org/10.1300/J145v9n04.
194. Grotevant HD (2009): Emotional distance regulation over the life course in adoptive kinship networks. In International advances in adoption research for practice. Edited by Neil E, Wrobel ECE . Chichester, UK: Wiley-Blackwell. pp. 295–316.
195. Farr RH, Grant-Marsney HA, Grotevant HD. Adoptees' contact with birth parents in emerging adulthood: the role of adoption communication and attachment to adoptive parents. Fam Process. 2014;53:656–71. https://doi.org/10.1111/famp.12069.
196. Von Korff L, Grotevant HD. Contact in adoption and adoptive identity formation: the mediating role of family conversation. J Fam Psychol. 2011;25:393–401. https://doi.org/10.1037/a0023388.
197. Daly KJ. Reshaped parenthood identity. The transition to adoptive parenthood. J Contemp Enthnogr. 1988;17(1):40–66.
198. Daly KJ. Towards a formal theory of interactive resocialization: the case of adoptive parenthood. Qual Sociol. 1992;15:395–417.
199. Lee JS, Twaite JA. Open adoption and adoptive mothers: attitudes towards birthmothers, adopted children, and parenting. Am J Orthopsychiatry. 1997;67(4):576–84.
200. Neil E. Contact after adoption: the role of agencies in making and supporting plans. Adopt Foster. 2002;26(1):25–38.
201. Neil E. A longitudinal study of contact with adult birth relatives after adoption of children under 4 at placement. School of Social Work and Psychosocial Studies: 2000–2003.
202. Kirk HD. Shared fate: a theory of adoption and mental health. London, New York: Free Press of Glencoe; 1964.
203. Kirk HD. Adoptive kinship: a modern institution in need of reforms. Toronto: Butterworth; 1981.
204. Wrobel GM, Ayers-Lopez S, Grotevant HD, McRoy RG, Friedrick M. Openness in adoption and the level of child participation. Child Dev. 1996;67:2358–74.
205. Smith J. Attitudes of prospective adoptive parents towards agency adoption practices, particularly open adoption. Paper presented at the meeting of the National Committee for Adoption, Washington DC 1991.
206. Kraft A, Palumbo J, Woods P, Mitchell D, Schmidt PM. Some theoretical considerations on confidential adoptions I: the birth mother. Child Adolesc Soc Work. 1985;2:13–21.
207. Berry M. Adoptive parents' perceptions of, and comfort with, open adoption. Child Welfare. 1993;77(3):231–53.
208. Etter J. Levels of cooperation and satisfaction in 56 open adoptions. Child Welfare. 1993;72:257–67.
209. McRoy RG, Grotevant HD. American experience and research on openness. Adopt Foster. 1991;15(4):99–111.
210. Grotevant HD, McRoy RG. Openness in adoption: exploring family connections. Thousand Oaks CA: Sage Publications; 1998.
211. Grotevant HD. Openness in adoption. Adopt Q. 2000;4(1):45–65. https://doi.org/10.1300/J145v04n01_04.
212. Von Korff L, Grotevant HD, McRoy RG. Openness arrangements and psychological adjustment in adolescent adoptees. J Fam Psychol. 2006;20(3):531–4.
213. Palacios J, Rolock N, Selwyn J, Barbosa-Ducharne. Adoption breakdown: concept, research, and implications. Res Soc Work Pract. 2019;29(2):130–42.
214. Berrick JD, Barth RP, Needell B, Jonson-Reid M. The tender years: towards developmentally sensitive child welfare services. New York: Oxford; 1988.

215. Barth RP, Berry M. Adoption and disruption: rats, risks and response. Hawthorne, NY: De Gruyter; 1988.
216. George RM, Howard EC, Yu D. Adoption, disruption, and dissolution in the Illinois child welfare system, 1976–94. Chicago: Chapin Hall Center for Children; 1996.
217. Lücker-Babel MF. Auslandsadoption und Kinderrechte. Was geschieht mit den Verstossenen? Freiburg: Universitätsverlag; 1991.
218. Lyttle E, McCafferty P, Taylor BJ. Experiences of adoption disruption: parents' perspectives. Child Care Pract. 2021; https://doi.org/10.1080/13575279.2021.1941767.
219. Goldberg AE, Garcia R. Predictors of relationship dissolution in lesbian, gay, and heterosexual adoptive parents. J Fam Psychol. 2015;29(3):394–404. https://doi.org/10.1037/fam0000095.
220. Barth RP, Berry M, Yoshikami R, Goodfield RK, Carson ML. Predicting adoption disruption. Soc Work. 1988;33:227–33.
221. Kasten H, Kunze HR, Mühlfeld C. Pflege- und Adoptivkinder in Heimen. Ifb-Materalien: Staatinstitut für Familienforschung an der Universität Bamberg; 2001.
222. Berry M. Adoption disruption. In: Avery RJ, editor. Adoption policy and special needs children. Westport, CT: Auburn House Press; 1997. p. 77–106.
223. Derdeyn AP, Graves CL. Clinicl vicissitudes of adoption. Child Adolesc Psychiatr Clin N Am. 1998;7(2):373–88.
224. Rosenthal JA. Outcomes of adoption of children with special needs. Future Child Adoption. 1993;3:1.
225. Rosenthal JA, Schmidt DM, Conner J. Predictors of special needs adoption disruption. An exploratory study. Child Youth Serv Rev. 1988;10(2):101–17.
226. Smith SL, Howard JA. A comparative study of successful and disrupted adoptions. Soc Serv Rev. 1991;65(2):248–65.
227. Rushton A, Dance C. The adoption of children from public care: a prospective study of outcome in adolescence. J Am Acad Child Adolesc Psychiatry. 2006;45:7.
228. Neil E, Beek M, Ward E. Contact After Adoption: A follow up in late adolescence. Published by the Centre for Research on Children and Families, University of East Anglia 2013.
229. Brodzinsky DM. Children's understanding of adoption: developmental and clinical implications. Prof Psychol Res Pract. 2011;42(2):200–7. https://doi.org/10.1037/a0022415.
230. Grotevant HD, Rueter M, Lynn Von Korff L, Gonzalez C. Post-adoption contact, adoption communicative openness, and satisfaction with contact as predictors of externalizing behavior in adolescence and emerging adulthood. J Child Psychol Psychiatry. 2011;52(5):529–36. https://doi.org/10.1111/j.1469-7610.2010.02330.x.
231. Neil E. Making sense of adoption: integration and differentiation from the perspective of adopted children in middle childhood. Child Youth Serv Rev. 2012;34(2):409–16. https://doi.org/10.1016/j.childyouth.2011.11.011.
232. McDonald TP, Lieberman AA, Patridge S, Hornby H. Assessing the role of agency services in reducing adoption disruptions. Special issue: research on special needs adoption. Child Youth Serv Rev. 1991;13(5–6):425–38.
233. Spring-Duvoisin D. L'adoption internationale. Que sont-ils devenus ? Enquête réalisée auprès de 282 jeunes adultes adoptés en Suisse dans leur petite enfance (p. 190). Lausanne: Ed. Advimark; 1986.
234. Tourbin RM. Caractéristiques sociales et médico-psychologiques des candidats à l'adoption. Neuropsychiatr Enfance Adolesc. 1995;43:10–1.
235. Maywald J. Die Position des Kindes stärken. Konsequenzen der Bindungsforschung für die Arbeit mit Pflege- und Adoptivkindern. Vortrag im Rahmen des Fachkongresses "Qailitätsentwicklung", Zürich, 03.11.2000; 2000.
236. Rushton A. A scoping and scanning review of research on the adoption of children placed from public care. Clin Child Psychol Psychiatry. 2004;9(1):89–106. London, Thousand Oaks: Sage Publ.

Chapter 5
Adoption Triangle: Biological Parents–Child–Adoptive Parents

It is not enough for parents to love their children. They often love them, but they also have all kinds of other feelings. Children need more than to be loved by their parents; they need something to sustain them even when they are hated and hateful [1].

For the child, adoption always represents a filiation breakup with the biological parents as well as a filiation creation with the adoptive parents. Adoption can be seen as a lifelong process of the persons involved in this triangle, namely the biological parents, the adoptive parents, and the child [2]. Adoption is inscribed in the biographical developmental history of a child and represents the source of a recurring theme of questions and concerns, which are expressed by adoptees in different ways in each life cycle. This is especially true during important life stages and events, such as adolescence, marriage, pregnancy, birth, and finally the death of a parent [3–5].

Vignette

"When my daughter was born, the world collapsed for me", said a mother, who was adopted as a child; she was completely overwhelmed by grief, by emotions associated with the losses of her birth- and adoptive mothers. She felt unable to assume the role and function of a mother for her child. When her daughter reached the age, at which she herself came from Asia to Switzerland to be adopted, she broke down and required psychotherapeutic help. "Why wasn't I asked, if I wanted to go away?" She exclaimed and: "Never could I give up my daughter, but I am afraid she might be taken away from me".

Love is the chain whereby to bind a child to its parents—Abraham Lincoln

© The Author(s), under exclusive license to Springer Nature Switzerland AG 2023
B. Steck, *Adoption as a Lifelong Process*, https://doi.org/10.1007/978-3-031-33038-4_5

Biological Parents

While more attention was paid to biological mothers than biological fathers, and investigations considered above all the impacts on birth mother having decided to place a child for adoption, there is today a greater acknowledgement of the significance of birth fathers in the adoption process.

Biological Mothers

The release of an infant for adoption represents an essential loss for the biological mother [6]. Childbirth is associated with intense emotions, increased physical and psychic vulnerability and permanent role change [7]; motherhood is an existential transition in life. Biological mothers, who gave their child up for adoption, often present with pathological grief, i.e., their grief may persist and even increase in intensity over time.

The following factors contribute to complicated or pathological grief: Biological mothers who give their child up for adoption often experience little emotional understanding and empathic support. Since the release of a child for adoption is seen as a voluntary choice, the grief reaction over the loss of the child is not acknowledged [8, 9]. The child's birthday and the date of release represent annual memories for biological mothers, associated with sorrow and pain. Mourning the child's loss is unrealizable, because the child is alive and phantasms of finding him again someday are maintained. Birth mothers deal in their phantasms—associated with feelings of guilt, depression, and anger—with the question of how the release of the child could have been prevented [10]; finally birth mothers' constant preoccupation with their child may lead to search for him, an attempt to fill an inner void and to recover the loss of a part of selfhood, caused by the loss of the child.

If a biological mother later creates a family of her own, her unresolved loss of the child given up for adoption can lead to relationship difficulties with her additional children. These mothers may tend to overprotect their children—for fear of a recurring loss—and experience separation anxiety during their children's development.

Vignette
A married mother brings Hannah, her second daughter, for a child psychiatric consultation, recommended by the pediatrician after Hannah's hospitalization for persistent therapy-resistant headaches, affecting her severely. She informs that Hannah's infancy and early childhood were burdened by illnesses, hospitalizations, and surgical interventions, needing continuously her availability and protection.

In the child psychiatric investigation, the relationship between mother and her teenage daughter reveals an overprotective maternal attitude; Hannah—with her symptomatology—seems satisfying her mother's need to constantly taking care of her.

In the following psychiatric interviews, the mother tells, that she still regrets, 25 years later, having given up her first child for adoption—at her own mother's insistence. She thinks about her daughter not only on her birthday, but every day. She had tried to get information about her—with the help of the placement agency—but the adoptive mother refused contact. Repeatedly she was confronted with questions about the well-being of her first daughter from persons who did not know about the adoption, which she had kept secret.

A review of studies, which surveyed 600 biological mothers from 4 months to 33 years after the release of their child for adoption, concludes that biological mothers suffer from long-lasting somatic, psychic, psycho-somatic and social effects [11, 12].

Of 75 interviewed biological mothers, all except two, were interested in their child's development and well-being and wondered whether their decision had been right and what has happened to their child [13]. They expressed the desire to explain some day to their child, why no other solution than his relinquishment had been possible. They were afraid of the child's judgement and wished the child would forgive them. None of the biological mothers interviewed expressed the desire to take back their child, knowing that they had no rights over the child, neither legally nor ethically.

In general, biological mothers who place their child for adoption are younger, have lower levels of education and professional training, and a lower socioeconomic status [14]. Their children are usually unwanted, and expecting mothers were abandoned by the biological father. Often, they recognized their pregnancy too late for an abortion. Only in a few cases, biological mothers were minors when they relinquished their child.

Processing grief over the release of the child, of his loss, may last for years. Preparation of the biological mother before the birth of the child is essential to support her in her decision. Providing biological mothers with the opportunity to co-select the adoptive family is recommended. Allowing birthmothers to have contact with the child after birth and 6 months later is considered helpful for initiating a grieving process. Open adoption is generally the better solution for biological mothers [15]. Yet birthmothers in open adoption need support with regard to their own families, and also in relation to the adoptive parents and their families, as a study of birth mothers' experiences of an unplanned pregnancy, followed by open adoption, describes [16, 17].

Semi structured interviews were conducted with six Irish first mothers, who had lost a child through closed adoption. The narrative analysis showed that all mothers suffered from prolonged and complex grief reactions and their coping strategies were characterized by affect dissociation. These findings demonstrate how essential the expression of grief feelings is for the processing of emotions associated with the traumatic loss in order to promote better coping skills. The reunification with their adult child was lived by all mothers as a positive and significant experience [18].

"Who is my father?" the water jug boy asked his mother.
"I don't know," she said.
"Tomorrow I will look for my father."

"You can't find your father," she said.
But the boy said, "I have a father, I know where he lives, I will go and see him."
He went to the southeast, where they called the source "waiyu powidi".
As he approached that source, he saw a man some distance from the source.
He asked the boy, "Where are you going?"
"I am looking for my father," he said.
"Who is your father?" the man asked.
"My father lives in this source."
"You will never find your father."
"I know you are my father."
"Yes, I am your father, I came out of that source to meet you."
And he put his arm around the boy's shoulder and
took him down with him into the spring.
Saga of the Pueblo Indians (in [19])

Biological Fathers

Vignette

In the 30th week of pregnancy, a 19-year-old mother learns that she is pregnant. She has to have an emergency delivery a week later. She does not wish to have contact with her child; she wants to give him up for adoption. She is separated from the child's father, a relationship, which lasted only a few months, but has informed him of the birth of a girl and her decision to release her for adoption. However, the father wishes to keep his child. Finally, the parents agree that their daughter will live with the father and his mother, while during daytime a maternal aunt will take care of their daughter.

Biological fathers used to play a minor role during the birth of a child, as well as in the decision-making process to place a child for adoption. However, in 1995 in the legal case of "Baby Richard", the biological father gained custody of his son whose adoption was revoked by the Illinois Supreme Court. The birth father had successfully reclaimed his child, which had been released for adoption by the biological mother [20].

Parental rights are based not only on biological and genetic ties, but on a lived relationship of care, commitment, and responsibility—from the beginning of pregnancy. Legal protection and psychological support are necessary conditions, which enable biological fathers to contribute to a greater extent to the deliberations to be made in a prospective adoption situation. Biological fathers are to be involved in the decision to give their child up for adoption; they have the right to oppose the adoption [21–23].

According to Clapton and Clifton [24], most biological fathers go through a grieving process over the loss of the child. Paying more attention to biological fathers is also in the interest of the adopted child, in case adoptees later seek knowledge regarding their biological family. Biological fathers of children relinquished for adoption are reported to have a higher propensity for dissocial behavior, delinquency, and alcohol and drug dependence [25–27]. In recent years biological fathers' significance and legal rights are better acknowledged [24].

> Those who educate children well are more to be honored than they who produce them; for these only gave them life, those the art of living well—Aristotle

Adoptive Parents

> Despite all their efforts and multiple attempts at treatment, they would not conceive a child; so, they tried to get adopted. They trusted so little in the value of their own race that they first turned to a black child, for they were white. Then, for reinforcement, they called for a second child, who came from Asia. The two youngsters considered the prognosis to be relatively good, and they took over the treatment, which lasted four years and was a complete success. The reluctance of these parents was essentially due to their fear and insecurity, which the children were able to reduce by showing the greatest kindness and obvious well-being. In addition, they increased physical contacts. Thus, the mother built a more lovable image of her own womb, which gradually became habitable again. A fetus nestled inside and developed under comfortable and satisfactory conditions. Finally, it was born into a family that was perfectly prepared for its arrival. Today, the three children seem to have no more annoyance with their parents than the average 'normal' child [28].

> A primary task for the prospective adoptive parents is gradually letting go of the biological parenthood identity in preparation for taking on the identity of adoptive parent. At the heart of this process is 'working through' the deeply personal and painful experience of infertility. Although it is unlikely that infertility is ever completely resolved, it is important for the individual or couple to find a comfortable way of incorporating this painful loss into a healthy and functional sense of self ([29]: p.22).

Adoptive parents are confronted with very specific challenges for realizing their desire for a child as well as on the common life path with their adopted child [30]. Many parents of adopted children experience a high degree of worries and stress situations, associated with great psychic burden for them and their children. The results of studies on the influence of genetic risk for children and for the parent-child interactive relationship [31]. suggest that the challenge faced by adoptive parents is substantially different from the one of biological parents.

Kirk [32–34] summarizes the difficulties faced by adoptive parents as follows: Feelings of deprivation resulting from the procreation incapacity; few experience of similar family situations to serve as models; no pregnancy to provide a framework for emotional preparation; no sympathy from friends and family regarding prospective parenthood; dependence on the placement agency; adoptive parents are usually older and have often lived without children for years; the period before the legal adoption is associated with uncertainty, insecurity and fear that the child may be taken away again; lack of traditional or religious ceremonies to announce the arrival of the new family member; parents, relatives and also society show little support and understanding; revelation of the adoption status to the child is difficult for most parents: the circumstances of the birth of their child out of wedlock may contrast with the moral beliefs and the sexual and reproductive education, which the parents will later provide to their child; discussions about the biological parents are frequently perceived as threatening.

Adoption is a planned project; it carries a certain risk and requires actions; social parenthood [1] may involve a potential vulnerability [35]. The physical strangeness of their adoptive child may complicate the attachment and relationship building for the prospective adoptive parents. They experience not only a long period of uncertainty during the adoption procedures, but also the revelations of their personal lives, which may lead adoptive parents to draw rigid boundaries to the outside world. In case they encounter difficulties with their child, they may also question their adoption decision.

In a study of prospective adoptive parents [36], infertility was in 70% the reason for adopting a child, others were an experience of miscarriage, a hereditary disease or humanitarian reasons and religious beliefs. Adoptive parents have to deal with infertility, the parent-child attachment, the child's early individuation and separation process with the associated ambivalent feelings and the identity and separation process in adolescence. Of great importance and significance is the ability of adoptive parents to acknowledge and recognize differences [36].

Adoptive families who are living highly centered on their nuclear family and closed to the outside world, tend—especially when their children are small—to deny differences. Individuation and separation processes in infancy take hardly place. Contrarily during their children's adolescence, certain adoptive parents emphasize differences very strongly, for example by blaming the adoption for their family disharmony. As a consequence, family members do no longer invest their relationships with each other and engage in each other's care. Acknowledging and respecting their child's origin and recognizing the difference between biological and social parenthood by adoptive parents has an essential impact.

Study results of adopted Swiss adolescents show that—according to the adolescents' assessment—57% of the adoptive parents have a favorable attitude towards the biological parents, 31% are indifferent and 5% devaluate biological parents [37].

The following intrapsychic conflicts appear to be particularly problematic in the process of developing and building their role as adoptive parents [38]: The discovery of infertility and the subsequent decision to adopt a child; the establishment of early parent-child dialogue; the management of the individuation and separation phase in infancy; the child's emotional and cognitive confrontation and coping for understanding the fact that he is adopted; and the process of individuation and separation in the adopted child's adolescence phase.

> We must assume … that the very impressions which we have forgotten have nevertheless left the deepest traces in our psychic life and acted as determinants for our whole future development ([39]: p.175).

---

[1] Social parenthood is a permanent, intimate relation between an adult and a child that is not based on blood ties but on social-emotional ones and includes the adult's economic responsibility for the child.

Motivations

In the period around 1970, a greater openness about adoption evolved. More and more married couples, who already had one or more biological children wanted to adopt a child for humanitarian reasons. Their motivation was and is still influenced by the great misery and plight of children in countries affected by wars, poverty, and hunger. The focus is less on satisfying a desire for a child, but rather on ethical-moral or religious backgrounds, leading to the adoption of a child.

The following remarks center on motivations influenced by intrapsychic factors. The conscious motivation to adopt a child—one of the most important being sterility [40]—obscures the unconscious motivations, which are often only revealed with the arrival of the child or come to light with the child's presence. Certain authors see the adoption motivation as a reflection of an abandonment syndrome in the adoptive parents [41]. The adoptive parents' desire to provide parents and a family for an abandoned, rejected child comes from their need to be a restorative parent to their own intrapsychic child [42]. However, the integration of an adopted child into the parental relationship may lead to the emergence of repressed, unconscious psychic conflicts, sometimes to such an extent resulting in a psychic breakdown of one of the parents or in the rejection and expulsion of the child from the family.

Numerous motivations are unconscious, for example, the desire to have a substitute child for one's own deceased child. A mourning process may thus be avoided. The lost child is usually idealized. The adoptive parents' guilt feelings with regard to their dead child complicate their affective investment of the adopted child. The adoptive mother may fall into the role of an "evil stepmother". The adopted child often evokes—compared to the lost child—aggressive feelings and resentment, which an adoptive parent denies and expresses with a disproportionate concern. The overprotection of the child by a mother reflects her inner conflict with her unconscious aggressiveness.

Furthermore, the future child can be expected to be a "therapeutic or healing child", when parents hope, he will solve their personal difficulties, compensate for emotional deprivations suffered in their childhood, save the marriage, help overcome personal loneliness or fill an inner void. These adoptive parents hope to be confirmed by their child in their parental competence. They harbor (un)conscious expectations that the adopted child will make up for disappointments and dissatisfaction suffered on a professional, relational, or social level.

These idealized and unrealizable expectations contrast with the adoptive parents' feelings of insecurity in their rights towards the child. Disappointments and disillusions are unavoidable and even more serious, the greater the expectations of the child were [43]. The difficulties the child presents are then perceived by the parents as a kind of betrayal on his part. Adoptive parents express their deepest disappointment of their child who does not fulfil the unconscious contract, namely, to be an ideal child. Parents may manifest their disappointment by openly rejecting their child, perceived as a stranger, i.e., expelling him from their family, as he is suddenly felt as a foreign body. For their part, the parents have withdrawn their emotional investment of their child.

In the less severe cases of rejection, the child is often labelled as a carrier of unacceptable character traits and his behavioral disorders are associated with his origin or inheritance. In this case, the parents are relieved of any personal responsibility that could underlie the child's disturbances. They deny a conscious rejection of the child, describe him as mentally ill and in need of treatment in a psychiatric institution. These reactions of the parents show that they do not perceive any personal problem, but project onto the adopted child thoughts or feelings that they themselves are unable to bear. They often overreact to aggressive or sensual feelings of their child and tend to blame genetic and family factors as the main cause of any behavioral disorder. Even if they identify with their child's behavior, often representing their own inacceptable drive impulses, they may attribute these to the child's constitutional factors or to the so-called "bad blood" of the biological parents.

Transition from the Imaginary to the Real Child

Like all parents, adoptive parents imagine a future child. The idealized and unrealistic expectations are often followed by great disappointments [43]. The real child does not correspond to the desired child. But it is the real child who reveals his adoptive parents' phantasms about the biological parents, his origins, and his heritage. It is harder to be a parent of an adopted than of a biological child, not because of the lack of biological attachment, but because of the phantasms projected onto the adoption event [44]. Such phantasms can be troublesome if they interfere with the process of parenting. Adoptive parents may project onto the child the knowledge they have of his biographic history: the child of a neglected mother is at risk of neglecting himself, that of a brutal father is prone to outbursts of rage. Parents ought to avoid using vague information about their child's biological origin as a projection screen for their own unresolved conflicts.

The same holds true for adoptive parents and for biological parents: the more flexible their phantasms and ideas, the greater the chance for their child to benefit from an autonomous developmental space and from the emotional investment [2] by his (adoptive) parents and to be integrated into their family. In the confrontation with their child, adoptive parents frequently need to process again and again their own intrapsychic conflicts, what helps them to build an emotional bond with their adopted child in such a way that all three succeed in developing a sense of belonging, of filiation. [3]

Original, or biographical features and characteristics of the child's personality may be perceived negatively by the adoptive parents and therefore disliked and rejected. However, these shape the image that the adoptive parents have of their

---

[2] In psychoanalysis, emotional investment or cathexis is defined as the process of allocation of mental or emotional energy to a person, object, or idea.

[3] Filiation is the relationship which exists between a child and the child's parents.

adopted child and are important components of the adoptive relationship. The child's personal identity may thus be maintained in the family with negative connotations, in an unfortunate way. At the same time however, it allows the child, to maintain a continuity with his origins. Thus, the specific conditions of adoption can lead to an entanglement of certain unacceptable characteristics or ways of being of the child with unresolved problems of the family or individual family members [45].

Adoption then becomes the bearer of intrafamilial communication disorders and the revealer of intrapsychic and interpersonal conflicts. The child with his fear of again experiencing abandonment and rejection, and his anxiety to adapt to the family, offers himself to the parental needs for gratification. He may even make himself available to harmonize certain problematic family structures or to stabilize family constellations and strengthen communication structures. To a certain extent, the child serves to prevent alternative solutions to personal and family conflicts. However, he pays the high price of being unable to continue his personal development. Both adoptive parents and adoptive children need to mourn the loss of their fantasized biological child and their fantasized biological parents—only then an authentic significant relatedness may be built up [38].

Edward Franklin Albee (1928–2016) American Playwright

He and his adoptive parents seem never have fulfilled a grieving process over their losses; their relationship ended in a breakup.

Albee has learnt about his adoption at around 6 years of age. However, it was only after his adoptive mother's death in 1989 that he learnt that his biological father had abandoned his mother Louise Harvey, who gave her son Edward up for adoption 2 weeks after his birth. Reed and Frances Albee became his foster parents when he was only 18 days old; they officially adopted him in 1929 and changed his name to Edward Franklin Albee III. His adoptive mother is described as emotionally cold and authoritarian, his adoptive father as distant and unengaged in his son's development. As a young adult, Albee left his home, and the relationship with his adoptive parents was interrupted for almost 20 years.

Albee's immensely creativity led to an outstanding literary oeuvre and illustrates what Moro [46] describes as the destiny of abandoned children; they are faced with a breakup of family ties and are confronted with an extremely threatening event. They preserve memories of these lived experiences in the form of interactive phantasms between themselves and their surroundings. The abandoned child develops in an environment that shares the child's conviction of radical strangeness. Their phantasmatic productions often demonstrate an oscillation between two poles: an extreme psychic vulnerability or the development of an extraordinarily creative potential, the latter being the case for Albee.

Albee's play *Who's Afraid of Virginia Woolf* (1962) represents an impressive example of parental phantasms: the "son" of the two protagonists George and Martha reveals himself as a phantasm. In these phantasms the "son" wonders whether he might have been adopted. For Martha and George fulfilling the parental role is the most noble task of all humanity's endeavors, their sterility being their mutual failure, a narcissistic injury, a tragedy. They create an imaginary idealized child who has all the most wished for qualities, some of which even differed: George giving the baby blue eyes and Martha green eyes like her father's.

Edward Franklin obviously did not represent this idealized child for his adoptive parents Reed and Frances Albee; he was not able to assume the task of healing his adoptive parents' narcissistic wounds due to their infertility. In the play Albee shows the game of Martha and George around their fictional son and demonstrates their defensive strategy of intellectualization against their feelings of narcissistic rage, sadness, and despair. They avoid facing, sharing, and engaging in a mourning process in order to work through their own loss of a biological child.

We are born, so to speak, provisionally, it doesn't matter where; it is only gradually that we compose within ourselves our true place of origin so that we may be born there retrospectively and each day more definitely. Rainer Maria Rilke.

The Adopted Child

Pediatricians pledge for children who are placed for adoption a comprehensive health evaluation to assess their medical condition and development stage in order to provide the necessary long-term care [47].

Winnicott [48] considered it necessary for adoptive parents to be knowledgeable about child development: "Adoptive parents have a need to be aware of what child development is about, much more so than parents who are caring for their own children. With their own children they can allow intuition full sway except when … a child is showing symptoms of illness. Adopted children need to be thought about, even when they are healthy" (p: 129).

Adoptive parents bear the consequences of a child's negative experiences, e.g., his lived emotional deprivation in his early childhood development. They are expected to cope with the disadvantages their child presents, for which they are not responsible. The better-informed adoptive parents are of the personal history of their future child, the more likely they can prepare for future difficulties and anticipate potential challenges.

An individual is not capable to build his history on his own, because he is always rooted in a family history that precedes him and where he occupies a place as a subject. The fundaments in this psychic transmission process are transferred to him by the preceding generations. The transgenerational inheritance, which consists of psychic experiences—phantasms, images, identifications—creates a mythical narrative from which each individual draws the necessary elements to form his personal family history. Infants need for their construction a history, not only a biological or genetic history, but a relational history. The infant is inscribed in the midst of his dual, maternal, and paternal filiation; this allows him to enter here and now into the current family group, but thereby also to be inscribed in the family history [49].

Development in Adolescence

Normal intrapsychic development in adolescence involves a mourning process over the loss of childhood and the transformation of self- and object representations (the significant primary relational representations). In accordance with his development, the adolescent has to grieve his primary love relationships, and giving up his familiar way of being, experiencing, and functioning in childhood. Simultaneously adolescents invest increasingly their self in a narcissistic retreat, a developmental period often accompanied by depressive moods and insecure self-perception.

In stressful situations around puberty, children or adolescents who have lived adversities in infancy or childhood, react with the emotional intensity they felt at the time of the traumatic experience, as if the traumatic event would repeat itself. They are not able to understand what is happening to them, as the biographical reference is unconscious. Long-lasting traumatic situations with additional injuries or losses lead to persistent pathological grief or chronic depression, which are accompanied by feelings of inner emptiness, meaninglessness, and lifelessness.

Puberty is closely associated with amplification of intensive drive impulses, needs, and feelings, as well as with the reactivation of infantile conflicts. This process may lead to confrontation with narcissistic, libidinal, [4] and aggressive impulses. Adopted adolescents may be overwhelmed by strong emotions of anger, sadness, and pain, they did live in critical life events in their early childhood. These past experiences cannot be remembered by conscious awareness and therefore cannot be expressed in words. The genital sexual maturation at the beginning of adolescence changes the relationship of the young person with his own body, a process that is often particularly conflictual for adolescent adoptees. The body represents—for adoptees—the only relatedness with their biological parents and is often ambivalently invested. Taking responsibility for one's body is not obvious. This transition period may be associated with numerous conflicts, sometimes leading to irresponsible behaviors of adolescents with respect to their own body. These are auto-aggressive behavior manifested by repetitive accidents, by substance abuse (alcohol, nicotine, drugs), by neglecting bodily care, or by promiscuity.

The autonomy aspirations of the adolescent adoptee are sometimes perceived by adoptive parents and adopted child as "rejection" or "abandonment" and the process of individuation and separation may be experienced as something destructive, remembering earlier relational disruptions. Both adoptive parents and adopted child bear in mind mostly unconscious ideas of not being able to suffer any further losses in life. Children remain then attached to their parents, incapable to leave the family, nor to accomplish a grieving process, necessary to engage into a love relationship of their own.

The failure of the parents to fulfill a mourning process, respectively their denial of grieving over experienced critical life events or suffered losses in their personal

---

[4] Libido, a Latin term meaning desire, want, amorous desire, is defined as the instinctual sexual energy underlying all mental activity.

history, contributes to their children's inability to grief and therefore to establish significant love relationships outside their family [50].

Individuation, detachment, and separation processes are then inhibited by conflicts of dependency, feelings of loyalty and guilt. In the absence of a stable incest taboo (the incest barrier has no biological basis), adoptive parents and adopted adolescents and youth [5] are faced with the challenge of maintaining sexual boundaries. The development of the adolescent adoptee's sexuality ought to evolve without interfering prejudices and phantasms regarding illegitimacy or inherited promiscuity. The adopted adolescent's oedipal [6] exploration, resolution and integration represent a complex process and may complicate the engagement of (heterosexual) relationships outside the family.

For the five children in the family, there are five different families [51]

Siblings

Biological Children

Parents considering adoption are worried about the impact that the adoption of a child might have on their biological children. In this regard, few studies investigated the stressful situation for biological children in adoptive families [52–56]. Biological children's reactions during the latency period to a sibling to be adopted or adopted in the past year, were mainly insecurity and fear, e.g., of being abandoned by their parents. In adolescence, the main reaction might be resistance to adoption, often accompanied by moral indignation and anger directed at the adopted child's birth mother. In young adulthood, characterized by desires for independence, the most common responses were either distancing or identification with the parental role. Siblings were mainly interested in the biological mother of the child to be adopted; questions concerning the biological father were not asked. Sibling rivalry was observed in some children but did not represent a major problem. It is essential to maintain communication between biological children and their parents, not only during the adoption process, but for a long time afterwards [57].

Biological children of a family sometimes sense or anticipate their parents' unconscious motivations (such as the unconscious desire to avoid dealing with their own losses by adopting a child) and oppose—out of fear—the adoption project, or

---

[5] The United Nations understands adolescents to include persons aged 10–19 years and youth as those between 15–24 years.

[6] Oedipus complex: the positive libidinal feelings of a child toward the parent of the opposite sex and hostile or jealous feelings toward the parent of the same sex; the Oedipus complex is reactivated in adolescence and needs to be resolved and integrated.

support it, hoping that their parents unfulfilled intrapsychic expectations might be realized.

When adding an adoptive child to children already living in the family (birth, adopted, or foster), it is important to maintain the seniority and sequence of siblings. Therefore, it is favorable to adopt a child who is younger than the children living in the family. The older siblings usually find it easier to accept a younger child and to show understanding for his needs for attention and care. The younger child will have enough time to integrate into the family and catch up on developmental steps without having to compete with siblings living in the family, especially siblings of the same age who may be more advanced in their development. An age gap of at least 3 years between the children is recommended. During the first intensive care period, which serves to build up an affective relationship between adoptive child and parents, no other children ought to be admitted into the family [58]. Simultaneously meeting the needs of all the children living in the family, places high demands on adoptive parents. The participation of all family members in the decision-making process to adopt a child and the preparation for his admission are important prerequisites for ensuring that the children already living in the family contribute to the integration of the adopted child.

Vignette
Julien, 13 years old, was adopted from an Asian country at the age of 5 years. His adoptive parents have adopted four other children, including two with disabilities, in the last 8 years and wish to adopt a sixth, disabled child.

According to the information of his adoptive parents, Julien presents severe behavioral problems, refuses to work for school and shows a selective mutism at home. The child psychiatric investigation concludes that Julian suffers from a pronounced depressive state.

Comment
With his drawing (Fig. 5.1) of a bird's nest with three baby birds fed by their parents, Julien expresses his need and desire for a greater presence and availability of his adoptive parents, a wish he does not dare to tell his adoptive parents, neither, out of loyalty to his parents, to the child psychiatrist.

Children adopted as infants in a family with biological children were twice as likely to have a psychiatric or behavioral problem in adolescence compared to children raised in adoptive families without biological children [59]. Whereas the presence of other adopted children acted as a slight protective factor, the presence of birth children appeared to double the risk of problem behavior. However, the results are controversial. The presence of biological children in the adoptive family does not seem to have a favorable or unfavorable effect on the adoption relationship [60, 61]. The breakup rates of the adoption relationship were lower in some studies and higher in others; when adoptive parents already had biological children the breakdown was more frequent.

Fig. 5.1 Julien, 13-year-old, a bird family

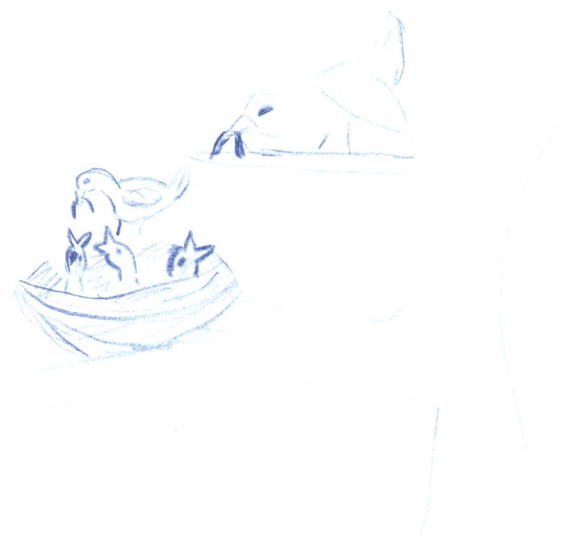

Adoption of Siblings

The joint reception of siblings creates great demands on future adoptive parents. Often there is a strong mutual dependency among the siblings, whose relation to each other is usually characterized by the adversities they have lived together. The roles and functions of the individual children are in most cases already well-established; the older sibling is usually parentified, i.e., he takes over tasks or responsibilities trying to replace the missing adult caregivers, respectively the parents. Children may therefore find it more difficult to open up to a new family situation and to engage in new relationships. Sibling rivalries may also intensify due to the individual child's efforts to win the love and affection of the adoptive parents.

Conversely, sibling pairs or groups that are torn apart and placed separately, experience additional losses and separations, what may interfere with their formation of new emotional attachments in the adoptive family; for this reason, the adoption of sibling groups is also endorsed [62, 63]. Children placed without their siblings showed a higher risk of psychosocial adjustment difficulties [62]. Sibling placements are usually discouraged when there are already biological children living in the family, as the likely formation of two competing sibling groups may impose insurmountable stressful strains.

Clinical experience shows that certain adoptive parents succeed in integrating several adopted children or a sibling group in addition to biological children into their family, and in meeting at the same time the individual developmental needs of the biological and adopted children, despite highly stressful conflicts. It is the adoption agencies' responsibility to assure the wellbeing of already adopted children, to limit the number of children to be adopted and especially of children with special needs.

The members of the adoption triangle (adoptive parents, biological parents, adopted children) ought to be mutually aware of their conscious and unconscious relationships and of their lived significant experiences, in reality as well as in fantasy, in the past and in the present.

References

1. Winnicott DW. The maturational processes and the facilitating environment. International Universities Press. New York; 1965.
2. Sorosky AD, Baran A, Pannor R. The adoption triangle. Garden City, New York: Anchor Books, Anchor Press; 1984.
3. Geller M. Biographien erwachsener Adoptierter. Westarp Wissenschaften; 1992.
4. Lifton BJ. Lost and found: the adoption experience. New York: Dial Press; 1979.
5. Rowal R, Schilling MK. Adoption through the eyes of adults adoptees. Am J Orthopsychiatry. 1985;55(3):354–62.
6. Howe D. The loss of a baby. Midwife Health Visitor Community Nurse. 1990;26:25–6.
7. Simkin P. The experience of maternity in a woman's life. J Obstret Gynecol Neonatal Nurs. 1996;26:247–52.
8. Davis CE. Separation loss in relinquishing birth mothers. Int J Psychiatr Nurs Res. 1994;1(2):63–70.
9. Lauderdale JL, Boyle JS. Infant relinquishment through adoption. Image J Nurs Sch. 1994;26:213–7.
10. Lancette J, McClure BA. Birth mothers: grieving the loss of a dream. J Mental Health Services. 1992;14:84–96.
11. Askren HA, Bloom KC. Postadoptive reactions of the relinquishing mother: a review. JOGNN Rev. 1999;28(4):395–400.
12. Blanton TL, Deschner J. Biological mother's grief: the postadoptive experience in open versus confidential adoption. Child Welfare League of America. 1990;75:525–35.
13. Swientek C. Wer sagt mir, wessen Kind ich bin? Von der Adoption Betroffene auf der Suche. Freiburg/Basel/Wien: Herder; 1993.
14. Klein-Allermann E. Adoptierte Kinder und ihre Eltern: Familien eigener Art. In: Hofer M, editor. Klein-Allermann E, Noack P: Familienbeziehungen. Göttingen: Hogrefe; 1992. p. 250–65.
15. Cushman LF, Kalmuss D, Namerow PB. Placing an infant for adoption. The experience of young birthmothers. Soc Work. 1993;38(3):264–72.
16. Clutter LB. Open adoption placement by birth mothers in their twenties Copyright © 2017. Wolters Kluwer Health, Inc; 2017.
17. Coleman PK, Garratt D. From birth mothers to first mothers: toward a compassionate understanding of the life-long act of adoption placement. Issues Law Med. 2016;31(2):139–63.
18. McNamara D, Egan J, McNeela P. 'My scar is called adoption': the lived experiences of Irish mothers who have lost a child through closed adoption. Adopt Foster. 2021;45(2):138–54.
19. Lifton B. Twice born. New York: McGry-Hill, dt. 1981, Stuttgart: Klett-Cotta 1975.
20. Kermani EJ, Weiss BA. Biological parents regaining their rights: a psycholegal analysis of a new era in custody disputes. Bull Am Acad Psychiatry Law. 1995;23:261–7.
21. Menard BJ. A birth father and adoption in the perinatal setting. Soc Work Health Care. 1997;24(3/4):153–63.

22. Tomlinson PS, Rothenberg MA, Carver LD. Behavior interaction of fathers with infants and mothers in the immediate postpartum period. J Nurse-Midwifery. 1991;36(4):232–9.
23. Westreich R, Spector-Dunsky L, Klein M, Papgeorgiou A, Kramer M, Gelfand M. The influence of birth setting on the father's behavior towards his partner and infant. Birth. 1991;18(4):198–202.
24. Clapton G, Clifton J. The birth fathers of adopted children: differences and continuities over a 30-year period. Adopt Foster. 2016;40(2):153–66.
25. Cadoret RJ, Troughton E, Bagford J, Woodworth G. Genetic and environmental factors in adoptee antisocial personality. Eur Arch Psychiatry Neurol Sci. 1990;239:231–40.
26. Cadoret RJ, Yates WR, Troughton E, Woodworth G, Stewart MA. Adoption study demonstrating two genetic pathways to drug abuse. Arch Gen Psychiatry. 1995;52(1):42–52. https://doi.org/10.1001/archpsyc.1995.03950130042005.
27. Peters BR, Atkins MS, Kay MKM. Adopted Children's behavior problems: a review of five explanatory models. Clin Psychol Rev. 1999;19(3):297–328.
28. Van den Brouck J. Handbuch für Kinder mit schwierigen Eltern. Stuttgart: Klett-Cotta; 1981.
29. Brodzinsky AB. Surrendering an infant for adoption: the birth mother experience. In: Brodzinsky DM, Schechter M, editors. The psychology of adoption. New York and Oxford: Oxford University Press; 1990. p. 235.
30. Derdeyn AP, Graves ChL. Clinicl vicissitudes of adoption. Child and Adolescent Psychiatric Clinics of North America. 1998;7(2):373–88.
31. Plomin R, Fulker DW, Corley R, DeFries JC. Nature, nurture and cognitive development 1 to 16 years: A parentoffspring adoption study. Psychological Science. 1997;8(6):442–7.
32. Kirk HD. Shared fate: a theory of adoption ans mental health. London, New York: Free Press of Glencoe; 1964.
33. Kirk HD, Ionasson K, Fish AD. Are adopted children especially vulnerable to stress. Arch Gen Psychiatry. 1966;14:291–8.
34. Kirk HD. Adoptive kinship: a modern institution in need of reforms. Toronto: Butterworth; 1981.
35. Schleiffer R. Adoption: psychiatrisches Risiko und/oder protektiver Faktor? Prax Kinderpsychol Kinderpsychiat. 1997;46:645–59.
36. Kirschner D. The adopted child syndrome: considerations for psychotherapy. Psychotherapy on Private Practice. 1990;8(3):93–100.
37. Keller-Thoma P. Adoption aus der Sicht des Adoptiv"kindes". Zürich: Schweiz. Gemeinnütziger Frauenverein/Adoptivkinder-Vermittlung; 1987.
38. Brinich PM. Adoption from the inside out: a psychoanalytic perspective. In: Brodinsky MD, Schechter MD, editors. The psychology of adoption. New York: Oxford Press; 1990. p. 42–61.
39. Freud S. Psychopathology of everyday life. New York, NY, USA: Macmillan; 1915.
40. Cottereau MI. Les adoptants à travers l'examen psychologique préliminaire de l'adoption. Ann Méd Psych. 1977;135(1):S. 624-644.
41. Hayez JY. Un jour, l'adoption. Paris: Fleurus; 1988.
42. Landerholm EK. The experience of abandonment and adoption, as a child and as a parent, in a psychological motivational perspective. Int Forum Psychoanal. 2001;10:12–25.
43. Cramer B. L'adoption vécue. Seuil: J Adler; 1988. p. S. 123-131.
44. Lévy-Soussan P. La parentalité adoptive: problèmes spécifiques ou universels ? J Pédiatr Puériculture. 2001;14:201–4.
45. Huth W. Psychoanalytische Reflexion und therapeutische Verfahren in Adoption und Familiendynamik. Pädagogik, Band 11 1982.
46. Moro MR. L'enfant exposé. Grenoble, Editions La Pensee sauvage, 1989.
47. Jones VF, Schulte EE. AAP COUNCIL ON FOSTER CARE, ADOPTION, AND KINSHIP CARE. Comprehensive Health Evaluation of the Newly Adopted Child. Pediatrics. 2019;143(5):e20190657.
48. Winnicott DW. The child and the family. London: Tavistock Publ; 1957. p. 129.
49. Golse B. In la Parentalité, défi pour le troisième millénaire sous la direction de L. Solis-Ponton. Paris: PUF, le fil rouge; 2002.

50. Kernberg OF. Barrier to falling and remaining in love. J Am Psychoanal Assoc. 1974;4:743–68.
51. Winnicott DW. Home is where we start from. New York London: WW Norton & Company; 1986.
52. Alstein H, Simon RJ, editors. Intercountry adoption: a multinational perspective. New York: Praeger; 1991.
53. Jacobs TJ. On having an adopted sibling: some psychoanalytic observations. Int Rev Psychoanal. 1988;15:25–35.
54. Markovitch S, Cesaroni L, Roberts W, Swanson C. Romanian adoption: parents' dreams, nightmares, and realities. Child Welfare. 1995;74:993–1016.
55. Ward M, Lewko JH. Problems experienced by adolescents already in families that adopt older children. Adolescence. 1988;23:221–8.
56. Westhues A, Cohen JS. Intercountry adoption in Canada. Final report. Ottawa: Division of Human Resources and Development, Canada 1994.
57. Phillips NK. Adoption of a sibling: reactions of biological children at different stages of development. Am J Orthopsychiatry. 1999;69(1):122–6.
58. Nienstedt M, Westermam A. Psychologische Beträge zur Sozialisation von Kindern in Ersatzfamilien. Münster: Votum; 1989.
59. Howe D. Parent reported problems in 211 adopted children: some risk and protective factorss. J Child Psychol Psychiatr. 1997;38(4):401–12.
60. Festinger T. Necessary risk: a study of adoptions and disruptive adoptive placements. Washington, DC: Child Welfare League of America; 1986.
61. Festinger T. Adoption disruption: rates and correlates. In: Brodzinsky DM, Schechter MD, editors. The psychology of adoption. New York: Oxford Press; 1990. p. 201–18.
62. Rushton A, Dance C, Quinton D, Mayes D. Siblings in late permanent placement. London: British Agencies for Adoption and Fostering; 2001.
63. Timberlake EM, Hamlin ERII. The siblings group: a neglected dimension of placement. Child Welfare. 1982;61:545–52.

Chapter 6
Filiation Breakup

"I desire so much, one day in the future,
    to see you with my own eyes,
    caress your faces with my hands,
    to become your child, just for a moment.
    But to be the child of a love relationship and not only of a sensual one.
    I wish so much to know your faces,
    to know at last, to no longer be in doubt,
    to stop living with ghosts.
    I want to understand, I want to know why.
    I want the truth, your truth and not the one of my record.
    Have you ever loved me?
    Will I one day be allowed no longer to be hurt?
    To no longer suffer when I think of you .
    Will you not stop persecuting me?
    I want this wound to be closed one day,
    over the years it has become burning, oversensitive.
    A tensioned rope, ready to tear at any moment.
    I know it's there, even when I'm not thinking about it.
    My wound feeds on my ignorance and on the time that passes.
    I don't want to suffer any more because of you,
    but I know that my path to the truth is sown with suffering.
    Unknown, what are you preparing for me?"
    young woman.

© The Author(s), under exclusive license to Springer Nature
Switzerland AG 2023
B. Steck, *Adoption as a Lifelong Process*,
https://doi.org/10.1007/978-3-031-33038-4_6

Psychic Trauma

Introduction

The significance of psychic trauma in the emergence of diseases has been anchored since ancient times in human awareness, the epic poems Iliad and Odyssey of the ancient Greek poet Homer bear witness to this time. The child psychiatrists Donovan and McIntyre [1] were the first to characterize children's traumatology as a distinct field of research, in describing the psychic injuries of children. The occurrence of post-traumatic disorders in children, as a result of severe psychic distress, was recognized only in the nineties; school children and even preschoolers may suffer from post-traumatic stress reactions, similar to those of adults and persisting for many months, even years [2].

Major research questions today address how adverse experiences or somatic illnesses affect mental health and how mental illnesses lead to physical consequences.

Psychic trauma (in Greek the word τραύμα means injury, wound), which unlike organic trauma leads to no externally recognizable lesions, nevertheless leaves wounds, which heal poorly, whose scars are often "visible" for the rest of a person's life and which suddenly, seemingly unexpectedly, begin to "bleed" again.[1] These wounds are engraved as memory traces in the individual's personal history, even if they are lost in his consciousness [4].

Psychic trauma is "an event in the subject's life, defined by its intensity, by the subject's incapacity to respond adequately to it and by the upheaval and long-lasting effects that it brings about in the mental organization" ([5] p. 465).

Traumatic experience is defined as a vital discrepancy between threatening situational factors and individual coping capacities, accompanied by feelings of helplessness, abandonment, and defenselessness, resulting in a permanent shock of self-understanding and comprehension of the world [6].

Difference Between Extra- and Intrafamilial Trauma

Extrafamilial trauma are adversities due to human aggression, atrocities such as war, terrorism, displacement, disasters caused by human error in technical matters, for example, aircraft accidents and industrial disasters, and natural disasters such as earthquakes, floods, hurricane, or fire.

---

[1] What is revealed from the hidden (ληθη, laethae in Greek), the Greeks called ἀλήθεια, a-laetheia, meaning truth. For Parmenides, the ancient Greek philosopher, truth is well rounded, ἀλήθεια ευκυκλέος, alaetheia eukukleos, a circle without beginning or end, just like the psychic trauma repeats itself; neither its origin is seen, nor its end is predictable [3].

Trauma within the family framework includes abuse, neglect and deprivation, the loss of loved ones through abandon, separation, death or suicide, multiple placements, parental chronic somatic or mental illness, accidents, operations, serious injury, or life-threatening or chronic illness, violence, witnessing cruel acts, and cultural uprooting.[2]

According to the data of the Child Maltreatment 2020 report of the US National Child Abuse and Neglect Data System,[3] 76.1% of victims are neglected, 16.5% are physically abused, 9.4% are sexually abused, and 0.2% are sex trafficked. The majority of victims (76.1%) suffered neglect defined as "a type of maltreatment that refers to the failure by the caregiver to provide needed, age-appropriate care although financially able to do so or offered financial or other means to do so" (http://www.acf.hhs.gov/programs/cb/research-data-technology/statistics-research/child-maltreatment).

Developmental Trauma Disorder (DTD)

"The traumatic stress field has adopted the term 'complex trauma' to describe the experience of multiple and/or chronic and prolonged, developmentally adverse traumatic events, most often of an interpersonal nature (e.g., sexual, or physical abuse, war, community violence) and of early-life onset. These exposures often occur within the child's caregiving system and include physical, emotional, and educational neglect and child maltreatment beginning in early childhood" ([7] p. 227). Developmental trauma disorder is the result of multiple interpersonal traumatic experiences (abandonment, betrayal, physical or sexual assaults, or witnessing domestic violence) with long lasting consequences in different functioning areas.

Children suffer intense affects such as rage, betrayal, fear, resignation, defeat, and shame and present with multiple somatic problems. They use defense mechanisms against recurrent unbearable emotions, trying to control or avoid—i.e., flight—imaginary, anticipated or potential threats. Children tend to reenact their traumatic lived events with aggressive or sexual acting out—i.e., fight—against other children, as perpetrators, or present with frozen watchfulness.[4] Flight or fight reactions are active defense responses, using the motor system, while freezing causes physical immobility [8]. Children's cognition is affected by reminders or flashbacks[5]; therefore, they may be confused, dissociated, and disoriented when

---

[2] Cultural uprooting represents social mutation, discontinuity from ancestry, and loss of family identification references.

[3] Child Abuse and Neglect is defined as "any recent act or failure to act on the part of a parent or caretaker which results in death, serious physical or emotional harm, sexual abuse or exploitation; or an act or failure to act, which presents an imminent risk of serious harm."

[4] The state of a child who is unresponsive to its surroundings but is clearly aware of them.

[5] Flashbacks, a form of dissociative state, are defined as involuntary, vivid images that occur in the waking state; these memories may be felt as if the traumatic experience would take place at the present moment.

faced with stressful stimuli. They easily misinterpret events as a return of the trauma and their helplessness; subsequently, they are constantly on guard, frightened, and overreactive. Finally, the child's expectation that the trauma will return, permeates his relationships, and leads to negative self-attributions, loss of trust in caretakers, i.e., of his belief that someone will care and protect him. Children organize their relationships with the assumption to reexperience abandonment or victimization and, at the same time, with efforts to prevent such situations. These beliefs are expressed in behaviors of excessive clinging, compliance, oppositional defiance, and distrust; children may be preoccupied with thoughts of retribution and revenge.

Research findings show that DTD results from an addition of interpersonal traumatization and disruption of primary attachment, leading to children's biological, somatic, emotional, cognitive, attentional, behavioral, and relational dysregulation, thus impeding crucial steps for their psychosocial development, such as emotion- and self-regulation, autonomy- and learning processes and identity formation [9–11]. Efforts for effective diagnostic and treatment are imperative for the prevention of the severe consequences these children may suffer.

Developmental Trauma Disorder (DTD) represents consensus among leaders within the National Child Traumatic Stress Network and other leading researchers in the area of Developmental Psychopathology.[6] DTD overlaps partly with PTSD.

Developmental Trauma Disorder (DTD)

A. Exposure.
- Multiple or chronic exposure to one or more forms of developmentally adverse interpersonal trauma (e.g., abandonment, betrayal, physical assaults, sexual assaults, threats to bodily integrity, coercive practices, emotional abuse, witnessing violence and death).
- Subjective experience (e.g., rage, betrayal, fear, resignation, defeat, shame).
B. Triggered pattern of repeated dysregulation in response to trauma cues.
   Dysregulation (high or low) in presence of cues. Changes persist and do not return to baseline, not reduced in intensity by conscious awareness.
- Affective.
- Somatic (e.g., physiological, motoric, medical).
- Behavioral (e.g., re-enactment, cutting).
- Cognitive (e.g., thinking that it is happening again, confusion, dissociation, depersonalization
- Relational (e.g., clinging, oppositional, distrustful, compliant).
- Self-attribution (e.g., self-hate, blame).
C. Persistently Altered Attributions and Expectancies.
- Negative self-attribution.

---

[6]See [12].

- Distrust of protective caretaker.
- Loss of expectancy of protection by others.
- Loss of trust in social agencies to protect.
- Lack of recourse to social justice/retribution.
- Inevitability of future victimization.
D. Functional Impairment.
  - Educational.
  - Familial.
  - Peer.
  - Legal.
  - Vocational.

Developmental trauma results from prolonged and cumulative interpersonal trauma during sensitive periods of infant and child development and disrupts the development of secure attachments to caregivers, as well as of social cognition, physiological and behavioral regulation; it also alters assumptions and beliefs about one's vulnerability to danger in the world. Developmental trauma disorders are often characterized by poor self-identity development, high interpersonal sensitivity, and constant relationship problems with adults, primary caregivers, and peers. The traumatic stress adaptation can contribute to emotional numbing, low frustration tolerance, emotional outbursts, and an incapacity to adjust behavior to changes or demands. The extreme fear- and anxiety tendency disrupts self-awareness, information processing, interpersonal communication, and mastery of age-appropriate developmental competencies leading to learning problems, social and behavioral difficulties [13].

Concepts of Trauma

The notion of trauma corresponds to a conceptual bridge between an event and its impact. Accordingly, it attempts to connect the external reality, the life events, with their consequences on the inner world of an individual, thus establishing a relationship between the inner and outer reality experience of a subject.

The following questions do not find definitive answers due to the complexity of the human nature, such as the individual genetic makeup, the manifold interconnectedness with the environment in which the subject grows up: When does a trauma occur, which external, which internal factors are crucial for triggering it? What are the short-term and long-term effects of traumatic events? What do children experience and how do they try to deal with psychic trauma? Why are certain children, who have been exposed to severe psychic stress for many years, psychically less affected than other children who are traumatized by less severe adverse experiences?

Janet [14], a contemporary of Freud, described the connection between symptoms and unprocessed memories of traumatic experiences already in 1889; he wrote that "…certain events would leave indelible and distressing memories—memories to which the sufferer was continually returning, and by which he was tormented by day and night "(p. 589).

Freud [15–17]) dealt throughout his life with the question whether the perceived reality, i.e., the external influences, or the phantasmatic configuration and the internal processing of the external influences were primarily responsible for the psychic consequences of a traumatic experience. Freud concluded that all memories were above all phantasmatic constructions. Not the trauma itself, but its subsequent processing, the retranscription[7] of memory, does represent the pathogenic factor, especially if early childhood traumatic experiences remain unassimilated and unmodified in the present. "The traumas of childhood operate in a deferred fashion as though they were fresh experiences; but they do so unconsciously." ([21] (1896): pp. 166–167). For Freud the traumatic situation is characterized by the encounter of external and internal danger, of a threat in the reality and the internal drive impulses, resulting in the subject's feelings to be helplessly exposed.

For some authors, however, the direct impact of traumatic experiences on the inner psychic world with its phantasms and libidinal investment should not be underestimated [22].

Winnicott [23] considers any event, which interrupts the subjects experience of continuity, as a psychic trauma. "Trauma means the breaking of the continuity of the line of an individual's existence. It is only on a continuity of existing that the sense of self, of feeling real, and of being, can eventually be established as a feature of the individual personality" ([24]: p. 22).

For Shengold [25], overwhelming psychic trauma is synonymous with soul murder.

Nathan [26] considers the unthinkable and unspeakable loss of one's cultural environment as a psychic trauma since each individual relies on his cultural environment to decipher reality. He sees the identity of a subject as a kind of memory, a memory that gives the subject a temporal continuity and a spatial unity.

Khan [27] developed the concept of cumulative trauma, i.e., multiple, or repetitive traumatic events. He considered the lack of the motherly shield function as traumatic and hypothesized a kind of short circuit between psyche and soma. What cannot be integrated psychically is imprinted in the body and manifests itself in psychosomatic phenomena, which are always recuring. It is as if the body "remembers"; a child inscribes into his body what is psychically not endurable, not bearable to feel.

For Barrois [28], psychic trauma is always subject to secrecy and absolute senselessness, because it is based on the experience of total non-communicability, even if taking place in a relationship. It is the result of an emotional overflow which cannot be mastered by the individual psyche, as a panic anxiety, generated by a given situation, or as the creation of a dead-living enclave, a "psychic crypt". An individual

---

[7] Retranscription of memory" according to Modell [18] or deferred action is a concept that refers to Freud's original term Nachträglichkeit [19], conceived as early as 1895 in the Project for a Scientific Psychology [20].

has no interest to repeat emotionally overwhelming experiences. He splits such experiences from conscious awareness, "hiding" them in form of crypts, by means of encapsulation. Whenever the loss of a loved person is denied, the "abandoned" individuum may incorporate the lost loved one and turn into a crypt carrier [29].

Non-integrated, unprocessed traumatic experiences of a parent are transferred to the child by unconscious, non-verbal communication [30]. Through identification with the lived experiences by persons of the previous generation, a child assumes unconsciously intrapsychic, transgenerational conflict configurations [31]. The parents' past may be transmitted to the child's present. For some individuals there seems to be no processing of psychic trauma: The nightmare of the past is then lived in the present and is the unique perspective of the future.

Vignette

A young woman, adopted in infancy, is pregnant and desires a girl. After giving birth to a boy, she is very disappointed and neglects her infant, whose condition deteriorates. She refuses to seek help and wants to let nature deciding the fate of her son.

Comment

In a double identification, on the one hand with the aggressor, i.e., with her own biological mother, who did not care for her as an infant, she exposes her child, as her own mother had done, to an uncertain fate. On the other hand—in the identification with the victim—she lets her child suffer her own fate; she herself was in a very poor nutritional state when she arrived for adoption.

Neurobiological Aspects

Even if children have great adaptive capacities, traumatic experiences can change the psychological and biological balance of a child in such a way that he is no more able to pursue his developmental steps or certainly no longer with pleasure. The basic neuroanatomical structure of the brain is determined by genetic factors. During the first stages of development, patterns of experience influence the specific shape of neuronal circuits and connection networks, following the principle of "use it or lose it". Sensory signals are translated into neurochemical and cellular processes that affect brain structure and function [32]. Neuronal connectivity and functions are of extraordinary plasticity at all levels of brain organization. Neurobiological changes take place throughout life in a complex interplay with surrounding forces and continuously shape an individual's behavior, knowledge, and skills. Brain and environment communicate interactively and influence each other. Mental processes are ultimately all biologically based and changes in mental processes are associated with corresponding organic modifications [33].

The plasticity of the brain holds a considerable adaptability but makes infants and young children particularly susceptible to long-term effects because of disruptive influences. Perception and awareness of bodily sensations and emotions are fundamental building blocks in the development of self-awareness and self-image, as well as of cognitive processes and creativity. These basic patterns of experience are built up in the earliest relationships with primary caregivers [34]. Any disruption in the early adjustment of primary caregivers to the infant's needs or any event that interrupts the continuity of the infant's experience and development may act as a traumtogenic factor [35].

Early childhood traumatic experiences affect the normal development of the cerebral cortex and the limbic system and lead to long-term changes in multiple neurotransmitter systems [7, 32, 36–39].

"The thalamus, amygdala, hippocampus, and prefrontal cortex are all involved in the stepwise integration and interpretation of incoming sensory information. This integration can be disrupted by high levels of arousal: moderate to high activation of the amygdala enhances the long-term potentiation of declarative memory, mediated by the hippocampus, while extreme arousal disrupts hippocampal functioning, leaving the memories to be stored as affective states or in sensory-motor modalities, as somatic sensations, and visual images" ([7]: p. 294) (Fig. 6.1).

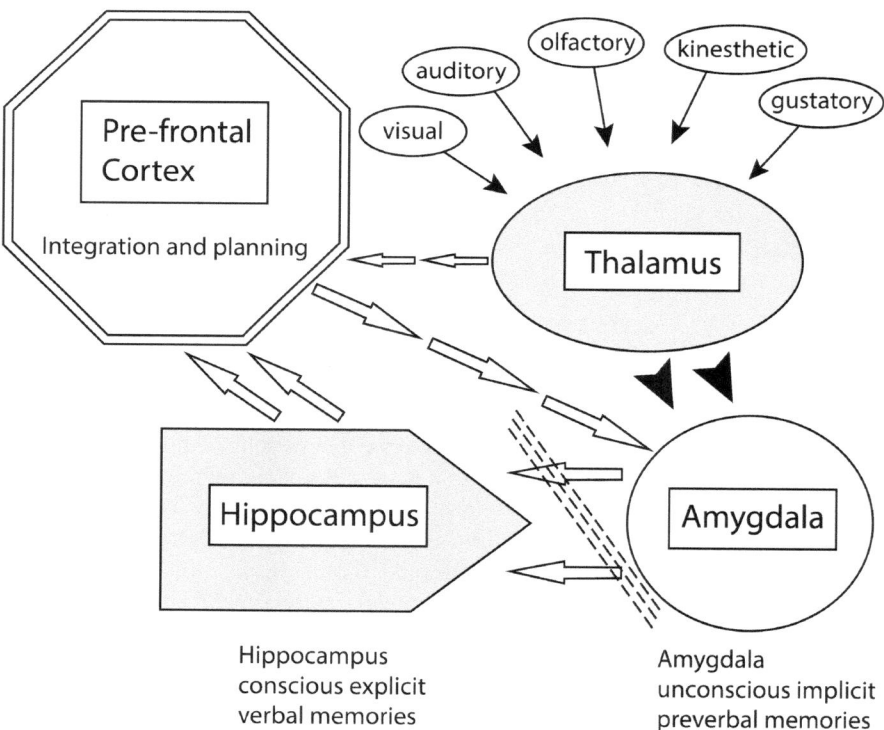

Fig. 6.1 Central nervous structures such as the prefrontal cortex, thalamus, amygdala, and hippocampus are involved in the stepwise integration of incoming sensory, visual, auditory information (after [32])

The amygdala holds a privileged position as emotional guard [40]. It is a hub for emotions and for emotional memories. Sensory, visual, or auditory signals arrive first to the thalamus and then to the cortex; the signal eventually passes to the amygdala and activates the emotional centers. Alternatively—in an extreme threatening situation—a portion of the original signal passes directly from the thalamus to the amygdala, bypassing the cortex. This transmission is faster, allowing a quicker, although less accurate response. In this way, the amygdala can trigger a reaction even before the cortical centers have fully understood what is going on.

The hippocampus, part of the temporal lobe of the brain, is essentially responsible for memory, with the function to transform unconscious preverbal memories (procedural or implicit memory), mediated mainly by the amygdala system, into conscious verbal memories (explicit or declarative memory) [40]. At the time of recollection, the hippocampus integrates the various aspects of memory and localizes the recollection according to time, place, and context [36]. Excessive emotions prevent adequate evaluation and categorization of the experience by inhibiting hippocampal function. Memories remain thus stored in the amygdala as affective or sensorimotor states of physical sensations and visual images and are indelible. Adequate assessment and integration of emotional experiences do not take place. Therefore, trauma-related memories remain timeless and self-alien. The hippocampus has a high concentration of receptors for glucocorticoids. Increase of serum cortisol is a physiological response to acute stress, present already in infancy [37]. The limbic system controls the activity of the pituitary gland, which in turn controls the production of hormones in the thyroid and adrenal glands. Dysfunctions of this hypothalamic-pituitary-adrenal axis (HPA) are among the main impairments with psychopathological consequences in adults, for example depression.

Psychobiological Aspects

Events occurring before the age of three are rarely consciously remembered. Memory traces or connections may either be lost or remain if constantly reactivated. The "use it or lose it" principle is essential in early brain development but is, according to Solms and Turnbull [41], a lifelong process which takes place without conscious awareness.

Preverbal affective and emotional experiences in the child's primary relations are stored in implicit unconscious memory (explicit memory is conscious remembering) in the amygdala [42]. Emotions that are expressed exclusively by the body in the form of pain, for example, often correspond to somatosensory sensations felt in early childhood. Such reactivated early childhood memories of traumatic events can be very strong but are consciously not retrievable as they are stored as implicit memories; however, they may influence a person's affective, emotional, sexual, and cognitive life.

The frontal cortex is poorly developed in the first 2 years of life; there are two growth spurts around 2 and 5 years; but the frontal cortex is crucial for the retrieval of memory in a realistic, rational, and orderly way. Current neurobiological theories suggest that there is a lower level of neurocognitive processing of memory traces in early childhood, compared to a higher level in later childhood. This transformation reflects a maturation process in memory circuits in the hippocampus and cortex.

The parent–child interaction plays an important role in the way painful experiences in early childhood are "remembered." Children of parents who deny these events may later manifest the traumatic experience with emotional or behavioral expressions, whereas this is not the case for children whose parents are available to engage in a supportive dialogue about the negative incident. A durable long-term autobiographical memory is dependent on social interaction. This necessitates the construction of a narrative through parent-child conversation and the formation of a significant parent-child attachment. Memory development is therefore as much an external as an internal process. Narrative memory appears around age 2–3, when children begin to talk. Memories of early infancy may be recovered if they are "translated" from immature, mostly emotionally tainted images, to adult-like narratives. This physiological developmental perspective does not rule out the possibility of "unconscious forgetting" in the case of intense emotional trauma in early life. The very rapid increase in narratives occurring after 2 years of age is linked to the formation of new cognitive patterns and developmental achievements such as language and the establishment of an autobiographical self [43].

The most lasting effect of traumatic experiences on the psyche is the inability to regulate states of arousal, to control feelings of anger, fear, sadness and express these emotions with words, as well as to perceive stimuli appropriately and to adjust to the environment. The younger the child at the time of traumatization and the longer the trauma lasts, the greater is his vulnerability [32, 44]. The loss of self-regulation manifests itself in various ways: as an attention problem (loss of ability to focus on specific stimuli) or—in a state of arousal—as an inability to inhibit acts (loss of impulse control), in other words, to react with uncontrollable fear, anger, or sadness.

If the traumatic origin of these intense emotions is not known, traumatized children will repeatedly live their own emotional outbursts as well as the emotional reactions of others as re-traumatization. Thus, feelings associated with the original trauma are continuously re-experienced on an interpersonal level.

Adverse experiences at critical or sensitive developmental phases during early childhood influence on a great degree brain development and may have long-lasting impacts, but brain development maintains its malleability until adulthood [45, 46]. The risk of negative effects of stressful experiences can be modified, thanks to emotionally available caregivers, who are capable of strengthening the resilience of abused children, even in the presence of a genotype responsible for increased vulnerability to mental disorders [47, 48].

Traumatic events in early childhood, leading to epigenetic modifications that alter gene expression, play an important role in the development of stress-related psychiatric illnesses and other health problems in later life. These changes are often enduring, but do not have to be permanent [46, 49]. Some neurobiological changes can be reversed by treatment interventions, for example, in providing secure attachment relationships. Various studies demonstrate that the negative consequences of early environmental stress or traumatic exposure can be alleviated by preventive interventions, such as offering a continuous and meaningful relationship with alternative care persons and addressing parent-child psychopathology. An essential task is to provide for children—in a safe, supportive environment—developmental opportunities for learning and practicing healthy adaptive responses to adverse experiences. These interventions show their efficiency up to adult life.

A study of over 2000 children aged 2–9 [50] confirmed that emotional maltreatment (without physical aggression) and hostile, rejecting, or inconsistent parenting are among the highest risk factors for children's physical and mental development. In addition, various negative impacts have subsequently cumulative effects.

Cumulative Trauma

Multiple or repeated traumatization in childhood have severe outcomes and affect multiple developmental domains such as regulation of affect and impulses, memory, attention, consciousness, self-perception, interpersonal relations, somatization, and systems of meaning. They result in complex symptoms and disorders also in adulthood [9, 39, 51].

Children are particularly vulnerable to compulsively reenacting traumatic experiences, as they have no conscious memory of the traumatic event(s), leading to repeated suffering either for themselves as victims or for others as perpetrators. Their behavior can be traced back to adversities encountered with primary caregivers in infancy or early childhood. If caregivers are absent or their reliance is existentially failing, children experience extremes of under-stimulation and hyperarousal, longing for and simultaneously fearing the caregiver's presence and intimacy. Violence and hostility of caregivers overwhelm infants or young children's inner lives, which are then filled with chronic anxiety, wariness, rage, anger, and finally retaliation [52].

Vignette

Benjamin, an eight-year-old adopted boy, suffers—according to the information of his adoptive parents—from sleep disorders, anxiety and nightmares, nocturnal enuresis, and chronic coughing. In the sessions with the child psychiatrist, Benjamin verbalizes his fears of separation, annihilation, and death. In his imagination, anger—his own or the one of his adoptive parents—results in physical injury. In his two drawings, Benjamin expresses his fears: he draws a robber with his leg cut off (castration anxiety) (Fig. 6.2) and a little boy waving goodbye to life for fear of death (Fig. 6.3).

Fig. 6.2 Benjamin,
8-year-old, a robber with
his leg cut off

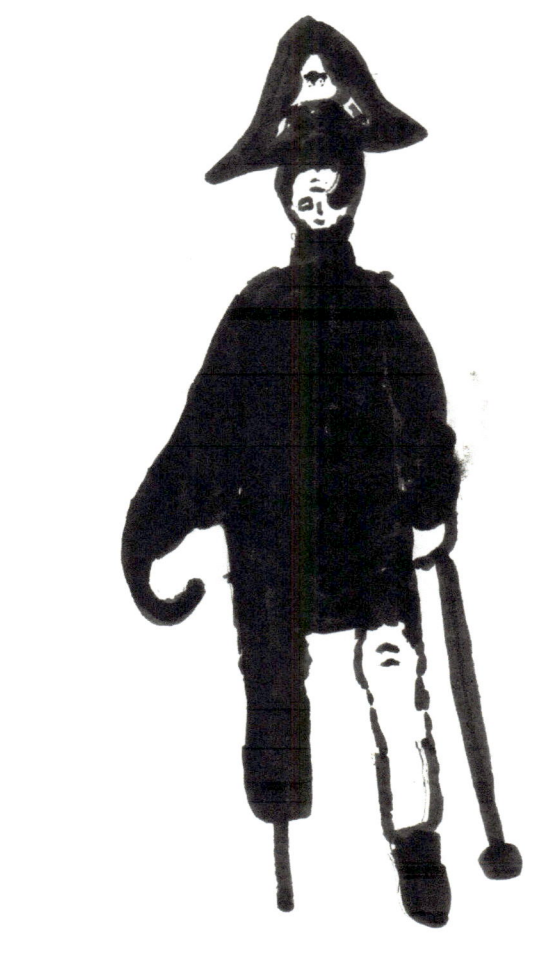

Fig. 6.3 Benjamin,
8-year-old, a little boy
waving goodbye to life

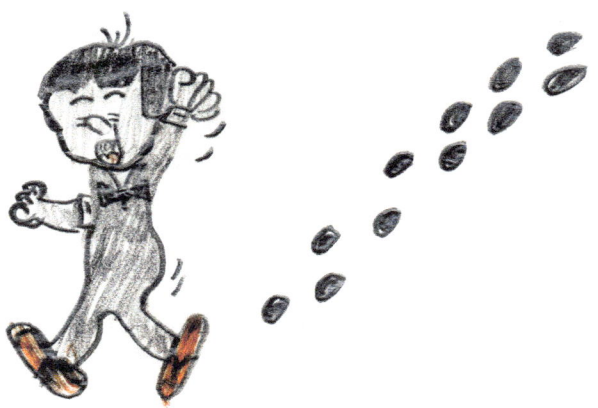

Assessment of a Traumatic Situation

The interactions of developmental processes and traumatic stress are complex. The child's cognitive and affective stage of development and his interpersonal relationships, his family and social situation, have to be considered. Maturity of defense and coping mechanisms, resources such as temperament, humor, and good cognitive abilities, which influence the meaning-attribution of traumatic experiences, belong to protective factors. In contrast, pre-existing physical and emotional vulnerability are risk factors.

Often several causes and circumstances are involved in a traumatic event or may interact simultaneously or successively. Psychosocial stresses are classified according to their severity: Acute events, such as the death of a parent, are distinguished from longer-lasting life circumstances, such as a parent's chronically disabling illness.

In the case of acute events (abuse, acute physical or psychic aggression), the excessive arousal is too intense for the child's coping skills; in the case of chronically stressful life situations (neglect, deprivation, chronic illness), i.e., repetitive, or cumulative traumatic events [27], the child's fundamental needs—essential for his development—are not met.

Symptoms and Characteristics of Psychic Traumatization

The appearing symptoms as a result of psychic stress are manifold and, in addition to emotional and behavioral disorders, include also physical functions and psychosomatic reactions—the expressions of unbearable feelings for which there are no words.

Symptoms and characteristics of psychic traumatization

- Behavioral disorders, regression
- Great neediness, clinging behavior
- Depressive mood, irritability
- Loss of previously acquired developmental skills, e.g., language skills
- Eating and sleeping disorders,[8] enuresis
- Anxiety disorders: separation anxiety and phobias
- Nightmares with threatening content, such as monsters and ghosts
- Psychosomatic symptoms such as headaches and abdominal pains
- Attention and hyperactivity disorders
- Fantasized feelings of guilt and responsibility
- Feelings of a limited future, e.g., life is too short to grow up.

---

[8] Parents of adopted children, aged 2–10, were asked to complete questionnaires with regard to their children's sleep: most frequent disorders were bedtime resistance, parasomnias, sleep-onset delay, and sleep anxiety. Neither the personal child history nor the adoptive family structure was significantly related to the sleep problems [53].

Vignette

Amara, a three-and-a-half-year-old girl from Africa (placed for adoption at the age of 18 months) was brought by her adoptive parents for a child psychiatric consultation because of her sleep disorders. While drawing, she explains to the child psychiatrist that she stays awake out of fear of all the monsters, lions, and phantoms who at night live in her room with her and who threaten to eat her parents. "I'm afraid to be left alone, I should go back to Africa to be reborn there." Amara is very much scared of being taken back to Africa, her country of origin, because her biological mother did not want to keep her.

Vignette

A ten-year-old adopted boy, Gael, constructs—in play scenes—families of animals; to the tiger family he narrates his wish to be the little tiger, who is 10 years old and who suckles his mother and defends her.

Comment

Gaels regressive desire to be a baby and suckle his mother, goes hand in hand with the progressive desire as a grown-up to defend his mother. This represents the characteristic situation so often found in adopted children who have never really been able to live a latency phase.

Vignette

Pedro, 16 years old, arrived at the age of 13 years from South America, where he had lived since the age of three in different orphanages. In the child psychiatric session, he tells in accompanying a squiggle game[9] [54] his adoption story (summary):

"A plane brings children from another country; the family will build a house where the children live forever. They are happy there."

Next squiggle: "A car, which broke down, because it was left in the rain. It belonged to a gentleman who didn't want it anymore. Another man felt sorry for the car and painted it; the car is now moving well, and the man keeps it".

Pedro would like to become a mechanic like his adoptive father to repair cars, which do no longer move. Therefore, he says, I need to have keys.

Pedro suffers from nightmares, in which someone wants to kill him; in this horror dream he can no longer stand up and the doctor tells him that there is no treatment for him and that he is going to die.

Comment

Pedro arrived in Switzerland with walking difficulties because he had been kneeling for most of the time in an orphanage. He seems to say that it takes a key, a phallic symbol to be able to repair him, that is the car,[10] his self. His nightmares reveal his

---

[9]The Squiggle Game was described by D. W. Winnicott (1896–1971) pediatrician and psychoanalyst.

It corresponds to a modality of diagnostic and therapeutic dialogue and is a way of maintaining contact with the conscious and unconscious personality interests of a patient. Winnicott conceived his game as interactive, as a form of therapeutic communication with children.

[10]Car = Auto in French and in German, from Greek αυτο = self

orphanage situation where he could not get up and where he suffered from death anxieties.

For Terr [55], "traumatic anxiety *is* a ghost! It moves through the generations with the stealth and cunning of a most skilled specter" (p. 528). He summarizes the characteristics of childhood trauma as follows [55]:

- recurrent, intrusive memories (most often visual, but also auditory, tactile, and olfactory).
- repetitive behaviors: the traumatic experience is repeated in playing and some aspects of the traumatic experience are (re)enacted in behaviors.
- trauma-specific fears, which are linked to the original traumatic situation.
- changed attitude towards people, to one's life and to the future; expectations are negative, and confidence is lost. The child is terrified by feelings of helplessness, horror, and despair. The younger the child, or the greater his vulnerability, the more he is overwhelmed by annihilation- and death anxieties.

Phases of Psychic Traumatization

Fischer and Riedesser [6] describe four phases of the traumatic reaction (Fig. 6.4). However, they do not always occur sequentially but may exist simultaneously. Working through trauma or trauma processing is influenced by coping and adaptive skills, as well as by age, developmental-phase, defense mechanisms and critical life events.

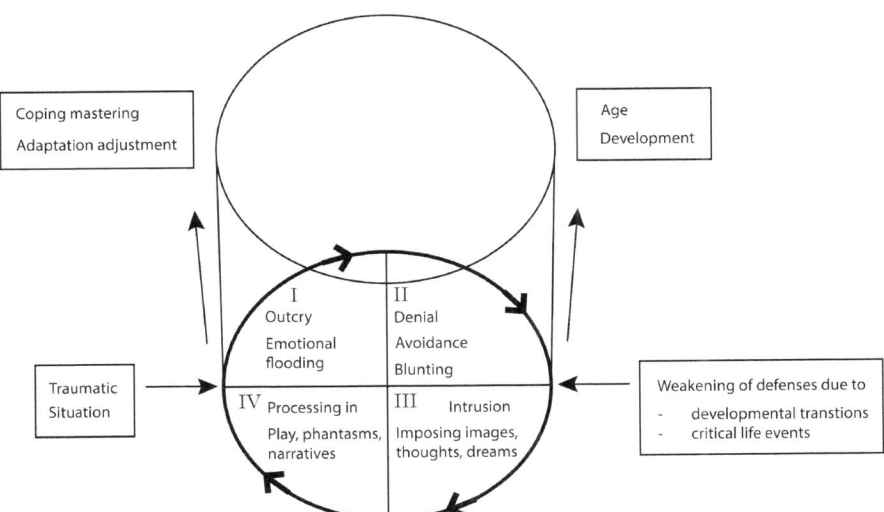

Fig. 6.4 Cycles of trauma processing (after [6])

Phase I corresponds to the experienced traumatic situation: the emotional disturbances are characterized by hyperarousal with manifestations of motor hyperactivity, explosive aggressiveness, or panic anxiety states. The primary defense reaction corresponds to fight or flight tendencies with subsequent immobilization. Children and adolescents may reexperience the same, recurring defensive response, linked to the lived threat of their traumatization event(s), in other critical or stressful life situations [8].

Subsequently (phase II), the traumatic event is denied, banished from waking consciousness, the memory of the event is repressed. The original feelings of fear, helplessness and despair are split off. Children in this phase are dysphoric, withdrawn, listless and joyless; simultaneously, they often remain very vigilant, attempting to anticipate threatening situations. They try to maintain emotional distance and avoid emotionally charged situations, which might relate to the trauma.

The transition to the intrusion phase (phase III) occurs when defense mechanisms decrease. Representations and thoughts associated with the traumatic experience overwhelm the child's mind. Since the memory traces are not erased, they emerge as nightmares, spontaneous images, sounds or even smells.

In playing and storytelling, children attempt to cope with and process their lived traumatic experience (phase IV). The child's play is characterized by repetitive scenes of the traumatic event. Children lack the ability—in pretend play—to try out interactive social roles and situations and to tell corresponding stories. Traumatized children's narratives are often chaotic and involve threatening topics. Working through traumatic events in a psychotherapeutic process facilitates the integration of such experiences.

Vignette

Eight-year-old Aron, adopted from Africa, suffers from violent tantrums and jealousy since the arrival of his sister for adoption. The adoptive parents were informed that Aron's birth mother had died when her baby boy was some weeks old and that his father was too poor to raise his son.

In the child psychiatrist consultation with the adoptive parents, Aron says: "When I am mad, I am no more able to think and can no longer control my heart." He gets very angry when playing games, as he does not tolerate to lose; this is especially the case when he plays the game in which one is "thrown out". Aron wants to know what makes him so angry.

Then, Aron speaks of his birth father and wonders, if the game makes him so angry because it reminds him of having been "thrown out" by his birth father.

Regarding the disputes with his recently adopted younger sister, Aron thinks she is being jealous because she believes that he was in his (adoptive) mother's womb. But, he says, they both do not need to be jealous of each other, since they were both not in the belly of their (adoptive) mother.

Aron wants to learn to control his heart so that his thinking does not turn off, and this without the help of his adoptive parents, this is his "aim", as he explains.

Comment

Aron's wish shows that he wants to appropriate the containing function of his adoptive parents and integrate it into his intrapsychic world.

In an individual interview, Aron recounts his nightmares, in which he is persecuted and attacked and wakes up with terror. At first confused and anxious, he narrates "his legend", i.e., the meaning he attributes to these nightmares: he sees himself as a baby fleeing with a man, dressed in black with a hood—whose face he cannot see. "The man is only dangerous for me, he directs his lightning against me; he is so powerful that if I am touched by him, I will die. He is a ghost that emerged when my birth mother died; this ghost possesses powers, which originate from early and modern times."

Comment

Aron seems to feel guilty for the death of his biological mother after his birth and to fear her and his biological father's revenge. The figure of the ghost or black man may be fantasized representations of his birth parents.

The greatest terror a child can have, is that he is not loved, and rejection is the hell he fears. John Steinbeck.

The Attachment and Relationship Breakup

The disruption of attachment and relationship with birth parents or significant caregivers can be considered as a psychic trauma. Abandonment is often seen as the central issue in the adoption process [56], as the words of a young adoptee attest: "To be abandoned is murder". The statements of adopted children, adolescents and adults illustrate how being abandoned is felt as rejection, expulsion, and exposure to an unknown fate. The resulting wounds heal poorly and leave scars that may reopen unexpectedly in a stressful life event or during a developmental transition. The memory traces of traumatically experienced events are imprinted in the personal history of an individual, even if they are lost from the subject's consciousness.

Depending on his age, a child has a conscious or unconscious memory of his biological family or primary caregivers, as well as of the separation and the attachment relationship breakup. The child suffers a personal loss, and often also a loss of love and protection, which he essentially needs in his dependence and deprivation [57–59]. "At this early stage the infant does not register what is good or adaptive, but reacts to, and therefore knows about and registers each failure of reliability. Reacting to unreliability in the infant care process constitutes a trauma, each reaction being an interruption of the infant's 'going-on-being' and a rupture of the infant's self" ([23]: p. 97). Good enough maternal holding creates a sense of reliance on the human environment; it guarantees continuity of personal experience, supported by preverbal communication. A child is deprived when he has not known this experience of reliance, or if the continuity in his life and development has been interrupted.

The experience of being rejected or expelled by parents is associated with feelings of being exposed and deprived of fundamental love. These emotions are often regarded to be the most responsible factor for children's psychic traumatization [60]. The smaller the child or the greater his vulnerability, the more he is overwhelmed by fears of annihilation and death.

The adopted child cannot talk about the separation with and loss of his affectively significant primary caregivers—if any were present—, i.e., there is a simultaneous communication loss and communication failure. In this light, the trauma always arises in the relationship with another emotionally significant person. However, infants and toddlers do not possess the necessary perceptual functions and structures to record experiences with overwhelming feelings in an organized way. But even the older child is submerged with feelings of helplessness, powerlessness, and despair, which may plunge him into a state of annihilation, bewilderment, and confusion.

As Ferenczi already described in 1933,[11] a child expects tender play in his exchanges with the adult caregiver, yet the adult sometimes responds with sexual or aggressive impulses. Anxiety and fear compel the child to surrender to the adult, to identify with the aggressor, and to introject the guilt feelings of the adult. "The most important change, produced in the mind of the child by the anxiety-fear-ridden identification with the adult partner, is the introjection of the guilt feelings of the adult…" [61].

As a kind of survival strategy, children imagine and build a fantasy world; their phantasms, which they construct after their traumatization, i.e., retrospectively, can be understood as an attempt to find meaning and coherence for what happened. Children look for an "explanation" on the fantasy level to understand the event. These fantasy formations represent inner-psychic conflicts and are often expressed by symptoms. The meaning children attribute with their affective response to these challenges, represents the basis of their post-traumatic adjustment.

Clinical Vignette

Aurelia, eight-year-old, came with her adoptive mother for a child psychiatric consultation. The adoptive mother informs that 6 years ago, she and her husband went to Aurelias country of origin in southern Europe and brought her back to Switzerland for adoption. Aurelia's symptoms consist of opposition behavior, slowness and apathy, masturbation, eating- and learning disorders; Aurelia refuses to learn reading.

Aurelia did not speak in the first session with the child psychiatrist, but played for half an hour, commenting her play scene summarized as follows: "This is a poor family that does not have enough money, and the children have nothing to eat. The oldest girl left with other people to get money; she will come back. Her mother (she is standing in the play-scene on a terrace to which a staircase leads) looks at her and knows that she will come back.

---

[11] The original paper was *The Passions of Adults and their Influence on the Sexual and Character Development of Children* published in Int. Z. f. Psa. (1933; 19: p. 5–15).

To the question by the child psychiatrist "when will the girl go back?" Aurelia answers: "The girl will have the same height, when she will be back with a lot of money."

When this scene was told to the adoptive parents, they were shocked; they informed the child psychiatrist, that the biological mother had waved from a terrace with stairs to Aurelia, at the moment they took her – 6 years ago—for her adoption.

Comment

Aurelia lost her biological mother, her first love relationship. What happened to her at this moment of the permanent separation, why she was abandoned by her mother, Aurelia was never able to ask her birth mother, as the communication with her was forever interrupted. Her personal fantasy construction of this traumatic experience, "the girl will have the same height" became pathogenic for Aurelia, prohibiting her to grow up, which she expressed by her symptomatology of eating- and learning disorders. Simultaneously, thanks to her fantasies, Aurelia maintained her loyal attachment to the biological mother.

This example shows that traumatic experiences, even if they are not consciously remembered, leave memory traces in the unconscious.

Consequences of the Attachment and Relationship Breakup

Adopted children need all their energy after the breakup with their birthparents or significant caregivers to adapt to circumstances, unknown for them, to learn to live with people they have never met and whose language they very often do not understand, in conditions, which are foreign to them. A study of adolescent adoptees – 10 years after their arrival in Switzerland for adoption—reveals that these young persons have no longer accurate memories of the traumatic moments of their arrival [62]. Adoptees are obliged to "invent" a new origin and a new destiny in a few weeks, being confronted with the question of their survival. In addition, they are faced with the expectation to transfer their love for birth parents or primary caregivers to unknown prospective parents. Transforming emotions of fear, longing, anger, sadness, and hatred, felt in the moments of separation from their previous attachment figures or care persons, into love, trust, and confidence, is a challenge with which adopted children are again and again confronted in future meaningful relationships.

Additional Losses

In addition to the loss of both biological parents, international adoptions involve the losses of ethnic, cultural, racial, and linguistic ties. Nathan [26] considers the unthinkable and unspeakable loss of the cultural environment as a psychic trauma since every individual depends on his cultural environment to decipher reality. He sees a subject's identity as a kind of memory, a recollection that gives the subject a temporal permanence and a spatial unity. Adopted children are uprooted from familiar places, language, ethnicity, religion, rites, and traditions; therefore, the development of their identity, the formation of a coherent self, is a complex process.

Vignette

Beatrice, an adopted girl from Africa, draws—in the child psychiatric session—spontaneously a house and a bridge inside the house, a tree without roots but bearing twelve fruits and a girl without legs and feet (Fig. 6.5).

Comment

With the drawing Beatrice seems to reveal her desire to integrate her dual parenthood and dual cultures by connecting the two parts of her intrapsychic house with a bridge. Her experience of having been deprived of her origin are expressed by the tree without roots; does she indicate her age by drawing the tree bearing 12 fruits? Legs and feet of the girl are missing in the drawing, respectively replaced by a kind of clothes rack. Does Beatrice communicate her feelings of helplessness and attentive immobility, a frozen hyperalert state[12]?

The date and year of her birth were unknown when Beatrice came to Switzerland for adoption. Based on the medical examination, her age was estimated at 10 years.

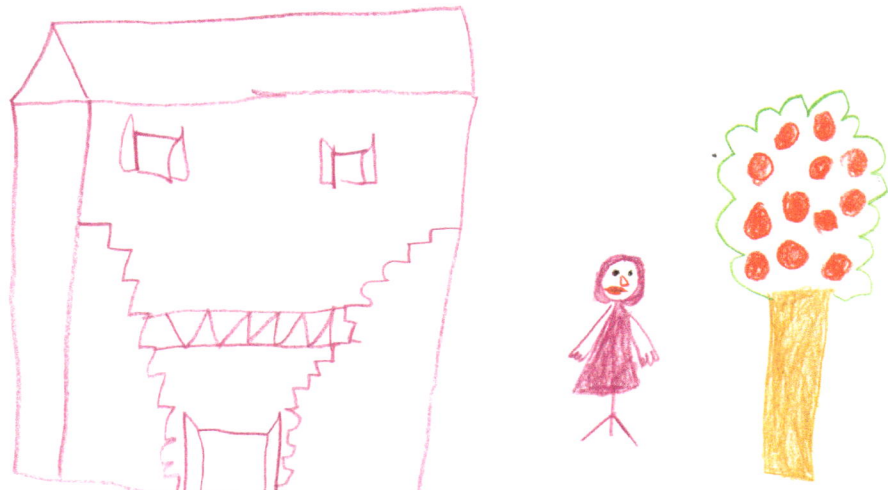

Fig. 6.5 Beatrice, a bridge inside a house, a tree without roots

---

[12] Freezing is a defense response.

Specific Disorders

Adoptive children may be carriers of specific disorders resulting from poor conditions during pregnancy or lack of stimulation in the first months or years. Older children often suffered severe trauma such as sexual, physical, or emotional abuse, neglect, and privation/deprivation.[13]Many have experienced multiple relationship breakups, various placements in different homes or war situations.

Post-Traumatic Consequences

Post-traumatic consequences result from complex dynamic interactions between the child's inner and outer world, between facts and their subjective meaning, between the traumatic event and the post-traumatic processing capacities. Trauma has different effects depending on age, developmental stage, and context. During the developmental process, various ego functions acquire a relative and secondary autonomy and defense, adaptation, and coping mechanisms attain a greater degree of maturity. The effects of traumatization depend therefore on the extent the child has been able to build up a fundamental trust in himself, in his own body and in meaningful persons of his outside world [63].

Helping their adopted child to work through injuries of the past, requires from adoptive parents almost infinite availability, great personal affective resources, and a solid marital relationship. Adoptive parents are being asked to function rather like psychotherapists than as parents, depending on the stress severity to which their child was exposed in his early affective development [64].

Vulnerability to Separation

Numerous studies (Bertocci and Schechter 1991; [65–67]) confirm that adopted children remain particularly vulnerable to any kind of separation. Any separation, emotionally so painful, seems to remind the child of his past relationship disruptions. Fears of separation are mostly expressed through aggressive or regressive behavior.

Adopted children often ask for exclusive, possessive love and have little tolerance for frustration, because any "no" from their adoptive parents seems to question the relationship again and again. Simultaneously, adopted children often have difficulties establishing affectively lasting, sustainable relationships. Because they have emotionally been poorly or inadequately invested and not taken seriously before their adoption, they did not learn to live closeness in a trusting relationship;

---

[13] Privation: lack of what is needed for existence. Deprivation: losing what one once had.

therefore, out of fear, they quickly retreat in any relationship and provoke their repeated rejection [68].

Vignette

Ela, a seven-year-old girl from India, whose adoptive parents live separately—the father has a girlfriend—suffers from asthma attacks, school performance difficulties and emotional problems. She experiences each end of the psychotherapy sessions and every interruption in her treatment as extremely painful: she hates the word "end" (the end of the therapy session), and always wants to stay with the therapist or threatens her to never come back. Ela insists, that her psychotherapist is only allowed to talk to her and not to anyone else: "You are here for me alone and privately". In playing, Ela expresses her wish to be the therapist's daughter and never leave her again.

She fantasizes that her adoptive father will have a baby by his girlfriend and will no longer love her; she would like to live with her adoptive father. In her play scenes and narratives, Ela portrays her adoptive mother as an unhappy woman who keeps everything for herself; in playing, Elsa locks her mother up in prison.

Comment

Ela's emotions, which she experienced at the moment of her relationship breakup with her birthparents, were reactivated by the separation of her adoptive parents, and seem to emerge at each separation. Ela has to endure these intense painful feelings when visiting and then again leaving her father, e.g., each time she moves from one parent to the other, as well as at the end of each psychotherapeutic session. These most violent and painful feelings of disappointment—each time her lived injuries in the "continuity of her being" are reawakened—seem for Ela too overwhelming to endure and are expressed through her body by asthmatic symptoms.

Traumatic experiences have—depending on the developmental level—different effects on cognitive, affective, and biological self-organization [44]. Early childhood adverse experiences lead to various developmental disorders and disease symptoms; the complex interconnections between the different brain regions evolve and mature in the course of early development [69]. Growth arrest, developmental delays, functional disorders, and structural changes always affect brain, body, and mind and impact in multidimensional interactions on psycho-neuro-endocrine-immunological pathways. Trauma-related psychopathology results from an overload on different systems including a dysregulation of the hypothalamus-pituitary-adrenal axis [70].

Neuroendocrine-Immunological Effects

Separating an infant from his mother leads to long-lasting neurobiological changes at the level of neurotransmitters (such as serotonin and catecholamines), which cause disturbances in heart rhythm, body temperature and sleep [37, 52], as well as changes in neurohormones such as oxytocin, known to increase empathy and bonding. Oxytocin, a "resilience-hormone" plays a central role in stress regulation; it reduces anxiety in psychosocial stress situations [71]. Children who experienced traumatic separations remain vulnerable because disturbances in neurotransmitters and neuroendocrine systems are long-lasting and can be reactivated later in other stressful situations, such as the loss of affective relationships.

Children with traumatic experiences are more prone to somatic disorders and especially infectious diseases. The child's body seems to take over the function of expressing unbearable emotions. The somatic symptoms must be taken seriously as a cry for help and often have symbolic meaning, such as the occurrence of asthma attacks or flare-ups of skin manifestations (eczema) in the context of traumatic or painful separation experiences.

Anzieu [72] speaks of a "toxic function" of the skin-ego[14]; he considers the outburst of eczema as an attempt of the subject to feel the somatic surface layer of the self, torn in a most painful, self-destructive conflict. The subject seeks a substitute for physical pain or psychic anxiety, wrapping himself in suffering ([73], in [74]). Separation anxiety disorders in childhood are a risk factor for developing panic- or anxiety disorders in adulthood [75].

Deprivation experiences in early childhood may lead to various addictive behaviors Opiates have the ability to alleviate feelings of separation and alienation, by increasing pain insensitivity [76]. It is well known that stressors elevate endogenous opiates [77]. Children, who have experienced separation anxiety in early childhood, later try to behave in a way that stimulates their opiate system to calm their arousal and unbearable anxiety states. In a compulsive way, they tend to expose themselves repeatedly to traumatic situations [78–81]. According to the findings of the American National Institute of Drug Abuse, dependence is a consequence of repeatedly disturbed regulatory processes in the brain's reward system—in which the neurotransmitter dopamine plays a major role—with effects on motivation, memory and impulse control [82, 83].

Effects on Motor and Language Development

Based on psychotherapeutic observations of abused infants and toddlers, Green [84] described the occurrence of developmental disorders. He noted that these children avoided eye contact with their parents, kept their distance, and approached their parents only from the side or from behind. They sat around often motionless but were highly alert. This state of hyper-vigilance prevents normal learning of language and motor skills.

Children, who are mistreated when they cry, or even vocalize, learn to suppress their verbal expressions, what inhibits and delays their language development. They

---

[14] The skin envelopes the body; the skin-ego is a psychic envelope with the function of containing and consolidating the subject.

begin to speak later, and articulation and expression difficulties are common. In a similar way, they abstain from motor activities such as crawling and climbing, if this behavior disturbs their caregivers, leading to transitory motor and coordination disorders. These children are often motor-wise very clumsy and hurt themselves easily.

Infants and toddlers, who are left alone in a state of extreme fear and helplessness, eventually cry themselves into an exhaustion sleep what may be regarded as a physiological protective mechanism, an avoidance of "psychic death".

Emotional Effects

The emotional response to various psychic traumas such as abuse, deprivation, kidnapping, incest [85] has been described as biphasic: first characterized by hyperarousal and overwhelming of emotions, then by apathetic encapsulation and emotional isolation and numbness [86–88]. Any physiological, emotional, sensory stimulus can later arouse and overwhelm a child to such extent that he reacts with motor hyperactivity, explosive hetero- and/or auto-aggressiveness, or with a panic state, less frequently with weeping and screaming. These are extreme reactions to external and internal stimuli. Deprived children are incapable of regulating their feelings of fear and aggression against others or themselves and unable to modulate their excitability and hyperarousal state.

Another inner response is characterized by the child's apathy and joylessness, a state of anhedonia. Trauma or overwhelming stress increases endorphin secretion and triggers numbing of certain feelings [89], resulting in emotional numbness and dissociation with a perception to be cut off from life and from sharing feelings with others. Children are dysphoric, isolate themselves, and withdraw emotionally completely; they are apathetic, but simultaneously over alert; they remain in a state called frozen watchfulness or attentive immobility.

Vignette
Sabine, an eight-year-old adopted girl, presents herself with an opaque mask-like face, remains sitting, motionless, stiff in her body, hardly responds or with "I don't know". With great difficulty, she begins several times to draw houses, which are cut in two parts and burning. Sabine comments: "No one will come out alive of these houses, only a cat." Sabine would like to be this cat. Her greatest fear is to be blind.

Comment
Sabine is terrified that she might no longer be able to foresee and control the imminent disasters awaiting her, namely the return of unbearable feelings of her past traumatic experiences. Sabine was 18 months old when hospitalized for the first time in a state of severe neglect with a development delay of 11–12 months.

A significant feature of a post-traumatic state is the behavior of a child who no longer smiles, nor responds to laughter, nor imitates a smile, and does no longer engage in exchanges of joy, pleasure, and gratification with others. Affective self-isolation often hides a chronic depressive state and/or a repression of anger and hate feelings. Children are incapable of sustaining an affective tonality; their emotional communications are unpredictable, marked by high ambivalence and ambiguity and often very superficial.

The question is not always easy to answer whether neglect and abuse create disturbed emotional communications, or whether this affective climate favors neglect and abuse to occur. Both parents and children find themselves in a relation of "malignant embrace" [90], which they are unable to change.

If psychic traumata are not integrated into a subject's life experiences, the victim remains with fixed memories to the trauma. Splitting, a major defense mechanism, allows exteriorizing the traumatic experiences from conscious awareness, repressing the memory of the event, and cleaving the initial feelings of fear, helplessness, and despair. In later stress situations, children react with the emotional intensity they felt at the time of traumatization, as if the traumatic event is repeating itself. They cannot understand what is happening to them because the historical, biographical references remain unconscious. Even if children try to keep emotional distance and avoid emotional situations which might be related to the trauma, memory traces cannot be erased. Often split-off elements of the traumatic experience emerge again, triggered by memory traces, such as nightmares, but also by spontaneous images, sounds, noises or even a certain smell.

Transition periods, such as adolescence, or life events such as a first love relationship, the onset of an illness, losses, or other stressful situations, reactivate traumatic infantile events; this can lead to an outburst of such overwhelming feelings that a mental breakdown may follow. The consequences are panic anxiety, escape reactions, confusion- and depersonalization- or severe depressive states with hetero- or auto-aggressive behavior.

Cognitive Effects

The developmental delays resulting from acoustic and visual perception disorders lead to cognitive dysfunctions. Traumatized children are incapable of using mental images to solve problems and must rely on sensomotoric actions to cope with change. One of the most significant sign is the rigidity of cognitive structures and functions, so that dynamic changes no longer take place. Autonomic nervous system alertness and the permanent anxiety state prevent the ability to plan and play with alternatives. Children show a lack of essential curiosity, necessary for exploratory behavior and learning processes [44, 52]. Traumatized children function by far the worst in perception and awareness of themselves and others compared to control groups. They have great difficulties in recounting narratives and feel no joy in storytelling. The content of their narratives often reflects terrifying events such as murder, kidnapping, abandonment, and rejection and rarely has a happy ending, as it is the case in control groups.

The longer a traumatic situation lasts, the less the child can adapt to his environment and the more energy he will spend creating an intrapsychic world with multiple omnipotent identities; in this inner world, the child is no longer confronted with the reality of the outside world and no longer exposed to criticism, comparison, or judgment.

Vignette

Luc, an 11-year-old adopted boy, "leads a dialogue" in an infantile language with his "clown", who dictates him with a quiet voice commands, which Luc must absolutely carry out. It is the clown, says Luc, who commits all the stupidities for which he is unjustly accused. The clown is linked to the meaningful persons Luc knew in his country of origin.

Comment

Luc has been sexually abused in his childhood. What he experienced as a powerless victim, he now reenacts as an active perpetrator with his clown, thus allowing him—in identification with the aggressor—to express his feelings of rage and revenge. His detachment from reality, i.e., a dissociation, permits Luc to maintain his desire to be a kind child and to be loved.

Gender Differences

Different psychological developmental tendencies are described for boys and girls: Girls are more likely to suffer from depression and show self-destructive behavior, thus identifying with the victim position. They are more vulnerable, manifest chronic feelings of helplessness, and the danger is considerable that they will be exploited and victimized again. Boys identify themselves more with the aggressor position; they behave destructively as far as to commit delinquent acts. In their relationship with younger children, they are aggressive and let the weaker ones suffer what they had to endure. Both representations of victim and aggressor are probably intrapsychically present in girls and boys, only the behavioral manifestations are different, whereby socio-cultural factors play a role.

Post-Traumatic Stress Disorder PTSD

PTSD is a disorder occurring after exposure to traumatic events associated with a significant stress response. There seems to be a genetic susceptibility for the formation of persisting aversive memories [91] and thus an increased risk of developing symptoms of PTSD. The response to traumatic events has many individual facets. Jones et al. [92] emphasizes the fact that response to trauma has changed over time and is influenced by culture. PTSD symptoms are variable and must be viewed in the context of a continually evolving picture of human reaction to adversity [93].

Intense emotions, particularly triggered by traumatic exposure, activate distinct brain regions such as the amygdala, hippocampus, anterior cingulate gyrus, orbito-frontal and prefrontal cortex. The amygdala is one of the structures, which determines the emotional significance of an incoming stimulus. The "rational" brain—before reacting to an emotional challenge—will contextualize the information by comparing it to an existing internal map. Children and adults confronted with acute or chronic psychic trauma lose the capacity to handle their emotions and feelings in an appropriate way and—as van der Kolk rightfully says—people who suffer from PTSD "seem to lose their way in the world" ([94]: p. 280).

The neurobiological disturbances of PTSD involve many of the stress-induced changes such as alterations in the limbic system, especially the amygdala [95]. Significant changes also arise in the locus coeruleus, which regulates the release of catecholamines and mobilizes the body for an emergency situation. If PTSD is already present, there is overreaction by parts of the limbic system with symptoms of fear, anxiety, hypervigilance, irritability, and flashbacks,[15] as well as involuntary overwhelming recollections of traumatic scenes, vivid images that occur in the waking state with reactions to fight or flee. "Victims of a devastating trauma may never be the same biologically." "It does not matter if it was the incessant terror of combat, torture, or repeated abuse in childhood, or a one-time experience, like being trapped in a hurricane or nearly dying in an auto accident. All uncontrollable stress can have the same biological impact" (Charney, cited in [96]).

The US Substance Abuse and Mental Health Services Administration (SAMHSA) describes individual trauma as resulting from "an event, series of events, or set of circumstances that is experienced by an individual as physically or emotionally harmful or life threatening and that has lasting adverse effects on the individual's functioning and mental, physical, social, emotional, or spiritual well-being." Complex posttraumatic stress syndrome (Complex PTSD) may be diagnosed in adults or children who have repeatedly experienced traumatic events, such as violence, neglect, or abuse. Complex PTSD is thought to be more severe if:

- the traumatic events happened early in life
- the trauma was caused by a parent or carer
- the person experienced the trauma for a long time
- the person was alone during the trauma
- there's still contact with the person responsible for the trauma

As it may take years for the symptoms of complex PTSD to be recognized, children's development, including their behavior and self-confidence, can be altered as they get older.[16]

---

[15] Flashbacks, a form of dissociative state, are defined as involuntary, vivid images that occur in the waking state.

[16] Adults with complex PTSD may lose their trust in people and feel separated from others. The symptoms of complex PTSD are similar to symptoms of PTSD, but may include: feelings of shame or guilt, difficulty controlling emotions, periods of losing attention and concentration (dissociation), physical symptoms, such as headaches, dizziness, chest pains and stomach aches, cutting

Post-Traumatic Stress Disorders in Children

Children, unlike adults, do not have the same skills to understand and manage stress. The child's post-traumatic consequences result from complex dynamic interactions between inner and outer worlds, facts, and their subjective meanings, and between the traumatic event and the post-traumatic processing capabilities. They are always related to the child's developmental stage and the familial and social context. Increased vulnerability, chronic persistent anxiety, and emotional numbness are all features of PTSD in children.

Research in the field of post-traumatic consequences of cumulative traumata or poly-victimization of children and youth has centered on the developmental aspects and family context in order to assess the multiple and serious mental health problems in children, youth, and adults[17] and to propose earlier preventive and therapeutic measures [9, 39, 50, 51, 85, 97].

A national survey of trauma exposure and PTSD in adolescents in Switzerland concluded that, in the general population, about half of the adolescents had experienced at least one traumatic event. Higher risk of trauma exposure was found in adolescents who did not live with both biological parents, who were not of Swiss origin or who had parents with lower education. The occurrence of PTSD was higher in females. Adolescents having witnessed domestic violence had the highest occurrence of PTSD [98].

Do not judge me by my success, judge me by how many times I fell down and got back up again. Nelson Mandela.

Resilience

Resilience[18] is an interactive concept and refers to the relative resistance of a subject to environmental risk experiences or to his overcoming of stress or adversity. Underlying psychosocial and biological processes, risk and vulnerability, as well as gene- environment interactions are all factors contributing to resilience. Good intellectual functioning and parenting resources are associated with good outcomes across competence domains, even in the context of severe, chronic adversity.

---

oneself off from friends and family, relationship difficulties, destructive or risky behavior, such as self-harm, alcohol misuse or drug abuse, suicidal thoughts.

[17] Adults who have experienced multiple or cumulative traumata in early childhood often present not only symptoms of PTSD, but additional symptoms, including difficulties in affective and interpersonal situations and disturbances in self-regulation skills. Psychotherapeutic interventions for adults with such complex symptomatology have therefore to consider failures of reliance in early relationships with primary care persons and the resulting developmental, emotional, and interpersonal problems.

[18] "Act of rebounding" from Latin resilire "rebound, recoil."

Children having different temperament styles seek out environments that may increase risk or promote resilience.

The quality of interpersonal relationships between the infant and his caregivers, parental attachment models, and the child's attachment security play an essential role in the development of resilience and in intergenerational transmission. Preventive and therapeutic interventions at both individual and family levels are important measures promoting resilience [99, 100].

Resilience is responsible for the individual variation in the response of children and adolescents to similar experiences. The exposure to stress and not its avoidance may in certain circumstances strengthen the resistance to later stress, the so-called "steeling" effect, in other words when risk experiences have been mastered by successful coping. "... resilience can be defined as reduced vulnerability to environmental risk experiences, the overcoming of a stress or adversity, or a relatively good outcome despite risk experiences" ([101]: p. 336). Resilience leads to successful adaptation and integration despite high risks, chronic stress, and psychosocial adverse conditions [102]. Positive adaptation is usually defined as social skills or as successful passage through distinctive phases of specific developmental tasks. In spite of experiencing significant discriminatory conditions or trauma, resilient children, adolescents, and young adults show positive adaptation [103].

Resilience is not constant, but can fluctuate during life, depending on situations and context. Traumatic life experiences can trigger maturation processes, particularly in three areas: self-awareness, interpersonal relationships, and attitude toward life (Tedeschi et al. 1998). Resilient children are generally very early able to establish relationships with surrogate persons and use them for their development, having a high interactive capacity. Temperamental differences rooted in infancy are important for understanding individual discrepancies in vulnerability and resilience [105]. Changes in manifestations of resilience take place especially during developmental transitions, such as adolescence [106], in which new risk factors arise and protective factors will be challenged.

Children who have high levels of positive emotionality, emotional access, and activity, are more likely to use active and flexible coping mechanisms to deal with stress and are therefore more resilient, while children with low scores in these items tend to use avoidance strategies [107].

The psychological and biological processes of reactivity to psychosocial stress and the related nature of confrontation and coping, as well as the recovery from stress, are fundamental to the understanding of the extent of the emotional and physical consequences of long-lasting chronic stress. Stress not only contributes to somatic illnesses and emotional and behavioral problems but also interferes with the functions in the brain that are primarily responsible for effective coping and self-regulation; stress impairs hippocampal integrity resulting in diminished cognitive functioning and affects the development of frontal regions implicated in emotional regulation [36]. The direct effect of chronic stress is thus reinforced by the impairment of the ability to effectively cope with stress.

The effects of single environmental burdens become quite strong when accumulated into multiple risk scores; they may even affect the development of offspring in the next generation, yet resilience research clearly shows that children and adolescents growing up in stressful situations or exposed to critical life events do not necessarily develop psychopathological symptoms. The quality of parental functions, the parent-child relationships, and the family milieu constitute effective mediators and moderators in unfavorable stress situations. Children's and adolescents' vulnerability can be compensated by mediating early, protective, and long-lasting interventions. Treatments for children at risk prove to be particularly advantageous at the time of developmental transitions, such as starting school, adolescence, or entering the world of work. Reduction of risk impact, promoting self-reliance and self-efficacy, and opening new opportunities and prospects through available stable and supportive relationships or successful task accomplishment are crucial measures to foster resilience. Resilient families often have strong value systems; reliable relationships; clear forms of communication based on trust, empathy, and tolerance; they dispose of flexible social and economic resources and have the ability to find solutions and adapt to new challenges [102].

Greenacre [108, 109] speculates for the gifted child an "innate equipment," which consists of a special degree of sensitivity, empathy, and perceptiveness. He believes that this peculiar capacity of perception is inborn, but that the sensitivity may be increased by early traumata. An inherent richness of stimulation with corresponding responsiveness may be confusing or even overwhelming but leads to an abundance, variety, and diversity of spontaneous symbolism and imagery. Personal relationships are invested with great interest; however, if these are not available, gifted children are able to use alternative figures (other people or even animals) and shapes (e.g., from sensory perceptions such as smells, sounds, light and shadow). These represent some sort of contemplated animation and meaning and are linked with lived earlier subjective experiences. Children's creative work does not express nor represent a solution but is a relief of emotions associated with lived traumatic experiences. In a highly creative person experiences are multifold, resonating with intuitively inspired imagery and presenting a relationship between creative and personal lives.

Give sorrow words: the grief that does not speak whispers the o'er-fraught heart, and bids it breaks. William Shakespeare [110].

Grief

Grief has been described since ancient times, among all nations, and finds expression in religion, literature, philosophy, and art. Grief can be defined as the process of giving intrapsychic significance to the experience of loss.

In the context of bereavement, loss, trauma, or deprivation there is always a potential crisis of meaning and a necessity for mourning. Grief work is a lengthy process of dealing with three different themes of mourning. The *first* is mostly concerned with loss, such as the death of a loved person but could also relate to the loss of one's health or the loss of one's homeland. The *second theme* in the mourning process addresses the fact that the experienced loss cannot be replaced. Adults who were emotionally deprived in their childhood often ask, with infinite longing and deep yearning, for all they feel having missed: love, attention, care, being held and contained. Also, sometimes health cannot be recovered or the return to one's homeland is impossible. There are manifold questions around grief: Why did I had to suffer these events? Am I responsible for what happened to me? Do I need to feel guilty about this situation? Would it have been possible to avoid or prevent the event? Could I have been aware of this situation earlier and changed the outcome? These questions are the *third theme* to be elaborated in grief work.

There are situations where a traumatized person enters a mourning process by asking all these questions—often becoming desperate and disappointed not to find the expected answers. This is the case for adoptees with traumatizing lived experiences in their early childhood, often representing an accumulation of multiple deprivations, of personal loss of biological parents, homeland, culture, ethnicity, and language.

In other situations, these questions may partially be answered when the traumatized subject begins to understand his mother's or father's lived experiences in their respective families. The comprehension of the subject's implication in a transgenerational transmission may favor mourning work, yet for adoptees to understand the situation of their birthmother and birthfather's personal and familial history is hardly ever possible.

In each mourning process, it is essential to elaborate the adoptee's subjective lived experiences of his past, as infant and child, even if such experiences cannot be verbalized, but are expressed through nonverbal communication.

Process of Coping with Losses

The fundamental question arises whether it is essential for adopted children to grieve their experienced losses for being able to build up emotionally sustaining new bonds with their adoptive parents.

"That night, as I lay in bed, I had the eerie sensation that my real parents were standing in the darkness, watching me with compassion. They sent me strength to bear all the humiliations of this existence. Just one sign from me, and they would come forward and reveal themselves. All my love for them rose in me and then another feeling, fear. I was afraid to face these spirits: Death had taken away their humanity as it had taken away their life. In the face of these ghost parents, there was a danger…that my safe world was crumbling. As much as I longed for them, I turned myself away" (Lifton[19] 1981: p. 34).

According to Freud [111], the construction of the human personality is shaped by ongoing losses. Infant and early childhood development is accompanied by loss

---

[19] Betty Lifton is an adoptee herself.

and gain, i.e., growing up goes hand in hand with losing. During the growth process, the child gains an ever-greater autonomy. This simultaneous gain may allow in parallel a grieving process of experienced losses.

Infants and toddlers have no memories when everything goes well but do remember if the continuity in their lives has been interrupted, which leads to distrust [23]. Holding[20] creates a feeling of trust in the environment, of stability that allows the continuity of personal experience; a "silent" communication takes place long before speech develops.

In general, children's mourning is described as a mental process that a child goes through after a loss, allowing him to continue his development within the normal range. A child's grief is not comparable to the adult's mourning process. Grieving in the true sense occurs only after adolescence. A child is not able to accomplish a mourning process alone; he needs the help of an emotionally significant adult person, available in a continuous relationship, to fulfill grieving. The child understands a loss only according to his psychological development [112].

For a child, the loss of a meaningful relationship arouses existential fears: his needs for protection, security, care, and narcissistic gratification are threatened. The child has not yet developed the maturity to cope with intense feelings of pain, sadness, fear, anger, and longing; therefore, he denies the loss, which is an unconscious defense response. Very often, the child maintains—on a fantasy level—his attachment to the lost caregiver and continues an internal relationship with the lost person. Such fantasies and internal dialogues, if not excessive, might be temporarily helpful. The loss of a significant relationship creates persistent longing and profound pain. Therefore, the child may fend off these feelings, i.e., the emotions are suppressed or split off, until he has reached a developmental level, at which he can endure his psychic pain. The child needs external help much more than the adult, so that his psychophysical needs may be satisfied, his fears contained, and his feelings and fantasies shared with the meaningful person.

Losses hinder identification-, individuation-, separation-, and disengagement processes. Children cleave their feelings by maintaining a love relationship with and a longing for their biological parents and by building up aggressive relationships with their adoptive parents. Grieving the separation or the loss of loved still-living persons does hardly take place. Children engage—often repeatedly—in a new relationship, hoping the new relation will help them to be relieved from the internalized representation of the non-deceased but absent parent, mainly the birth mother.

However, children also mobilize resources and invent creative solutions and phantasms in relation to the lost caregiver; these can temporarily serve the child as transitional objects or fantasized companions in the period after the loss. A child may, for example, rely on a pet or animated object, such as a stuffed animal, with which he engages a dialogue. For children, animals serve not only as protectors and guardian angels, but as intimate confidants who are ready to hear every sorrow and

---

[20] Winnicott's concept of holding means safeguarding and maintaining the continuity of the infant's or child's experience of being and being alive over time.

receive all pain, always understanding and alleviating any feelings of distress and grief through their presence and their nonverbal communication, for example, their gaze.[21] According to Winnicott [114] personalization of an imaginary companion is an important part of the development of the self. "…this very primitive and magical creation of imaginary companions is easily used as a defense, as it magically bypasses all the anxieties …" (p. 151).

Daydreaming allows children to dissociate from an intolerable reality into their fantasy world. The fantasy creations often have omnipotent character and are expressed repeatedly in playing; they represent symbolic repetitions of preserving and losing to better cope with the traumatic experience. Imaginative fantasy must be differentiated from fantasizing [115]. Fantasy is part of a child's effort to deal with *inner* reality out of creative imagination, which provides meaning and furthers the developmental process. On the opposite side, *fantasizing* is, contrary to creative imagination, leading to omnipotent manipulations of *external* reality.

A child is unable to process a loss without the existence of a parallel new relationship because he is not able to give up the narcissistic gratification, which he seeks on a fantasy level in maintaining his attachment to the lost person. Children are able to express their affects in relation to the loss as well as work through their fantasies, but only according to their development stage. Building a relationship with a new person who satisfies the child's needs is no guarantee that a disinvestment of the lost, beloved person has taken place. Often it is only an attempt to shift the former love to a new person as a defense against a longing pain. Establishing new relationships remains a difficult task, since children have first to mourn their losses of previous bonds before they are able to form new attachments. Accepting the reality of the irretrievable loss is a precondition of grief work. The child's mourning process will be reactivated by inner developmental phases or by external events, necessitating that he resumes his grieving.

Vignette

Prospective adoptive parents ask for a child psychiatric evaluation for her 4 years old daughter Viviane, who arrived recently from South America. The parents describe a little girl who is crazy, sulks and has absences, is unattainable and does not respond; Viviane remains seated for hours, refuses to eat and does not react even to punishments, which go so far as to lock her up in the cellar. She does not want to hear anything about her country of origin. Her brother, biological child of the parents, says, during the family interview, in tears, "we must leave her alone". While the prospective adoptive parents are talking, Viviane plays with a bear; she spanks him, locks him up, because, as she says, he is mean and sulks. The parents tell

---

[21] Of 850 mentally healthy adolescents, 17.6% had an imaginary companion in their childhood. The results of applied psychometric measures showed that these teenagers experience a high degree of psychological distress, especially with regard to social interaction, feel emotionally vulnerable and utilize immature defense mechanisms such as projection, passive aggression and acting out in stressful situation [113].

Viviane: "You behaved like that in South America, but now, living with us, you can no longer present this behavior."

Comment

The parents negatively comment Viviane's earlier behavior and apparently wish to erase Viviane's past. The girl's depressive state and the fact that she does not want to hear about her country of origin, are the expression of her immense pain and sadness with regard to her losses. Through her massive opposition and refusal behavior she shows her anger and rage. Viviane demonstrates that she is not ready or willing to build up a relationship with her adoptive parents who respond by rejecting her behavior, which they claim being related to her past. Simultaneously Viviane is able to maintain loyalty ties with her past. The parents delineate her child as sick in her head and crazy. Only when significant relationships between the adoptive parents and Viviane are established, she will be able to begin mourning her losses and gradually give up her behavior.

Vignette

Lea, 9 years old, has been in the care of her adoptive family for the last 2 years; a child psychiatrist evaluation is required because of her repetitive forgetfulness and difficulty to learn reading and calculating. Lea forgets even own pleasures.

During the session Lea does not want to talk about her past experiences and says that her 2 years old brother has it much easier since he does not remember anything.

Comment

In her effort to forget the memories of her past, Lea tends to forget everything and is therefore unable to acquire any knowledge. She defends herself against a mourning process, as she fears that working through her losses will be far too painful.

Various authors observed that older children's capacity to build positive attachments in their adoptive family is connected with their ability to recount previous relationship and to share with their adoptive parents their lived feelings [116–118]. There are controverse opinions about the necessity of mourning previous relationships; some authors suppose that a final disinvestment of past ties is not necessary, (un)conscious forgetting being sufficient for memories not to interfere with the formation of new attachments to adoptive parents. Eagle [119] postulates that adoptive children are capable of building new emotional bonds while simultaneously maintaining persistent ties to their birth parents. Other authors estimate that children have first to grieve their losses from previous attachments before they are able to establish new relationships [120, 121]. The question of how long grieving is necessary remains unanswered [122], as mourning takes place individually, at different times, at its own rhythm and with varying degrees of completeness. This hypothesis is confirmed by adopted children, adolescents and even adults who—at the transition of a life period or during critical experiences—are again confronted with their adoption situation and then resume mourning.

Adoptees' grieving is complicated by their past experienced traumatization, but also by the incertitude about life or death of their birth parents and the absence of biologically related persons. Mourning can only be fulfilled when there is certainty about the death of the significant person. Reality testing thus is an essential part of grief. Mourning proves to be necessary, not only for the child's ability to continue his developmental process, but also to avoid that he re-enacts his traumatic past events and thereby experiences additional traumatization.

For many adopted children however, mourning does not take place. They deny the loss and maintain the bond with their birth parents on a fantasy level [123]. Their life happens in the past, in a very hidden way. They dialogue with the lost parent or imagine, before falling asleep, that birth mother or father are present, holding them in their arms; they tell them all their misfortunes and pray for them to God.

They fantasize a reunion with the lost parent to whom all their love is devoted. This helps the child to alleviate the painful loss of parental love and to maintain a much-needed narcissistic gratification. The emotional significance of the internal parental representation does not diminish, but on the contrary parental representations are idealized and overinvested. The denial of the loss of a parent exists simultaneously with the conscious and correct knowledge of the reality of the loss (Freud 1927–1931). If these children allow themselves to begin mourning, they must give up the hope of finding again a birth parent and being able to (re)establish a relationship with him. Information or knowledge are rarely available from absent or dead parent and there are no witnesses or testimony from family members with memories of the lost parent, no funeral, and no grave. Therefore, mourning for these children is impaired as the loss cannot be perceived and recognized as permanent and irrevocable. "It is only when the loss has been acknowledged and the mourning experienced that re-creation can take place" ([124]: p. 199).

Vignette

Alisha, a dark-skinned Asian girl of about 9 years (the date of her birth is not known) is addressed by the adoptive mother for a child psychiatric evaluation because of her reading- and writing difficulties; she attends the second-year elementary school.

Alisha expresses in projective materials such as squiggels, scenotest[22] and drawings her feelings of longing, homesickness, grief, anger, sadness, loneliness, and helplessness, associated with her adoption situation.

She remembers the moment when her birth mother took her to the institution, from where she was later adopted. She didn't understand what happened to her, she only wanted to stay with her mother. Today she wishes to ask her mother questions and to swap places with her older sister; she desires living with her mother in her country of origin, while her older sister stays with her adoptive parents. Alisha has an only wish: to be reunited with her mother and sister. She tries to love her birth mother and her adoptive parents the same way, she says, as she does not want to hurt

---

[22] The Scenotest by G. von Staabs is a projective instrument employed for diagnostic and therapeutic purposes. The standardized material of this test procedure is composed of flexible human figures and accessories: animals, trees, symbolic figures, and items from everyday life. The Scenotest arouses the natural desire to play, reveals unconscious thoughts in a non-stressful way, and the many figures offer patients the opportunity to relive their own experiences.

anybody, but this is very hard. At school, she often feels excluded from classmates because of her appearance, which reveals her adoption.

Alisha tells her repetitive nightmare in which her birth mother is imprisoned. She worries that her mother might be sick. She herself suffers from multiple fears: dying from an accident on the road, drowning in the sea, falling from a plane or ship, being stolen by a thief. Alisha desires to be 4 years old; at this age, she says, one does not die so soon. She would prefer being a boy, boys are much stronger and can defend themselves better.

Comment

Alisha—in dreaming that her mother is imprisoned or fearing, she might be sick— expresses an unconscious wish for her mother to be punished for having abandoned her; at the same time her fears of dying represent her anxiety to be punished for her aggressive feelings towards her birth mother.

The intense mourning of her losses (of biological parents, extended family members: siblings, grandparents, as well as her country of origin with cultural, ethnic, linguistic ties) represents a continuous stressful situation for Alisha, aggravated by her loyalty conflicts and non-admitted rejection of her adoption. Her wish to be 4 years old (Alisha lived the loss of her mother at the age of four, the moment when she was brought to the institution) shows the need of Alisha to go back to the moment of her traumatization—the breakup with her birth mother —, which would allow her to resume her development and permit her to "read and write" her biographical story.

Vignette

"I cannot accept the fact that my (biological) mother died, I do not want to believe that she is no longer alive; there is no reason for it. I have no explanation and I cannot ask God, or only when I am dead". Nine-year-old Emmanuel wants to return to the past to see his mother once more.

Grieving is also so hard, because children, who do not have contact with biological parents, are unable to explain why they were abandoned, felt as being rejected. They often ask the same question: why have *I* been abandoned, what is my otherness, my fault that my mother did not want to take care of me? The child is not satisfied with answers that explain the context, e.g., situations of war or poverty. The idea of having been rejected, given away, is associated with very painful, even unbearable feelings, as the statements of adoptees testify [125, 126].

Psychic Manifestations Due to Losses

Adopted children often manifest depressive symptoms in contexts, which are not related to the adoption situation. They confide in an animated object, e.g., a stuffed animal or a pet, and engage a dialogue. The animal serves as a kind of bond to the lost caregiver, is a confident, giving sympathy and reassurance. Children's desperate states of grief may suddenly be expressed through a crying crisis, e.g., when a beloved pet falls ill or the child suffers even a minor injury. If feelings of grief are suppressed, mourning can shift to the physical level and may manifest itself in somatic complaints.

Adopted children aged 8–12 years, for whom the loss of their biological parents was associated with pronounced negative feelings, showed higher levels of depression, and rated their self-worth lower than children for whom the loss of their biological parents was associated with fewer negative feelings [127].

The usually unconscious aggressive emotions towards the lost caregiver are caused by feelings of having been abandoned and rejected and are expressed in aggressive and destructive behavior towards the adoptive parents who are often blamed for the loss, since these emotions cannot be directed against the lost birth parents. Anger and rage are also manifested by destructive activities in playing, which allows to deny the strong feelings of guilt. The child's presumed guilt is to have caused the death or loss and therefore to deserve punishment and death.

Thoughts of death or even suicide attempts arise from fantasied wishes to be reunited with the lost parent, feared already dead; the desire to die may also express the need to be punished. Severe illness, injury, and separation are equivalent to death or loss, and in all these situations, the child is afraid of dying or wishes to die. These are excessive identifications, which lead to pathological consequences. Loss may become the core around which various conflicts crystallize.

Upon the death or loss of a parent, a child is deprived of his fundamental identificatory references. A child may fight against identification with a sick or lost mother; if it is a girl, she may behave like a boy and express her wish to become a father. Smaller children, contrariwise, may identify with the lost loved person and become ill like their mother or father. Some children identify with death as a person (personification) and not with the deceased person. They develop fears that death will call upon them or that the dead parent may come back for revenge; this is the way children express their phantasms of retaliation.

There is no secret that is not, in its origin, a shared one (Abraham 1987: p. 254).

Pathological Grief and Secret

The distinction between normal and pathological grief is complex and controversial. There is pathological grief when mourning is delayed, particularly long, unusually grave, suppressed, or even nonexistent. The assessment of pathological grief in children must consider the circumstances of the loss, the grieving process, subsequent events, and the personal developmental changes. Generally, one can speak of pathological mourning when the child expresses sadness in behavior and symptoms that—according to his level of development—can no longer be considered as an appropriate response to the loss. For a small child, this is the case when there is a breakdown of already acquired functions, such as walking or talking, or the loss of affect, i.e., an inability to respond emotionally, or a persistent regression, i.e., a return to earlier behavior and modes of experience. The preschool child and the child in latency may present a behavior of retreat, or a depressive state, or the abandonment of pleasurable functions or skills. In adolescence, the inability to accomplish mourning can seriously affect the engagement of relationships or learning processes [128].

A traumatic experience of a loss of a family member, which could not be processed and overcome, often represents the starting point for the development of family secrets. Such critical events are related to the parent-child bond or to the death of a significant person. A secret always arises in a meaningful relationship and is a shared experience [29]. The formation of a family secret seems to be comparable to the creation of a "void," a hidden space in the mind of an individual, which is subsequently often filled with bizarre intrapsychic fantasies [27].

In painful loss situations, such as breakups of relationships or origins, the child records and "integrates" a "picture" of the moment of the event and the persons involved, as well as their emotions the child perceived, together with his associated feelings of shock, fear, pain, anger, guilt, and shame. A child or adolescent may, under certain circumstances, later identify with these stored memories or express associated fantasies or feelings again [129].

A child has no organized representation of traumatic experiences occurring in early childhood, but they leave sensorimotor traces. Repression capacities or mental processing in infancy are insufficiently formed. Under certain circumstances, especially in adolescence, the traces of these events are re-actualized, expressed as somatic or motor manifestations, experienced as intense feeling states, or acted out as emotional outbursts. Events, which can mentally not be adequately represented, risk merging with the subject's archaic fantasies and fears [129].

The presence of a secret involves any meaningful relationship, where an individual depends on another person, as in the case of a child on his parents, or in a love relationship. The affective experience in the personal history of an individual is in such cases re-actualized. The reactivation harbors the hope that the meaningful person, for example, a parent, will open the secret, explain its meaning, and help the child to understand its importance.

When painful or violent situations of loss such as relationship-breakups are silenced in the family, and the child receives no help to cope with such an event, his emotional resonance will be partly cleaved or encapsulated so that the child does not perceive feelings of shock, fear, pain, anger, and shame associated with the event. At a later point in his life, a child or adolescent may again feel and sometimes express these emotions, which have been changed by the process of retrospective attribution. They are first felt as strange, sometimes even as a foreign body. "Enigmatic message" is "a perplexing and impenetrable implicit communication that is overloaded with significance. Such messages implant themselves as foreign bodies, haunting questions in the child's psyche" ([130]: p. 242).

According to Diatkine [131], a family secret leads to intellectual inhibition when a child incorporates the crypts of a parent who denies the loss of a loved person. Under these conditions, the child is not stimulated by the secret. On the contrary, such inherited mental representations oblige the child not to know and forbid him even to think.

Our memories are the fragile but powerful products of what we recall from the past, believe about the present and imagine about the future ([132]: p. 308).

Intra- or Transgenerational Transmission of Traumatic Events

Parents' biographical history cannot be dissociated from the child's personal history. Under certain conditions, the impact of critical events or psychic trauma can be transmitted from one generation to another. What happened in the parents' past is transmitted to the child and becomes his actual reality. Transgenerational and unconscious conflictual patterns of the child's parents or primary caregivers are internalized by the child, through his identification with their emotional experience. Thus, the history of earlier generations can be transmitted like a cultural heritage; this is particularly true when the mourning of losses never ends and the non-elaborated past of family members becomes the presence for their children, impacting their sense of time and continuity of being. A child's individual psychic traumatic experience may lead—especially in a psychotherapeutic process—to recognize an intergenerationally transmitted traumatic event.

Numerous authors studied the transmission of traumata and losses through the process of identification including Abraham and Torok [29] who speak of "endocryptic identification", Faimberg [31] of "telescoping", Kestenberg [133] of "transposition", Kogan [134] of "concretization", and Oliner [135] of "hysterical identification".

Abraham and Torok [29] contrast "introjection," a process that enriches the self, endowing it with certain features of the lost person, with "incorporation", the fantasy having ingested an external object, which is felt to be physically present inside the body. Incorporation functions according to the pleasure principle and the magic of hallucinatory wish-fulfillment. There is incorporation whenever loss is denied. The inclusion of another being through the process of "incorporation" turns the subject into a "crypt carrier".

Communication from unconscious to unconscious[23] [29, 30] takes place in the earliest preverbal interactions (whose variables are of tactile, visual, auditory, or of sensorimotor nature) between infant/toddler and the primary caregiver. Nonintegrated, unprocessed traumatic experiences of a parent can be passively transmitted by unconscious, nonverbal forms of communication to the child [30]. Through identification with life experiences of persons from the previous generations, the child unconsciously assumes intrapsychic, transgenerational conflict configurations [31]. These identifications are often alienating.

In the *adoption situation* unintegrated, unprocessed traumatic experiences of a biological or adoptive parent are transferred to the child by unconscious, non-verbal forms of communication; through identification processes the child incorporates the split-off parts of the parental representations into his own self-representation. The motivation of a birth mother to give her child up for adoption, or the one of prospective adoptive parents to adopt a child, may be related to critical events in their personal life history.

---

[23] As part of intersubjective processes, two minds transmit and receive unconscious messages.

In pathological grief—according to the theories of Abraham and Torok [29]—a person affected by a traumatically experienced loss of a love object—is not able to fulfill mourning; he then is a bearer of a secret crypt or enclave, which he sets up inside himself by incorporating the lost love object. Incorporation fantasies preserve a narcissistically and libidinally irreplaceable object, for example a parent or a child whose sudden loss must be radically denied. Incorporation fantasies keep the lost person in a state of dead-alive or dead-dying person.

However, if a parent is a crypt carrier, his child is at risk to develop symptoms, he may for example suffer from fears of monsters, phantoms, ghosts—which also appear in nightmares—and from sleep disorders, phobias, learning difficulties and memory disorders; he is a phantom carrier. The phantom is the unconscious processing of an unacknowledged secret of another significant person. The child's play represents not only the symbolic enactment of his own drive impulses and unconscious elements, but also secret suffering and hidden fears or anxieties of his parents. The child symbolizes what he is not able to understand and what he is incapable to name. Sometimes there is an enacting in play scenes, which represent a kind of phantasmatic solution to the parental burden; the child may suffer from serious psychic and intellectual inhibition. The clinical manifestations result from the child's psychic stress, his coping and processing attempts, combined with his hope to understand the parent and in turn to be better understood and loved by his parents. Simultaneously the child seeks to fill a void in his fundamental representations.

Vignette

Two orphaned and adopted siblings were referred for child psychiatric evaluation; their personal history revealed that Sandra, a nine-year-old girl and Andrew, her eleven-year-old brother, were abandoned by their birthmother, and shortly afterwards their birthfather was killed. Both the boy (referred for behavioral and psychosomatic disorders) and the girl (suffering from severe learning disorders despite good intelligence) shared these events in an individual initial interview. The children were integrated into different, psychoanalytical psychodrama group therapy.

Sandra suggests playing the story of a boy who is always hungry and wants to eat. During the psychodrama—play, Sandra, who assigned the role of the boy to someone else, explained what happened to the boy: "He was so hungry that he ate his mother, killed and lost her. Therefore, he is an orphan, always hungry and must eat."

Comment

Sandra's phantasms reveal that she has incorporated her mother and nourishes her but remains forever insatiable. Sandra maintains a loyal, vampire-like fantasy-bond with her biological mother.

Andrew repeatedly proposes stories involving violent death and chooses the role of the one who dies or is dead.

The adoptive father informs the psychotherapists that Andrew, sick with influenza, cried and screamed in his arms for hours, telling him that he is going to be killed and that he wants to die.

Comment

Andrew's play scenes show his identification with his murdered biological father and his extreme fear to suffer the same fate.

Sandra's symptom points to an encapsulated grief [136]. Incorporation fantasies assume that thoughts, feelings, ideas, or persons can be incorporated like objects into the body in a magical way. Incorporation fantasies tend to maintain—inside the subject—the lost loved person in a strange state between dead and alive. The actual fate of the person and the reality of the loss are denied.

The examples show that Sandra maintains her loyal bond to the lost loved person, her birth mother, in a state of an alive person, feeding her, while Andrew maintains his fantasy bond to his murdered father in a state of an ever-again dying person. Both incorporation fantasies allow a continuous connection to a loved person of whom the subject does not need to separate. The pain of the missing person is in this way alleviated. The subject does not have to admit the real pain of his narcissistic injury, which cannot heal.

Vignette

Oliver, an eleven-year-old adopted boy, acts his oral greed and aggressiveness compulsively in eating paper, rubber, Lego parts; he describes himself as an omnivore. The question arises, if Oliver was not able to mourn the loss of his biological parents, his country of origin, his ethnic, racial and language roots; his acting-out (incorporation of objects) points to an encapsulated grief: Oliver "feeds" his lost love objects, which he has incorporated in a secret enclave in the interior of his (body) self but remains always insatiable [29].

Clinical experience shows that adopted children often adapt to a great extent to their adoptive family. Intensive feelings to be abandoned and rejected again by adoptive parents lead to survival strategies. Psychic breakdowns happen usually during adolescence and suicide attempts are not uncommon. Adolescence is the time for individuation, separation, and detachment processes from parents; adoptees are simultaneously confronted with unresolved, unprocessed losses from their childhood.

In these often-tormenting transition period, adoptive parents and adopted adolescents may have the painful sensation not to be related by strong and sustaining affective ties. The adolescent is legally adopted but does not feel himself or herself as son or daughter of his or her adoptive family; he or she has remained a stranger and has maintained fantasized ties to his or her original family.

"I never considered my adoptive parents as my parents", adolescents may say, while their parents state: "We adopted a child, but he is not our son". The loneliness and emotional gap due to pre-existing injuries deepen. If healing is possible, it will be a long and distressing process resulting in the adolescent choosing the adoptive parents as *his* or *her* parents. Adoption takes place in these situations at two different times and is a mutual recognition of emotional belonging, i.e., adoptees adopt their adoptive parents in return. Adolescents need to have previously worked through their anger of not having been asked if they agreed to be adopted.

In certain adoptive families, processes of separation and detachment do not take place. Neither adoptive parents nor adopted children ever plan to part or leave; disengagement is avoided out of mutually unconscious fear of an individual, and/or a family breakdown [62].

References

1. Donovan DM, McIntyre D. Healing the hurt child. A developmental-contextual approach. New York: Norton; 1990.
2. Udwin O. Annotation: Children's reactions to traumatic events. J Child Psychol Psychiatry. 1993;34(2):115–27.
3. Kirk GS, Raven JE, Schofield M. Die vorsokratischen Philosophen. Einführung, Texte und Kommentare. Stuttgart, Weimar: Verlag J.B. Metzler; 1994.
4. Steck B. Psychisches Trauma und Trauerprozess beim Kind. Schweiz Archiv für Neurologie und Psychiatrie. 2003;154(1):37–41.
5. Laplanche J, Pontalis JB. The language of psychoanalysis. New York: Norton; 1973.
6. Fischer G, Riedesser P. Lehrbuch der Psychotraumatologie. München/Basel: E. Reinhardt; 1999.
7. Van der Kolk BA, Alexander C, McFarlane AC, Weisaeth L. Traumatic stress: the effects of overwhelming experience on mind, body, and society. New York: Guilford Press; 2007.
8. Kozlowska K, Walker P, McLean L, Carrive P. Fear and the defense cascade: clinical implications and management. Harv Rev Psychiatry. 2015;23(4):263–87.
9. D'Andrea W, Ford J, Stolbach B, Spinazzola J, van der Kolk BA. Understanding interpersonal trauma in children: why we need a developmentally appropriate trauma diagnosis. Am J Orthopsychiatry. 2012;82(2):187–200. https://doi.org/10.1111/j.1939-0025.2012.01154.x.
10. van Der Kolk BA, Ford JD, Spinazzola J. Comorbidity of developmental trauma disorder (DTD) and post-traumatic stress disorder: findings from the DTD field trial. Eur J Psychotraumatol. 2019;10(1):1562841. https://doi.org/10.1080/20008198.2018.1562841.
11. Spinazzola J, van der Kolk B, Ford JD. When nowhere is safe: interpersonal trauma and attachment adversity as antecedents of posttraumatic stress disorder and developmental trauma disorder. J Trauma Stress. 2018;31:631–42.
12. Van der Kolk BA, Pynoos RS, Cicchetti D, Cloitre M, D'Andrea W, Ford JD, Lieberman AF, Putnam FW, Saxe G, Spinazzola J, Stolbach BC, Teicher M (2009): Proposal to include a developmental trauma disorder diagnosis for children and adolescents in DSM-V.
13. Cruz D, Lichten M, Berg K, George P. Developmental trauma: conceptual framework, associated risks and comorbidities, and evaluation and treatment. Front Psych. 2022;13:800687. https://doi.org/10.3389/fpsyt.2022.800687.
14. Janet P. Psychological healing. New York: Macmillan; 1919/1925.
15. Freud S. New introductory lectures on psychoanalysis and other works, Standard edition, vol. XXII. London: Hogarth Press; 1932–1936.
16. Freud S. Analysis terminable and interminable. Int J Psychoanal. 1937;18:373–405.
17. Freud S. Moses and monotheism. An outline of psychoanalysis and other works, Standard edition, vol. XXIII. London: Hogarth Press; 1937–1939.
18. Modell AH. Other times, other realities. Toward a theory of psychoanalytic treatment. Cambridge: Harvard University Press; 1990.
19. Freud S. Project for a scientific psychology, vol. I. SE London: Hogarth Press; 1895.
20. Freud S. Studies on hysteria, Standard edition, vol. II. London: Hogarth Press; 1895.

21. Freud S. Further remarks on the neuro-psychoses of defense, Standard edition, vol. 3. London: Hogarth Press and the Institute of Psychoanalysis; 1962/1896.
22. Haynal A. L'histoire du concept de traumatisme et sa signification actuelle. In: le bloc-notes de la psychanalyse, Nr., vol. 8; 1988. p. 149–60.
23. Winnicott DW. The maturational processes and the facilitating environment: studies in the theory of emotional development. Int Psycho-Anal Library. 1965;64:1–276. London: The Hogarth Press and the Institute of Psychoanalysis.
24. Winnicott DW. The concept of the healthy individual. In: Winnicott DW, editor. Home is where we start from; 1986.
25. Shengold L. Soul murder. The effects of childhood abuse and deprivation. New Haven, London: Yale University Press; 1989.
26. Nathan T. Trauma et Mémoire. In: Métamorphose de l'identité. Nouvelle Revue d'Ethnopsychiatrie; 1986. p. 7–18.
27. Khan M. Le concept de traumatisme cumulatif. Distorsion du Moi, traumatisme cumulatif et reconstruction dans la situation analytique. In: le soi caché. Paris: Gallimard; 1976.
28. Barrois C. Les névroses traumatiques. Paris: Dunod; 1988.
29. Abraham N, Torok M. The shell and the kernel: renewals of psychoanalysis. Chicago: University of Chicago Press; 1994.
30. Nachin C. Les fantômes de l'âme. A propos des héritages psychiques. Paris: Editions l'Harmattan; 1993.
31. Faimberg H. The telescoping of generations. In: Birksted-Breen D, editor. The new library of psychoanalysis. London/New York: Routledge; 2005.
32. Van der Kolk BA, McFarlane AC, Weisaeth L. Traumatic stress. New York: Guilford Press; 1996.
33. Price BH, Adams RD, Coyle JT. Neurology and psychiatry, closing the great divide. Neurology. 2000;54:8–14.
34. Damasio A. Descartes' error: emotion, reason, and the human brain; 1995
35. Winnicott DW. Fear of breakdown. Int Review of Psycho-Analysis. 1974;1(1-2):103–7.
36. Bremner J, Narayan M. The effects of stress on memory and the hippocampus throughout the life cycle: implications for childhood development and aging. Dev Psychopathol. 1998;10:871–85.
37. Glaser D. Child abuse and neglect and the brain—a review. J Child Psychol Psychiatry. 2000;41:97–116.
38. Kaufman J, Plotsky PM, Nemeroff CB, Charney DS. Effects of early adverse experiences on brain structure and function: clinical implications. Biol Psychiatry. 2000;48:778–90.
39. Van der Kolk BA, Roth S, Pelcovitz D, Sunday S, Spinazzola J. Disorders of extreme stress: the empirical foundation of a complex adaptation to trauma. J Trauma Stress. 2005;18(5):389–99.
40. Le Doux J. The emotional brain. New York: Simon and Schuster; 1996.
41. Solms M, Turnbull O. The brain and the inner world. New York: Other Press; 2002.
42. LeDoux JE. Emotion circuits in the brain. Annu Rev Neurosci. 2000;23:155–84.
43. Pillemer DB. What is remembered about early childhood events? Clin Psychol Rev. 1998;18(8):895–913.
44. Van der Kolk BA. Zur Psychologie und Psychobiologie von Kindheitstraumata. Praxis Kinderpsychologie und Kinderpsychiatrie. 1998;1:19–35.
45. Weder N, Kaufman J. Critical periods revisited: implications for intervention with traumatized children. J Am Acad Child Adolesc Psychiatry. 2011;50(11):1087–9.
46. Weder N, Zhang H, Jensen K, Yang BZ, Simen A, Jackowski A, Lipschitz D, et al. Child abuse, depression, and methylation in genes involved with stress, neural plasticity, and brain circuitry. J Am Acad Child Adolesc Psychiatry. 2014;53(4):417–24.
47. Kaufman J, Yang BZ, Douglas-Palumberi H, Houshyar S, Lipschitz D, Krystal JH, Gelernter J. Social supports and serotonin transporter gene moderate depression in maltreated children. Proc Natl Acad Sci U S A. 2004;101(49):17316–21. https://doi.org/10.1073/pnas.0404376101.

48. Kaufman J, Gelernter J, Hudziak JJ, Tyrka AR, Coplan JD. The research domain criteria (RDoC) project and studies of risk and resilience in maltreated children. J Am Acad Child Adolesc Psychiatry. 2015;54(8):617–25. https://doi.org/10.1016/j.jaac.2015.06.001. Epub 2015 Jun 10

49. Nemeroff CB, Binder E. The preeminent role of childhood abuse and neglect in vulnerability to major psychiatric disorders: toward elucidating the underlying neurobiological mechanisms. J Am Acad Child Adolesc Psychiatry. 2014;53(4):395–7.

50. Turner HA, Finkelhor D, Ormrod R, Sewanee SH, Leeb RT, Mercy JA. Family context, victimization, and child trauma symptoms: variations in safe, stable, and nurturing relationships during early and middle childhood. Am J Orthopsychiatry. 2012;82(2):209–19.

51. Cloitre M, Stolbach BC, Herman JL, van der Kolk B, Pynoos R, Wang J. Developmental approach to complex PTSD: childhood and adult cumulative trauma as predictors of symptom complexity. J Trauma Stress. 2009;22(5):399–408. https://doi.org/10.1002/jts.20444.

52. Van der Kolk BA. Psychological trauma. American Psychiatric Press; 1987.

53. Rajaprakash M, Kerr E, Friedlander B, Weiss S. Sleep disorders in a sample of adopted children: a pilot study. Children MDPI; 2017.

54. Winnicott DW. Therapeutic consultations in child psychiatry. London: Hogarth; 1971.

55. Terr L. Remembered images and trauma: a psychology of the supernatural. Psychoanal Study Child. 1985;40

56. Steck B. Anmerkung zum intrafamilialen Trauma beim Kind. Schweiz. Archiv für Neurologie und Psychiatrie. 1997;148(6):229–38.

57. Colon F. The family and child placement practices. Fam Process. 1978;17(3)

58. Lifton BJ. Forward; in Benet MK: the politics of adoption. New York: Free Press; 1976. p. 2–3.

59. Trisiliotis J. In search of origins: the experiences of adopted people. London, Boston: Routledge and Kegan Paul; 1973.

60. Cifali M. Le traumatisme du nourrisson savant. Les traumatismes psychiques. 1993;12:7–22.

61. Ferenczi S. The confusion of tongues between adults and children. Int J Psychoanal. 1949;30:225–30.

62. Waber-Thevoz H, Waber JP. Le lien d'adoption à l'épreuve du temps. Neuropsychiatrie de l' Enfance et l'Adolescence. 2000;48:179–98.

63. Bürgin D. Children—war and persecution. In: Proceedings of the Congress in Stiftung für Kinder, Hamburg, 1993, Sept 26–29.

64. Winnicott DW. The child and the outside world. London: Tavistock Publ; 1957.

65. Bertocci D, Schechter MD. Adopted adults' perception of their need to search: implications for clinical practice. Smith Coll Stud Soc Work. 1991;61:179–96.

66. Brodzinsky DM. A stress and coping model of adoption adjustment. In: Brodzinsky DM, Schechter MD, editors. (1990) the psychology of adoption. New York: Oxford Press; 1990. p. 3–24.

67. Hersov L, Rutter M. Adoption: modern approaches. Oxford: Blackwell Scient. Publ; 1976. p. 136–62.

68. Stierlin H, Levi D, Savard RJ. Parental perceptions of separating children. Fam Process. 1971;10:411–27.

69. Kaudal ER, Jessel T. Early experience and the fine tuning of synaptic connections. In: Kaudal ER, Schwartz JH, Jessel TM, editors. Principles of neural science. New York: Elsevier; 1991. p. 945–58.

70. Cirulli F, Alleva E. The NGF saga: from animal models of psychosocial stress to stress-related psychopathology. Front Neuroendocrinol. 2009;30(3):379–95. https://doi.org/10.1016/j.yfrne.2009.05.002.

71. Heinrichs M, Baumgartner T, Kirschbaum C, Ehlert U. Social support and oxytocin interact to suppress cortisol and subjective responses to psychosocial stress. Biol Psychiatry. 2003;54(12):1389–98.

72. Anzieu D. The skin ego. New Haven: Yale University Press; 1989.

73. Anzieu D. Lost for words: difficulty expressing feelings in work with three adolescent boys. J Child Psychother. 1984;38(1):32–48. https://doi.org/10.1080/0075417X.2011.651842. 873/1989:102) in Tyminski R (2012)

74. Tyminski R. Lost for words: difficulty expressing feelings in work with three adolescent boys. Journal of Child Psychotherapy. 2012;38(1):32–48. https://doi.org/10.108 0/0075417X.2011.651842.

75. Kossowsky J, Monique PHD, Pfaltz C, Schneider S, Taeymans J, Locher C, Gaab J. The separation anxiety hypothesis of panic disorder revisited: a meta-analysis. Am J Psychiatry. 2012;AiA:1–14.

76. Schore A. Early organization of the nonlinear right brain and development of a predisposition to psychiatric disorders. Dev Psychopathol. 1997;9:595–631.

77. Cohen MR, Pickar D, Dubois M, Bunney WE Jr. Stress-induced plasma beta-endorphin immunoreactivity may predict postoperative morphine usage. Psychiatry Res. 1982;6(1):7–12.

78. Abercrombie E, Jacobs B. Systemic naloxone administration potentiated locus coeruleus noradrenergic neuronal activity under stressful but not non-stressful conditions. Brain Res. 1988;441:362–6.

79. Green AH. Self-destructive behaviour in battered children. Amer J Psychiatry. 1978;135(5):579–82.

80. Green AH. Child maltreatment and its victims. A comparison of physical and sexual abuse. Psychiatr Clin North Am. 1988;11(4):591–610.

81. Perry BD, Pollard RA, Blakley WL, Baker WL, Viglante D. Childhood trauma: the neurobiology of adaptation and use-dependent development of the brain. Infant Ment Health J. 1995;

82. Volkow ND, Fowler JS, Wang GJ, Goldstein RZ. Role of dopamine, the frontal cortex and memory, circuits in drug addiction: insight from imaging studies. Neurobiol Learn Mem. 2002;78(3):610–24.

83. Volkow N, Li TK. The neuroscience of addiction. Nat Neurosci. 2005;8:1429–30.

84. Green AH. Dimension of psychological trauma in abused children. J Am Acad Child Psychiat. 1983;22:231–7.

85. Finkelhor D, Ormrod RK, Turner HA. Lifetime assessment of poly-victimization in a national sample of children and youth. Child Abuse Negl. 2009;33(7):403–11. https://doi.org/10.1016/j.chiabu.2008.09.012.

86. Gaensbauer TJ, Sands K. Distorted affective communications in abused/neglected infants and their potential impact on caretakers. J Am Acad Child Adolesc Psychiatry. 1979;18:236–50.

87. Krystal H. Trauma and affects. Psychoanal Study Child. 1978;33:81–116.

88. Wilson JP. Trauma transformation and healing. An integrative approach to theory, research and post-traumatic therapy. New York: Brunner and Mazel; 1989.

89. Glover H. Emotional numbing: a possible endorphin-mediated phenomenon associated with post-traumatic stress disorders and other allied psychopathologic states. J Traumatic Stress. 1992;5:4. https://doi.org/10.1002/jts.2490050413.

90. Stierlin H, Rucker-Embden I, Wetzel N, Wirshching M. The first interview with the family. New York: Brunner/Mazel; 1980.

91. de Quervain DJ, Kolassa IT, Ackermann S, Aerni A, Boesiger P, Demougin P, et al. PKCα is genetically linked to memory capacity in healthy subjects and to risk for posttraumatic stress disorder in genocide survivors. Proc Natl Acad Sci U S A. 2012;109(22):8746–51.

92. Jones E, Vermaas RH, McCartney H, Beech C, Palmer I, Hyams K, et al. Flashbacks and posttraumatic stress disorder: the genesis of a 20th-century diagnosis. Br J Psychiatry. 2003;182:158–63.

93. Young A. Our traumatic neurosis and its brain. Sci Context. 2001;14(4):661–83.

94. van der Kolk BA. Clinical implications of neuroscience research in PTSD. Ann N Y Acad Sci. 2006;1071:277–93.

95. Charney DS, Deutch AY, Krystal JH, Southwick SM, Davis M. Psychobiologic mechanisms of posttraumatic stress disorder. Arch Gen Psychiatry. 1993;50(4):295–305. Review

96. Goleman D. A Key to Post-Traumatic Stress Lies in Brain Chemistry. In: Scientists Find. The New York Times; 1990.

97. Thoma MV, Rohner SL, Höltge J. Editorial: assessing the consequences of childhood trauma on behavioral issues and mental health outcomes. Front Psych. 2022;13:1101099. https://doi.org/10.3389/fpsyt.2022.1101099.

98. Landolt MA, Schnyder U, Maier T, Schoenbucher V, Mohler-Kuo M. Trauma exposure and posttraumatic stress disorder in adolescents: a national survey in Switzerland. J Trauma Stress. 2013;26:209–16.
99. Bürgin D, Steck B. Resilienz im Kindes- und Jugendalter [Resiliency in childhood and adolescence]. Schweiz. Arch Neurol Psychiatr. 2008;159:480–9.
100. Steck A, Steck B. Brain and mind, subjective experience and scientific Ob-jectivity. New York: Springer; 2016.
101. Rutter M. Resilience as a dynamic concept. Dev Psychopathol. 2012;24(2):335–44. https://doi.org/10.1017/S0954579412000028.
102. Welter-Enderlin R, Hildenbrand B, Heraus geber. Resilienz—Gedeihen trotz widriger Umstände. Heidelberg: Carl-Auer; 2008.
103. Luthar SS, Cicchetti D. The construct of resilience: implications for interventions and social policies. Review. Dev Psychopathol. 2000;12(4):857–85.
104. Tedeschi RG, Park CI, Calhoun LG. Posttraumatic growth: conceptual issues. In: Tedeschi RG, Park CI, Calhoun LG, editors. Posttraumatic growth: positive changes in the aftermath of crisis. Mahwah, NY/London: Lawrence Erlbaum; 1998.
105. Schwartz CE, Kunwar PS, Greve DN, Kagan J, Snidman NC, Bloch RB. A phenotype of early infancy predicts reactivity of the amygdala in male adults. Mol Psychiatry. 2012;17(10):1042–50.
106. Silk JS, Vanderbilt-Adriance E, Shaw DS, Forbes EE, Whalen DJ, Ryan ND, et al. Resilience among children and adolescents at risk for depression: mediation and moderation across social and neurobiological contexts. Review. Dev Psychopathol. 2007;19(3):841–65.
107. Compas BE. Psychobiological processes of stress and coping. Implications for resilience in children and adolescents—comments on the papers of Romeo & McEwen and Fisher et al. Ann N Y Acad Sci. 2006;1094:226–34.
108. Greenacre P. The childhood of the artist. Psychoanal Study Child. 1957;12:47–72. New York: International Universities Press.
109. Greenacre P. Discussion and comments on the psychology of creativity. J Am Acad Child Psychiatry. 1962;1(1):129–37.
110. Shakespeare W. The tragedy of Macbeth; 1623.
111. Freud S. An autobiographical study, inhibitions, symptoms and anxiety, the question of lay analysis and other works, Standard edition, vol. XX. London: Hogarth Press; 1925–1926.
112. Sekaer C. Toward a definition of "childhood mourning". Am J Psychother. 1987;XLI(2):201–19.
113. Bohman M, Sigvardsson S. Outcome in adoption: lessons from longitudinal studies. In: Brodzinsky DM, Schechter MD, editors. The psychology of adoption. Oxford University Press; 1990. p. 93–106.
114. Winnicott DW. Collected papers: through paediatrics to psychoanalysis. 1st ed. London: Tavistock; 1958.
115. Colombi L. The dual aspect of fantasy: flight from reality or imaginative realm? Considerations and hypotheses from clinical psychoanalysis. Int J Psychoanal. 2010;91(5):1073–91.
116. Kadushin A. Adopting older children. New York: Columbia University Press; 1970.
117. Nickman SL. The adoption experience: losses in adoption. Psychoanal Study Child. 1985;40:365–98.
118. Rosenberg EB. The adoption life cycle: the children and their families through the years. New York: Free Press; 1992.
119. Eagle RS. The separation experience of children in long-term care. Am Orthopsychiatr Assoc. 1994;64(3):421–34.
120. Kates WA, Johnson RL, Kader MW, Grieder FH. Whose child is this? Assessment and treatment of children in foster care. Am J Orthopsychiatry. 1991;61:584–91.
121. Steinnhauer P. How to succeed in the business of creating psychopaths without even trying. In: Dawson R, editor. Training resources in understanding, supporting and treating abused

children, vol. 1. Toronto: Ministry of Community and Social Services, Children's Services Division; 1979. p. 153–94.

122. Stroebe M, Gergen MM, Gurgen KJ, Stroebe W. Broken hearts of broken bonds: love and death in historical perspective. Am Psychol. 1992;47:1205–12.

123. Manzano J. La séparation et la perte d'object chez l'enfant. Une point de vue sur le processus analytique. Rev Franç Psychoanal. 1989;1:241–72.

124. Segal H. A psycho-analytical approach to aesthetics. Int J Psychoanal. 1952;33:196–207.

125. Delfieu F., De Gravelaine J. Parole d'adopté. Résponses, R. Laffont; 1988.

126. Schärer R. Adoptiert. Lebensgeschichten ohne Anfang. Muri bei Bern: Cosmos; 1991.

127. Smith SD, Grigorenko E, Willcutt E, Pennington BF, Olson RK, DeFries JC. Etiologies and molecular mechanisms of communication disorders. J Dev Behav Pediatr. 2010;31(7):555–63.

128. Bürgin D, Steck B. Indikation psychoanalytischer Psychotherapie bei Kindern und Jugendlichen. In: Diagnostisch-therapeutisches Vorgehen und Fallbeispiele. Stuttgart: Klett-Cotta; 2013. ISBN 978-3-608-94829-5.

129. Tisseron S. Tintin et les secrets de famille. Paris: Aubier; 1992.

130. Laplanche J. Essays on otherness. London: Routledge; 1999.

131. Diatkine G. Chasseurs de fantômes, dans: le secret sur les origines; problèmes psychologiques, légaux, administratifs. Paris: Editions ESF; 1986. p. 71–90.

132. Schacter DL. Searching for memory: the brain, the mind, and the past. New York: Basic Books; 1996.

133. Kestenberg J. What a psychoanalyst learned from the Holocaust and genocide. Int J Psychoanal. 1993;74:1117–29.

134. Kogan I. The cry of mute children. London: Free Association Books; 1995.

135. Oliner M. Hysterische Persönlichkeitsmerkmale bei Kindern Überlebender. In: Bergmann M, Jucovy M, Kestenberg J, editors. Kinder der Opfer, Kinder der Täter. Frankfurt a.M: S. Fischer; 1995.

136. Steck B, Bürgin D. Über die Unmöglichkeit zu Trauern bei Kindern trauerkranker Eltern. Kinderanalyse. 1996;4:351–61.

Chapter 7
Filiation Creation

"To my mother (adoptive mother).
   Why couldn't I enjoy my mother like other children?
   My mother was so beautiful.
   But like all beautiful things, she was ephemeral.
   She was a mother for far too short a time.
   And now I remain bitter and without a mother.
   But if you remain with bitterness, you will never succeed to build up your life.
   She desired me; more than another mother who abandoned me.
   Is it perhaps her so strong desire that has allowed me to build up what I have today?
   She may have left, but she did not abandon me.
   Our separation has allowed me to discover life by myself and has made me stronger.
   My mother was named after a flower: Camelia.
   And her life was so much like this flower; the camelias are very rare.
   My mother made every moment of my life a rare moment."
   Adopted female adolescent

Adoption Attachment and Relationship

The term filiation (from the Latin filius = son, filia = daughter) is used here as an expression of the bond between mother, respectively father and child. Filiation is the legal term for the recognized legal status of the relationship between family members, or more specifically the legal relationship between parent and child. The term legally includes an individual's lineage and family connection, and also contains a subject's related beliefs. Guyotat [1] defines the filiation bond as how an individual relates and is related to his real and imagined ancestors and descendants.

B. Steck, *Adoption as a Lifelong Process*,
https://doi.org/10.1007/978-3-031-33038-4_7

Three Axes of Filiation

The biological child and parenthood, whose references are procreation, pregnancy, and birth (the biological axis). The imagined child or parenthood, shaped by emotions, expectations, hopes and projections (the affective or psychic axis). The social or symbolic parenthood, which allows names and inheritances goods to be transferred and determines rights and obligations of the parent-child relationship and affiliation (the institutionalized, legal axis). Adoption is an instituted form of family formation and an established parent-child relationship; the biological axis is missing in adoption, yet the affective or psychic and the institutionalized or legal axis are sufficient for the cultural-social recognition of the family, the parental bond, and the affiliation[1] [2]. The following example shows how the lack of a biological filiation can be felt by adoptees.

Vignette
Matthew, a young adult adoptee considers the total dependence on the adoptive parents as his main difficulty in the adoption situation. Matthew thinks that the loss of personal characteristics, such as language and culture and of his biological family expectations towards him, leads to the fact, that he is, as an adopted child, merely a beneficiary of the adoptive parents' contributions. In this sense, the adoption relationship is not based on reciprocity, on an opportunity of mutual give and take. This reality, in addition to the experience of being abandoned, gives Matthew a sense of being dispossessed of his self, and is associated with feelings of shame: "Being adopted gives me the feeling of being worthless".

In adoption, the absence of the biological filiation may favor adoptive parents' unreal, non-sexualized or, on the contrary, promiscuous ideas of procreation. Adoptive parents often emphasize the priority of social and legal filiation. However, the adopted child needs to mentally elaborate his parents' personal encounter for his attachment building and identity formation. If the signification of birth is reduced to a sexual or legal event, the fundamental experience of the birth parents' human encounter (even if it is brief) is denied, and with it the associated feelings of desire or love. The silencing is linked to the risk that the original event is not transmitted to the child [3]. For adoptive parents, an additional challenge and mentally demanding task might be to affectively invest their couple relationship in such a way that for the child it will represent a "psychic birth" and become the place of his origin and his own history. Therefore, both adoptive parents are being asked to integrate the child in their own family history; simultaneously they gain awareness of the inner child they once were.

Vignettes
In her psychotherapeutic sessions, Nina, an eight-year-old girl adopted from India, whose adoptive parents live separately, creates, in her play scenes, repeatedly families, giving herself the role of a girl or a mother.

---

[1] Affiliation (family law), a legal form of family relationship

In one of her stories, the girl of the family lets her dog do its business every-where. Nina comments: "The girl is not real, that is why she cannot take care of her dog. She comes from outer space and from there she got into a belly, from which she was born."

Comment

Nina's statement demonstrates how difficult it is for her to imagine her origin from a generative sexual relationship of her parents (both biological and adoptive), reason for her difficulty to take care of herself.

Five-and-a-half-year-old John refuses to explain his adoption situation and to name his country of origin and declares: "An angel brought me to Mummy and Daddy; nobody gave birth to me." He imagines himself to be a child of God.

Comment

John prefers to deny his biological conception and origin; being a child of God renders him omnipotent.

Sebastian, an eight-year-old boy adopted from South America, imagines that his birth mother is being hunted by Eskimos in Alaska and must fight for her survival, the reason why she could not take care of him and gave him up for adoption. In his play scenes Sebastian repeatedly creates catastrophic stories, in which all characters die except a newborn baby who, left alone, has to fight for his survival.

Comment

Sebastian declares his biological mother to be innocent; her living conditions were too catastrophic for keeping him with her. His phantasms express his guilt of having survived, as well as his existential threats and loneliness.

Adopted children may omnipotently dramatize their biographical situation of origin in their phantasms, as the following example shows.

Vignette

Jonas' adoptive parents are very concerned by their nine-year-old son's daily dramatic scenes with his homework. They describe, how Jonas screams to be stupid and sobs violently, saying he wants to kill himself. These repetitive scenes are almost unbearable and incomprehensible for the adoptive mother, because Jonas - after these crises of rage and crying - completes his homework in a short time and usually without mistakes.

In the psychotherapeutic session, Jonas explains that he has first to let explode the diabolic inside him, his anger and malice, before he can concentrate on his homework. He says, he cannot bear being stupid, this would be reason enough to kill himself. He continues that his biological father has no job, is poor, can barely survive and has never been able to learn a profession.

Comment

Jonas fantasizes the same destiny for himself as his biological father and simultaneously imagines a tragic story of why his biological father gave him up for adoption. In his daily passionate phantasmatic dramatization, Jonas expresses his anger and profound sadness, what allows him to grieve the loss of his birth father, with the help of his adoptive parents. The narcissistic support and emotional affection of his adoptive parents contribute to the building up of Jonas attachment and their shared relatedness.

Summary

Attachment and relationship formation, i.e., the adoption filiation, is affectively nourished by the exchange of mutual wishes and needs of the parents and their child. It is the adoptive parents' desire to welcome a child and to recognize this particular child as their own, and the child's desire to have parents and to accept those very parents as his own. Such a parent-child relationship enables the child to fantasize the adoptive parents' sexuality as the place of his origin [4] and to build up a sense of descent from his adoptive mother and father. Filiation is based on a legal framework (institutionalized filiation) that appoints the parents and is formed within this framework on an intrapsychic and intrapersonal level through affective and imaginary exchanges in the parent-child triad. This psychic process allows each member in the triangle to build his identity, develop his subjectivity and contribute to his destiny.

> Who is my real mother? he shouted.
> I am, I said. I am your real mother by love and by law.
> Pearl Buck speaking to her child [5].

Loyalty Conflicts

Family loyalty is based originally on biological hereditary kinship. Etymologically, the word loyalty comes from the French (la loi = the law) and means law-abiding conduct.

The invisible phases of loyalty are anchored in consanguinity, in the preservation of biological life, in ensuring the family's continuity and in the acquired merits of the family members [6].

The fact that a child has been given up for adoption, the secret information about the biological parents and the required protection of the adoptive family often holds up strong features of denial [7]. Precisely this denial hinders the adopted child to resolve conflicts of loyalty towards his parents (both biological and adoptive). If a child prefers the one parents, he is disloyal to the others. The original loyalty to the biological parents continues to exist. Adopted children feel obliged to understand the reasons why they were given up for adoption by their birth parents. The adopted child does not accept that his birth parents acted out of ignoble motives; a deep, although conflictual, devotion to his biological parents persists. In his phantasms about the mystery of pregnancy, birth and further contributions by his biological parents, the child believes that the adoptive parents, without deserving it, have acquired exclusive rights and merits. Adopted children often tend to develop a special myth around their birth parents. A child may for example imagine his parents were forced to give him up and creates a strong imaginary-secretive bond without ever having met them. Throughout his life, the adopted child must try to find a balance between the myth about his biological parents and the reality requiring of him to fulfil relevant obligations towards his adoptive parents. The adoptive parents in turn must meet the challenge of reconciling the dichotomy between the rights and responsibilities of their parenthood and the fact that they have biologically made no contribution to this parenthood.

Vignettes
Mala, a nine-year-old girl from India says that she tries to love her birth mother and her adoptive parents equally, what is hard for her, but she does not want to hurt anybody. She recounts a recurring nightmare, in which her birthmother is sent to prison.

Comment
Mala's anger of having been given up for adoption finds expression in her nightmare; she seems to wish and fear at the same time that her birth mother will be imprisoned for having abandoned her.

A seven-year-old girl, Maya, whose country of origin is in South America, narrates that her birth mother is so poor that she has to feed herself from rubbish bags; she wishes so much to bring her food and toys.

Comment
Maya expresses her ambivalent feelings towards her birth mother: she desires that she is being punished for having abandoned her, e.g., obliged to eat rubbish; at the same time, she longs to be reunited with her mother and to repair her anger and resentment in bringing her food and toys.

Noah, an eleven-year-old boy, born in Africa, tells his birth phantasm: a baby bird - while being incubated by the mother - lost his father. The father bird was killed by his brother bird. The latter wanted to take the newborn bird with him as an accomplice to rob, and plunder black storks. White storks - Noah explains - give birth to children, while black storks curse children. Yet the mother bird defends her young and avenges the father by killing his brother.

Comment
Noah's narrative may be understood as his attempt to find a coherent meaning for what happened to him around his birth. His phantasm contains the wish that his mother would have protected him from being separated from her by a stealing third party. The narrative reveals clearly that Noah avoids feelings of guilt, caused by unconscious patricidal phantasms. He seems to split his parental representations into good, life-giving ones (the white storks) and bad predators who curse children (black storks). Are his biological parents the life-giving ones and his adoptive parents the stealing predators?

Adopted children take upon themselves responsibility and guilt of having been abandoned and rejected, what allows them to preserve intrapsychically "good, innocent" biological parents - representations they crucially need for their psychic survival. Phantasms that the child got lost and has not been found by the biological parents or even that it has been stolen by the adoptive parents are very common. Adopted children often find it inconceivable that a mother gives her child away, having carried it in her womb for nine months. Others imagine that their mother did not wish to take care of them, because they were ugly, nasty, dirty babies. The phantasm of being a "feces child", i.e., worthless, is expressed in various ways, for instance by a boy, saying: "You can flush me down the toilet, I am only excrement". A five-year-old girl acted out her fantasy of being a feces child by leaving her stool not only at any place at home, but also in playgrounds. These are regressive behaviors to an infantile (anal) stage of development.

Vignette

In his psychotherapy, a thirteen-year-old boy from Africa said: "I always think I'm stupid and silly, that's why I was thrown out".

It is evident that this proven intelligent adolescent carries the phantasm of having been expelled by his biological parents because of intellectual deficits - his "stupidity". He seems to hold on to his explanation and even wanting to prove it by behaving "stupidly and silly" at home and in school.

When adopted children fantasize being lost children, the biological parents bear no responsibility for giving them up for adoption and can be idealized as innocent parental figures; adoptees might then feel responsible and guilty for having been lost. When adopted children fantasize having been stolen by their adoptive parents, they are entitled to blame and justify their anger towards them. The phantasm of being a stolen child serves to establish a self-representation of being worthy, valued, and desired.

Vignette

Adoptive parents report that their ten-year-old son Samuel is preoccupied with the movie "Batman", of which he said, "it's like my story". He apparently identifies with the film's villain, a penguin who was born a monster (nose and fingers deformed), confined by his parents, and eventually thrown into sewers. A penguin family adopts the monster penguin, who is subsequently chosen as the king of the penguins. He wants to take revenge, i.e., kill his biological penguin parents, who threw him into the sewers, however, they are already dead. Then he wishes to blow up the city they lived in, but he is caught by the police and thrown again into the sewers.

Comment

In identification with the monster penguin, Samuel expresses his feelings of helplessness and hopelessness: despite his position as king - gained thanks to adoption - he fails to escape his original fate.

Common to both sexes are the unconscious or preconscious fantasies of bisexuality. Freud (1887–1904) coined the term unconscious bisexuality as early as 1898 (letter to Fliess No.81, 4.1.1898) and dealt with it throughout his life in a wide variety of works.

In male and female individuals both masculine and feminine drives are present and unconscious, when repressed. Throughout life the libido vacillates between the male and the female object [8].

Vignettes

A ten-year-old girl, Elisa, adopted from South America is completely fascinated by the Lion King story, the Walt Disney film, which she has seen several times. She narrates how the lost lion prince Simba, whose king father was killed by the father's brother, takes revenge as an adult lion, ascends his father's throne, and marries the lioness Nala.

Comment

Elisa wants to be both Simba and Nala. She expresses her omnipotent desire to own both sexes. She has not yet entered a process of definitive sexual identity formation, which includes the loss of fantasized bisexuality and acceptance of the fact to belong to only one gender.

The adoptive parents are very worried about the sexual identity of their eight-year-old son Joshua, who wants to be a girl, dresses like a girl and only plays with dolls.

Joshua, in a child psychiatric interview, draws a bee with a sting, with which the bee kills all other bees, as Joshua recounts, because the bee wants to be the only one and the strongest. The bee then takes the honey of all the dead bees to feed her children. Joshua wishes to be both a boy and a girl, like the bee (Fig. 7.1).

Comment

Equipped with a phallus (sting), Joshua fantasizes himself as a man who destroys all his rivals and at the same time as a woman and mother who nourishes her children.

Adopted children of both sexes very often tell that the reason for having been given away by their birth mother was the fact they were a boy or a girl, i.e., the fault was their gender.

Fig. 7.1 Joshua, 8-year-old, a bee with a sting

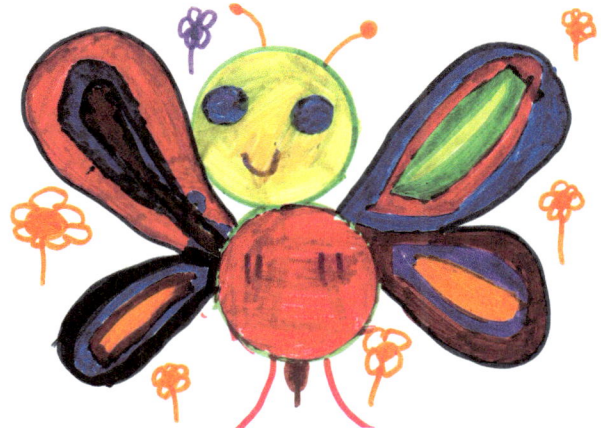

Vignette
A five-year-old girl, adopted at 13 months, believes that all children are born boys.
If the mother takes care of her child immediately, he remains a boy; if the mother
fails to do so, the doctor pierces the boy's penis and creates a vagina [9]. "Me and
my (adopted) sister were left in the hospital, that's why we are girls".

Comment
Being abandoned is synonymous with being castrated. Not being desired appears
in the self-representation as being castrated, analogous to biological parents who
are experienced as a lost part of one's self and analogous to infertile adoptive
parents.

Loyalty conflicts arise from the difficulties of the dual parenthood. Adoptees
develop specific loyalty ties to their unknown biological parents, which may be in
competition with those to their adoptive parents. The adoptees' interest in their parentage and the clarification of their own filiation serve to elucidate and determine
their own identity.

> Oedipus.
>> My father was Polybus of Corinth,
>> my mother Merope, a Dorian.
>> There I was regarded as the finest man
>> in all the city, until, as chance would have it,
>> something really astonishing took place,
>> though it was not worth what it caused me to do.
>> At a dinner there a man who was quite drunk
>> from too much wine began to shout at me,
>> claiming I was not my father's real son.
>> That troubled me, but for a day at least.
>> I said nothing, though it was difficult.
>> The next day I went to ask my parents,
>> my father and my mother. They were angry
>> at the man who had insulted them this way,
>> so I was reassured. But nonetheless,
>> the accusation always troubled me -.
>> The story had become well known all over.
>> And so I went in secret off to Delphi.
>> *Oedipus the King,* Sophocles (translation by Ian Johnston 2004: p. 928–945).

The Revelation of Adoption

One of the main tasks of the adoptive parents is to inform their child about his adoption and origin. The timing of revelation has been the subject of much controversy
in the literature [10–14]. Should the revelation take place before or after the child's
oedipal development phase? Providing information too early could be retraumatiz-
ing for the child and harm his psychosexual development. At a time when the child
does not yet clearly perceive the difference between fantasy and reality, information
of his adoption may lead to fears of being abandoned again. If the information is

given too late, there is a danger that the child will be informed by a third person. The secret about being adopted affects the child's self-image and complicates his identity development [15]. Similarly, the secrecy of adoption - both for the parents and the child - may be associated with emotional burdens and communication problems. There is probably no "right" time, but there are likely many wrong moments, for example when the adoptive parents are not yet ready to inform their child, or when the information about the adoption takes place in an aggressive, hostile atmosphere, or in a crisis situation (e.g., separation or divorce of the adoptive parents).

Vignette

Silvia was placed with her future adoptive family at the age of one month. The adoptive parents tell having informed their daughter about her adoption at the age of four. Silvia is brought for a child psychiatric consultation at the age of ten years because of her depressive state and pronounced learning disorders.

In the individual interview with the child psychiatrist, Silvia draws a cat (Fig. 7.2) and says that this is a four-year-old female cat who is sad because she no longer has a mummy; the cat - Silvia recounts - does not know how it lost its mummy.

Fig. 7.2 Silvia, 10 years, a cat who does not know how it lost its mommy

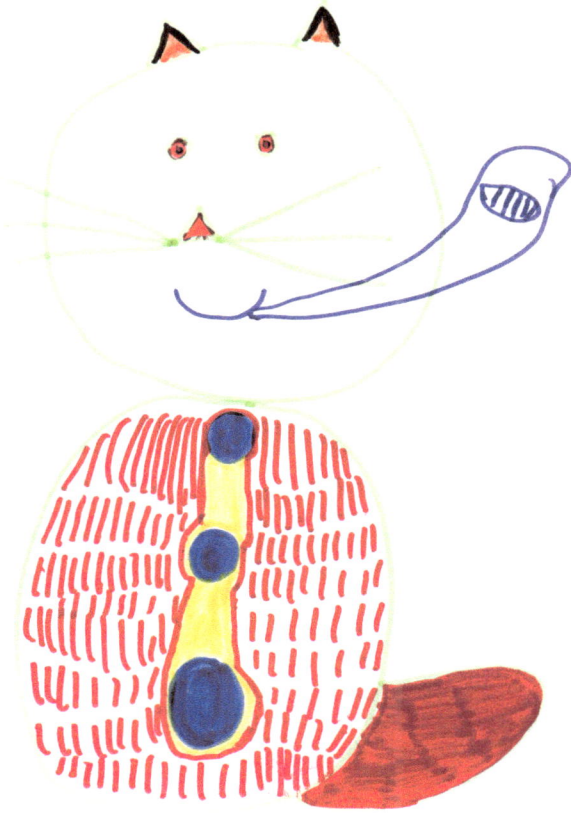

Comment

In the drawing, the cat is depicted with a happy face. Silvia fends off her grief over the loss of her birth mother, which she expresses in her depressive symptoms. The question is to what extent Silvia's learning difficulties are related to her ignorance of her origins. She seems to be identified with the cat, a four-year-old female. One wonders if the revelation of her adoption at the age of 4 years represented a traumatic experience.

Should the information be given before the child asks questions or only when the child asks questions [16]? A child who does not ask questions may not be developmentally ready to deal with the adoption information. Too early information could trigger overwhelming separation anxiety or regressive behavior, violating the child's basic trust, leading to phantasmatic distortions or even traumatization. When the child has reached the necessary age-appropriate development, he will ask questions on his own. The main reason for carefully informing the child, even if he does not ask any questions, is that the information should be provided by the adoptive parents and not by third persons, as the latter may be experienced by the child as a betrayal. When adoptive parents did not inform their child, he may react with feelings of mistrust, indignation and even despair to the disclosure by a third person.

Knowledge and Significance of Adoption Filiation

A large study investigated the understanding of the meaning of adoption.100 children, adopted in the first 2 1/2 years of life and a comparison group of 100 biological children of various ages (4–5, 6–7, 8–9, 10–11, 12–13 years) were asked about the difference between being adopted or being born by biological parents [17]. Results showed that the adopted children were only at the average age of 7 years able to clearly distinguish between the two situations. At an average age of 8 years and 8 months, adopted children were uncertain of the permanence of the relationship between parents and child. They believed that their biological parents could take them back or that the adoptive parents could give them away. It was not until the children were 10 years and 4 months old that they were certain of the permanence of the relationship between adoptive parents and adopted children, by referring to authority figures such as judges, doctors, or lawyers. Adopted children knew at an average age of 12 years and 5 months that adoption is associated with the transfer of parental rights and duties - grounded on a legal basis - from the biological parents to the adoptive parents. Only at an average age of 11 years and 11 months did the adopted children understand that the placement agency has the task of ensuring the welfare of the child placed for adoption and therefore of checking out the future adoptive parents. In the comparison group the results were the same; the understanding of adoption also developed in a long-lasting process among biological children. The 200 investigated children achieved better understanding at different points in time, but there were no significant differences between the two groups.

Based on these findings, it is easy to understand why eight- to nine-year-old adopted children may feel insecure in their adoptive family and ask questions about their family of origin. Before the age of 13–14, dual parenthood is a challenging reality to come to terms with, as this process, linked to the child's cognitive development, may take a long time.

Girls have a better understanding of adoption than boys [18]. This may be due to the different ways in which girls and boys socialize, as has already been shown in other studies on family concepts [19, 20]. Adoption is an important issue for girls, as they deal more intensively with the topic of motherhood or parenthood, than boys [21, 22]. A literature review on gender differences of adoptees shows that both biological and adoptive fathers occupy a marginal position; adoptive mothers and daughters are more involved in the emotional confrontation with the adoption situation than adoptive sons [23]. This may be a consequence of the greater need for emotional expression and social support of mothers and daughters, in addition to socio-cultural influences.

Revealing to the child his adoption is a process that takes years and is inscribed in the child's developmental history [24]. The questions the child will ask about his filiation will vary according to his age. The young child is concerned with questions of conception and birth and wants to know why the adoptive mother did not carry him in her womb and gave him birth. The information must be continuous, adapted to the child's age and ability to understand, and aimed at not harming his self-esteem. Even if the child knows that he is adopted, the significance of his specific status only becomes clear during the latency years. The information about origin and adoption is linked to questions from the child about the reasons for his release for adoption and about his own guilt and responsibility. This information transfer is thus a process that takes place over years, its meaning must be shared, which requires a great deal of empathy and emotional support from the adoptive parents towards their adopted child. Working through losses together brings parents and children closer to the specificity of their shared family bonds [15].

The fact that children sometimes do not ask questions about their origins is probably due to various reasons; their environment often assumes that the child is not interested in his origins and his biological parents. On the one hand, the child wishes to be able to forget his own past; on the other hand, however, he also feels the fear of his adoptive parents of being devalued in favor of the biological parents or of being questioned in their parental competence. In addition, infertile parents may find themselves in a conflictual situation regarding the transmission of sexual information to their children, as they find it difficult to explain to their child the difference between sexual activity and procreative capacity. The unconscious link between sexuality and procreation can be associated with insecure feelings about their own sexual competence. Their inability of procreation, pregnancy and birth often appears to infertile parents as a sexual failure [25]. Further, in the unconscious imagination of the adoptive parents, especially the adoptive mother, the adopted child may symbolize the transgression of a prohibition - given by nature or God - to conceive a child.

Often it seems to be easier for adoptive parents to remain silent or to present the biological parents as dead. Sometimes this corresponds also to statements of adopted children, who say it would be easier to know that the biological parents have died. Fears that the adopted child will love his biological parents more or prefer them or leave the adoptive parents one day are thus eliminated.

Vignette

Brigitte, a teenage girl who is thought to be mentally retarded and integrated in a school for disabled children, says in an individual interview with the child psychiatrist: "My mother claims that my birth mother is dead. But I know that's not true. I know she is alive."

The adoptive mother informed the child psychiatrist that - for the sake of "simplicity" - she had preferred to declare the biological mother dead.

Comment

The silencing of Brigitte's birth mother by the adoptive mother brought communications between her and Brigitte to a standstill and lead to Brigitte's intellectual inhibition, resulting in her mentally retardation.

It still happens that adoptive parents, in a moment of despair, reveal the filiation status to their adopted child: "Do whatever you want. You are anyhow not our child!" The revelation of the adoption filiation in such a form may have traumatic effects on children or adolescents: It is as if they suddenly lose their belonging and identity; unbearable feelings of being rejected and abandoned as well as of loneliness, forlornness and homelessness are then coupled with feelings of being deceived and lied to.

The disclosure may also be delicate for adoptive parents because they have the impression to be in a kind of double bind: on the one hand they are engaged doing all they can for their child's belonging to the family, on the other they are obliged to reveal that he is not their child, i.e., not of their blood.

I was a little ashamed, at night before I fell asleep, to rejoice in bringing the other (the birth mother) back to life, dead in my secret, under the always graceful features of an actress, a star, a dancer, or a princess, always of English descent. Marie Brunet [26], author of the book *L' amour adopté*, is herself an adopted child.

Family Romance

Adoption causes a particularly intense transformation of the "family romance", common to all human beings, i.e., of an internal scenic imagination of one' s origin [27–30]. The family romance appears in mythologies, legends, fairy tales and in novels.

According to the psychoanalytical Freudian theory [28], the family romance develops in different phases. After initially overestimating the value and authority of his parents, the child adopts a more critical attitude, motivated by sexual rivalry with the same-sex parent, the feeling of being excluded from the parental couple and intensified by sibling rivalry. The child tries to release this tension through phantasms, such as to descend from other parents or being a found or stolen child.

In prepuberty or in early adolescence the child dreams in his phantasm of parents with a higher social rank, less libidinal, omnipotent, ideal parents. The child thus replaces his own low-valued parents, gains distance from them and tries to avoid conflicts. While the child does not perceive the parents separately in the first phase of the family romance, he separates them in the second phase and denies the primal scene.[2] He thus creates omnipotent, parental figures. Through the narcissistic over-investment of these mythical fantasized parental figures, the child can feel loved again, a narcissistic gratification, which functions as a defense against drive tensions.

In the second phase of the family romance, the awareness of the differentiated sexual functions of the parents has the effect that the mother is no longer doubted as the procreative one, while the father continues to be fantasized as unknown and idealized (mater certissima, sed pater semper incertus est[3]). But the mother can only be approached at the price of her humiliation, she is secretly accused of infidelity or is perceived as a seductress; secret love affairs are attributed to her, why unconscious fantasies of an illegitimate, i.e., a "bastard" child, arise.

The first phase of Freud's family romance corresponds to a foundling who - trapped in the preoedipal world - can free himself only thanks to the omnipotence of his phantasms. The second phase corresponds to a "bastard" child who, because of his illegitimacy, arrogates for himself unique rights to attack the real world as if it were lawless, in search of the idealized father, carried by the ambition to replace or surpass him.

Freud [28] concludes his explanations of the family romance by emphasizing that in his phantasms the child maintains his first feelings of tenderness for his parents and gives expression to his longing for the time of childhood when his parents were perfect models.

The Family Romance from the child's Point of View

Fairy tales and legends tell us about children who are abandoned by their parents and left to their fate or live unhappily with their stepparents. Le *petit poucet* by the French author Charles Perrault, or *Hänsel und Gretel* by the German Brothers Grimm relate how, using a trail of pebbles they dropped to mark the route - an equivalent fairy tale of Tom Thumb - they find their way back home after being abandoned in the woods by their parents. *The Adventures of Tintin* by Georges Prosper Remi, better known under his pen name Hergé, a character from French

---

[2] The primal scene (German: Urszene) is the initial unconscious fantasy of a child of a sexual relationship between the parents.

[3] "The mother is always certain; the father is always uncertain".

comics, is a perpetual adolescent, who never has real parents and lives solely with family romance characters.

According to Anna Freud [31], most children between the ages of 6–10 years cherish a secret daydream, called family romance, in which they imaging to descend from royal or noble parents who have confined them to their real parents of low descent. These phantasms are attempts to deal with a whole range of conflicting emotions. The family romance allows the oedipal situation to be de-dramatized. The boy is allowed to love his mother - without coming in conflict with the incest prohibition - and to feel aggression towards his father without feeling guilty. Thus, the family romance serves for example to compensate for narcissistic offences and to ward off incest desires.

For certain adopted children, however, the creation of a family romance in their imagination seems impossible, as if the real existence of the biological parents prevents the inner fantasy process. Adopted children, according to Anna Freud, are usually deeply troubled in the latency period, at the time when all children experience the inevitable disappointment in their parents and the "family romance", i.e., the fantasy of not being the child of one's own parents, is heightened to a painful experience by the reality of adoption ([32]: p. 71). For a child, being loved and being given away are incompatible [33].

The family romance allows the adopted child to idealize his birth parents as being omnipotent and to split internal parental figures into good (e.g., the biological parents) and bad (e.g., the adoptive parents) representations [34, 35]. If this cleavage of parental representations persists, the child may unconsciously identify with one part of the parental representations. Adopted children, for example, identify with the fantasized bad or idealized characteristics of the biological parents and behave accordingly. In this way, they try to cope with the relational task of their dual parenthood (biological and adoptive parents) and thereby maintain an unconscious loyalty bond to the biological parents.

In a typical family romance situation of non-adopted children, the biological parents are disdained, while the desired fantasized "adoptive" parents are idealized. According to Blum [36], the adopted child, on the contrary, disdains both the adoptive parents and the (unknown) biological parents. However, adopted children also develop extended and changing family romance-fantasies that serve to build up self-representations and are maintained well into adolescence or even adulthood, always bearing traits of a possible reality. The length of the family romance period may reflect the extent of the subjectively experienced expulsion-, rejection-, abandonment feelings [37].

The Family Romance from the Point of View of Adoptive Parents

For certain adoptive parents, adoption seems to represent an opportunity to realize their own fantasized family romance in the current reality with their adopted child. The adoption project reawakens family romance fantasies of the prospective adoptive parents, triggered by the existence of their future child's biological parents. Adoptive parents identify with the all-powerful ideal parents they fantasized as a child, while the child's biological parents represent their low estimated parents.

When the family romance of the adoptive parents "meets" the family romance of the child, the intrapsychic dynamic of these family romances connects with the interpersonal family dynamic. Adoption then becomes the carrier of secret links between the phantasy worlds of adoptive parents and adopted child.

The adoption process may be understood according to the phases of the family romance described by Freud [28]: The foundling[4] child will be a royal child by adoption. Based on the family romance, one may hypothesize that adoptive parents unconsciously fantasized to be children of nobler parents, e.g., royal children. They project these phantasms on their adopted child, a royal child or ideal child, they honor as restorative parents.

An adoptive mother reports that she feels very indebted to the biological mother as she regards her son as a "royal child", who allowed her to become a mother.

Adoptive parents thus put themselves in the place of the omnipotent ideal parents they once fantasized and distance themselves from the biological parents whom they may reject since they did not care for their child but abandoned and gave him up for adoption. They believe in a reparation of the adopted child, representative of their own inner child, respectively their own self.

In practice these adoptive parents have troubles setting limits to their child, letting him live joyfully into the day, confronting him hardly with reality. The adopted child is receptive to the unconscious fantasies of his adoptive parents, adapts himself and lives by an inner motto, which conveys: "You desired me, you have chosen me, so I am entitled to everything".

Both, the adoptive parents, and their adopted child live then in a kind of shared family romance, which begins with the arrival of the child. This new start is like a birth. The adoptive parents may not only change the child's first name, but also register his arrival date as the date of his birth at the civil registry office and thus even change his age. The adopted child confirms the adoptive parents in their family romance, i.e., in the position of ideal parents. They represent for the child the ideal parents of his own family romance: King and Queen who rescue the rejected foundling and thus help repair his narcissistic injury. The adopted child adapts optimally, out of his feelings of fear of being abandoned and rejected again, a survival strategy. Thus, the past of adoptive parents and adopted child is canceled. These "problem-free" adoptions are generally seen in psychology or child psychiatry clinics only later, in prepuberty or adolescence of the adopted child, when the unconscious contract between ideal child and ideal parents, i.e., the joint family romance of the all-powerful foundling, collapses like a house of cards. The breakdown is a fall into the past. The shared idealization by the adoptive parents and the adopted child affects their inevitable adjustment difficulties, as well as the integration of natural

---

[4] 'Foundling' is an historic term applied to children, usually babies, that have been abandoned by parents and discovered and cared for by others.

ambivalence, resulting in intense feelings of guilt. The relatedness is carried by a powerful desire for harmony, yet in crisis situations great despair and severe dismay may arise. The unconscious narcissistic contract, which underlies the adoption bonds, allows the conflictual parts of the relationship and the associated feelings of hatred and resentment to be denied. These negative emotions of parents and adolescents are split off but are insidiously carried out by attacking the parent-child bonds, the self-image, and even the ability to think and act [38].

Vignette

A seven-year-old girl adopted from India is referred for psychotherapy because of learning difficulties (in spite of good intelligence), social integration difficulties, emotional outbursts, and behavioral problems (stealing and lying). During the sessions, Rebecca forbids her psychotherapist to write, paints over her own drawings, and destroys her play scenes. No one is ever allowed to know what she says or does in psychotherapy. In repetitive scenes (with the scenotest), she deals with her adoption situation and associated phantasms and emotions. In the transference relation with the psychotherapist, she expresses her hatred and murderous rage especially towards her adoptive mother, responsible - in her feelings - for the loss of her biological parents.

Before an interruption in her therapy, she is once again busy erasing everything (drawing, play scenes). To her psychotherapist's intervention that she does not want to leave any traces of herself, while she is overwhelmed by feelings of not knowing anything of her birth mother, she answers in crying "no, no", covers her ears and runs to the phone to ask her adoptive mother to pick her up immediately. She insults the therapist for being mean, stupid, silly, and too fat or too thin and never wants to see her again but destroy everything what the psychotherapist owns. The latter gently names her despair and pain over the loss of her birth mother and that she does not know what she looks like. Rebecca answers that she wishes so desperately to have at least *one* photo of her birthmother.

Comment

Rebecca harbors a self-image of being silly, stupid, a mean girl. She seems incapable to feel, perceive and build up her body image (too thin or too fat), her body being the only connection to her birth mother. Her intense preoccupation with her biological mother - in the transference with the therapist - is lived by her as an attack on the adoptive bond, therefore she has to erase all reminders of her therapeutic sessions. Her feelings of not being allowed to know, of not being able to inscribe traces of her past into her current psychic experience, is reflected in her learning difficulties.

If adoptive parents are no longer confirmed in their role as ideal parents by their child, they are confronted with their own family romance, which suddenly emerges into consciousness. This irruption of unconscious phantasms into consciousness may already take place during the encounter with the future adoptive child, i.e., at the moment when the imaginary and the real child are confronted with each other in a conscious way.

Phantasm of the omnipotent, phallic mother-figure becomes by projection the revengeful, persecuting biological mother who takes her child back, while phantasms of the birth mother being too poor or too ill to care for her child, helps an adoptive mother to avoid her feelings of rivalry or guilt. Finally, phantasms of a seductive mother, accused of infidelity, turns by projection into the prostituting biological mother whose illegitimate and unwanted child awaits the same fate.

Vignette
Adoptive parents ask for psychiatric evaluation of their adopted daughter Franziska. Her stealing of sweets led to her adoptive parents' breakdown and rejection of their daughter. In the family consultation session, the parents say that they obviously do not satisfy their child, that she never established an authentic bond with them, and that their daughter's behavior is not surprising if one knows the life of her mother. All their efforts and dedication would never compensate for the inheritance of their child. They find it inconceivable what their daughter will do in a few years when she reaches the age at which her birth mother got pregnant.

Comment
The adoptive parents relate her daughter's problems to heredity and believe in an inevitable repetition of the same fate of mother and daughter. However, with her stealing of sweets Franziska shows her despair and distress over her losses in the past and her imperative need to be loved and cared for by her adoptive parents.

At the time of prepuberty or adolescence, the adopted child usually fulfils no longer his parents' expectation and the adoptive parents' omnipotent reparative dream out of their foundling position as ideal, spiritual parents can no longer be maintained. Their rebelling "bastard" child then emerges and is projected onto the adopted child, and the adopted adolescent turns into an indignant refuser of law and order, attacking the world and society and trying to impose his willfulness. Here too, adoptive parents speak of heredity, of a child conceived by "lawless" parents, who defies social and legal norms, e.g., in the case of delinquency, toxicomania, promiscuity.

Vignette
A child psychological evaluation was requested by adoptive parents for their eight-year-old son Alexander, because of his extreme violent, destructive behavior, and his aggressive outbursts. Alexander rejects his adoptive mother, tells her to leave and beats her. The parents inform that her son was beaten by his birth mother. Alexander was taken away by the authorities and given up for adoption at the age of 3 years; the biological father is unknown, the biological mother was imprisoned.

An individual psychotherapy for Alexander and accompanying consultations for his parents were arranged. The desperate and helpless adoptive mother tells the psychotherapist, that she dreads her son's violence, and she expresses her fears that Alexander might be a criminal and end up in prison, thus enduring the same fate as his biological mother.

Family Romance and Adoption Motivations

The motivations of adoptive parents to adopt a child may be viewed from the perspective of the family romance.

The conscious motivation (one of the most important is sterility) to adopt a child obscures the unconscious motivations, which are often only revealed when the child arrives or come to light with the child's presence. The integration of an adoptive child may cause repressed, unconscious psychic conflicts to break open, sometimes to such a degree of severity leading to a parent's decompensation or the rejection of the child and his expulsion from the family. Adoptive parents' unprocessed losses or severe parentifications[5] seem to favor a continuity of the family romance fantasy into adulthood.

An adoptive mother's robbery fantasy expresses her family romance having been a stolen child herself. She seems to be identified with her own mother, to whom she attributes - in her experience or in her phantasms - having stolen her as a child or having robbed her of her childhood, as the following example illustrates.

Vignette
During the adoption of a second child, the adoptive mother met with the child's birth mother in the country of origin. After returning to Switzerland with her future adoptive child, she is haunted by the phantasm having stolen the child. These robbery fantasies evolve into intense, persistent obsessive thoughts that prevent the mother from caring for the child, and she demands that the child be taken away from her.

One may hypothesize behind the desire of single women to adopt a child a denial of the primal scene, i.e., the refusal of the phantasmatic perception of parental sexual activity and procreative function; phantasms of the omnipotent mother figure are perpetuated. Often these women are pious, and they believe that God will assume the father figure for their child, in referring to their Christian faith. However, a third person is excluded in this mother-child twosome; the single future adoptive mother - in her omnipotent phantasms - intends to take on both roles (mother and father). Simultaneously incest fears are probably hidden.

Vignette
An adoptive parental couple agrees to declare to the authorities that their child is a biological child, born of the adoptive mother's adultery; in fact, they adopted a child in a foreign country and kept this international adoption secret.

The phantasm of the mother figure, who can be seduced by anyone, is revealed in this situation.

Other phantasms, which belong to the unconscious adoption motivations, are to avoid a biological parenthood, as if a new established filiation might protect against

---

[5] Parentification is the process of role reversal whereby a child is obliged to act as parent to his own parents or siblings.

a genetic or blood filiation. Incest desires, phantasm of infanticide or patricide must be avoided.

The classic example of a prohibition-transgression - given by nature or God - is the tragedy of Oedipus: Laios, his father, transgresses the Sphinx's procreation prohibition. Oedipus, his child, is punished for his father's erroneous transgression. The transgenerational malediction is passed on to Antigone, Oedipus' daughter, and sister, who by her death renounces further procreation, i.e., brings the generation line to an end (see Annex:The History of Oedipus).

Unconscious fantasies sometimes also reveal the desire not to transfer one's heredity or one's painful past to a biological child. Adoption is supposed to ensure the generational leap from son/daughter to father/mother, but at the same time interrupts the biological generation line. Multiple fears, such as not being able to be a more competent parent to a biological child than one's own parents or burdening a biological child with the fate of a foundling or "bastard" child, may contribute to interfering with one's reproduction. The fact that adoptive parents do not let their parents become biological grandparents may perhaps be based on an unconscious need to avoid the confrontation of inner-psychic images with fantasized and real parents.

Vignette
A filiation based on social, relational, affective, and legal bonds may be preferred to consanguinity, as the example of a father shows who - on the same day - gives up his parental rights of his biological child and adopts the child of his second wife.

The event of adoption holds both misfortune and chance. Adoptive parents hope to create a new life story with the adopted child, which will provide memories of shared experiences and thus repair the continuity interruptions of both adoptive parents' and adopted child's past. Adoption represents a kind of mirror phenomenon of this unconscious hope and expresses the need to deny or repress the personal often so painful history. However, the desire to create a new history with the adopted child, devoid of individual burdened life experience, fails to be realized. The adopted child (very often a traumatized child) reveals the experienced, unprocessed traumas of his adoptive parents.

The desire of the adoptive parents to be "reborn" by the adopted child is reinforced by the fact that the adopted child has the same desire to be reborn in order to forget his painful traumatic history, as well as by the reality that adoptive parents often know little about the child's biological parents and his personal history.

When adoptive parents work through their intrapsychic conflicts in confrontation with their adopted child, they fulfil a mourning process of their own losses. In this situation, the parents speak of a chance. When they fail to use this interaction opportunity with the adopted child for their intrapsychic processing, they project their problematic past onto the adopted child. The supposed savior child may then be a disaster child. Between these two described extreme situations, the complexity of adoption and the resulting clinical manifestations are manifold.

The phantasm of the family romance is intended to avoid what Oedipus realizes in ignorance, namely the double crime of patricide and incest. The most sorrowful figure of the Greek theatre, the unfortunate Oedipus, has been understood by Sophocles as the noble man, destined to error and misery despite his wisdom, but who, in the end, through his immense suffering, exerts around him a magical blessing power which is still effective beyond his passing [39].

The intrapsychic dynamic of the family romance is linked to the interpersonal family dynamic. The fantasy life of a child is shaped by the interaction with the fantasy world of his parents, the latter being present before the child is born. The parents' imaginations about a future child originate in their own family romance. Every pair of parents, every future mother or father, is confronted with the question of their personal identity, result of the integration of the psychic process of identifications in relation to the real and the fantasized parents.

In adoption, not only family romance phantasms of the adoptive parents and the adopted child come to phantasmatic interaction, but also fantasy worlds of both the adopted child and the adoptive parents concerning the biological parents. For adoptive parents, the biological parents of the adopted child represent a source of imaginations, phantasms, and fears [30]. Biological parents may occupy space and time in the unconscious interactive play of the adoptive parents and the adopted child. These phantasms are to be taken "seriously", as they hold a rarely imagined importance when unspoken, all the more as the phantasms refer to parents who exist in reality but are often absent and unknown.

Adoptive parents' fears center around such questions as: will they or the biological parents be the true parents for their child, and will the biological parents represent the ideal parents, while they might be unwanted, rejected by their child? These are the adoptive parents' projections of their own family romance phantasms. Therefore, the integration of the family romance into the psychic dynamics of adoptive parents has great significance for adopted children.

In the social jungle of human existence, there is no feeling of being alive without a sense of identity. Erik Erikson.

Identity

Definitions

"Identity is the term used to describe the experienced unity of a person. It encompasses and integrates the diversity of experiences derived from the individual life history and from the various roles to be filled by each individual in a diversified society. Fixed characteristics of the person - for example, physical ones such as gender, age, height and attractiveness, but also others such as level of education, occupation, birth and origin, cannot be exchanged at will; these are elements of individual uniqueness." (Parsons and Goffmann, in [40]: p.61).

According to Breccia [41], "identity is a feeling of self which each individual is forming and transforming in the course of his own psychic and social life". "The feeling of identity forms and transforms itself over time…" and "encloses within the identity both the familiar and the foreign, oneself and alterity" (p. 17). Expressions of identity are continuously related to unconscious processes. The subject has to be able to "conserve a feeling of self through change" (p. 15), an equilibrium between being and becoming. The relationship with the other - not only in the earliest phases of development, but throughout time - contributes to the identity of a person. Earliest experiences are contained in the constitution of identity. Genealogical unconscious forces are part of an individual's identity formation and may be accompanied by uncanny feelings.

The formation of a personal identity includes genealogical aspects, through which each individual feels connected to previous and future generations, a dimension of identity, called psycho-historical by Erikson [42–44]; it embraces the existential interests that bind a person throughout the life cycle - from birth to death - to earlier and future generations and represents a continuity of his genealogical history, his ancestry or descent.

Erikson's [42] writes about identity: "At one time. .. it will appear to refer to a conscious *sense of individual identity*; at another to an unconscious striving for a *continuity of personal character*; and, finally, as a maintenance of an inner *solidarity* with a group's ideals and identity" (p. 57).

In Erikson's formulation, cultural considerations, particularly as revealed in differing childrearing techniques, influence the manner in which common problems such as autonomy and separation, or the generative demands of adulthood are coped with; the crucial issue is the extent, to which each individual can absorb and internalize the available cultural values and produce a set of ego functions that are at one with the surrounding society. Mental health is basically a product of successful adaptation to culture or, rather, a successful use of cultural resources to enable integration of the ego as a center of a coherent personal identity.

"The adolescent process … is conclusively complete only when the individual has subordinated his childhood identifications to a new kind of identification, achieved in absorbing sociability and in competitive apprenticeship with and among his age mates. These new identifications are no longer characterized by the playfulness of childhood and the experimental zest of youth: with dire urgency they force the young individual into choices and decisions which will, with increasing immediacy, lead to commitments 'for life'. The task to be performed here by the young person and by his society is formidable. It necessitates, in different individuals and in different societies, great variations in the duration, intensity, and ritualization of adolescence. Societies offer, as individuals require, more or less sanctioned intermediary periods between childhood and adulthood, often characterized by a combination of prolonged immaturity and provoked precocity"([43]: p. 155–156). "The final identity, then, as fixed at the end of adolescence, is superordinated to any single identification with individuals of the past: it includes all significant identifications, but it also alters them in order to make a unique and reasonably coherent whole of them "([43]: p. 161). In Western societies, significant events - ritualizing the transition from child to adult - are increasingly missing.

Vignette
The repetitive play of an eight-year-old adopted girl, Sarah, in psychotherapy clearly shows, how her identity development is shaped by the exploration and confrontation with her origins. In her play scenes, there are always two girls who experience various challenges: Sarah calls one girl with the name given to her by her adoptive parents, the other with her original name, which she received from her biological parents.

Identity Development Difficulties for Adoptees

Adolescence is a particularly dramatic developmental phase for adopted children. Preoccupations, deep concerns, and anxieties with regard to their origins intensify. The young adoptees' identity conflicts include curiosity and interest in their genealogical history, i.e., their ancestry. This psycho-historical dimension of identity [43, 44] encompasses the existential interests linking human beings - throughout the life cycle from birth to death - to previous and future generations, a continuity adoptees are missing in their identity development.

In all steps of individuation and separation in childhood and adolescence, adoptees are reminded of their adoption state and the related relationship breakups [45]. Such a gap in identity, the interruption in the continuity of generations, creates feelings that the future may again harbor disruptions. Existential fears and anxieties are accentuated: "I have no roots, therefore I have no center and no direction". "My past is cut off by a wall, which also rises up against my future". "I am identity-less." Such statements from young adoptees show to what extent their experience of the filiation-breakup can complicate the developmental process of their sense of identity [46].

On the one hand, adoptees feel shaken in their self-esteem, question and doubt their affective attitude towards themselves; on the other hand, their affective distancing from their adoptive parents is complicated since this process of individuation and separation is not only a symbolic loss, as it is the case for all adolescents, but this emancipation evokes their real losses in their past.

Adolescents - in their search for identity and during their individuation process - have a strong need to be "different" from what their environment or adoptive parents expect of them; some adoptees experience intensively and painfully their physical appearance, different from their adoptive parents.

The results of an analysis of various questionnaires filled by 135, 11–20 years old, adopted adolescents (72 girls, 63 boys) – inquiring about their identity - revealed that adolescents with a very high degree of preoccupation with their adoption showed significantly higher levels of estrangement from and significantly lower levels of trust towards their adoptive parents [47].

Identification with biological parents - who are often fantasized as dissocial or promiscuous - can result in adolescents acting out such behaviors, all the more since the adoption situation is associated for many adoptees with feelings having been victims of acting adults: they were born unplanned, given away by their biological parents, adopted - without being asked - by the adoptive parents; in addition, their adoption was handled by an intermediary agency. Some adoptive parents have difficulty tolerating biologically based differences or may hold their adopted adolescent's biological background responsible for his behavioral problems. To counterbalance biological strangeness with social familiarity is a demanding and complex task. Reciprocal sexual phantasms, conscious or unconscious, between adoptive parents and adolescent adoptees may trigger intense anxiety and guilt feelings because of the non-biological incest barrier and disturb, unsettle the relationships and interaction between parents and adoptees.

Ethnic Identity

Ethnic identity is a multidimensional construct, inseparable from familial and social relational interactions. Parents of international transracial adoptees need to be aware of the task their children face, namely, to identify with their country of origin and simultaneously with their family's national culture, and in addition to develop an identity as an adoptee [48]. To integrate these different identities into a sound sense of self is a challenging effort, complicated by the society's often discriminatory or discordant messages: rejected as immigrants, but welcomed by adoptive families and relatives [49].

Vignette
A young, adopted woman from Africa complains bitterly, that her white adoptive parents will never be able to understand her; since early childhood she felt being regarded as different, foreign, and suffered throughout her life from multiple discriminations, something her white parents in a predominantly white society never experienced. "My parents tell me they always loved me how I am; but this is not enough! Never there were discussions in my family how I felt as a black girl, surrounded by white persons, and nobody ever prepared or told me how to deal with discrimination. I feel very lonely and forlorn to build up my identity as a black person in a white society."

Ethnic Identity Development [50]

Developmental theories postulate that the formation of ethnic identity is based on cognitive development, i.e., on a progressive ability of the growing child to perceive, understand and distinguish ethnic signs. Four-year-old children compare their physical characteristics with those of their parents. The difference in skin color is the first sign to be consciously perceived and is often associated with adoption. This gives for example rise to the belief that only colored children are adopted. By the age of six-seven years, the child has a rudimentary understanding of reproduction and realizes that the different physical characteristics mean that he does not really belong to his adoptive parents. The double minority status - ethnicity and adoption - may be particularly painful for school-age children.

Vignettes
An eight-year-old adopted black boy from Costa Rica claims that his younger, also adopted, but light-skinned sister, has been carried by his adoptive mother in her belly (i.e., she was not adopted) and is boundlessly jealous. He maintains his conviction that only black boys are adopted. He wishes to be white like his sister and says, that black is ugly.

A nine-year-old adopted boy, born in Africa, complains bitterly that he is teased at school because of his skin color, e.g., he is called "chocolate". He draws the children, who are humiliating him, as monsters with horns, teeth, smoking cigarettes, without a heart, but with spiked chains on their arms and compares their behavior to the Nazis (Fig. 7.3).

Ethnic identification is composed of various overlapping components such as personal identification, self-esteem, and identification with different social groups [51]. The child's attitudes towards race and ethnicity crystallize by middle school age, a time when children begin to relate to, select and integrate into groups. The importance of ethnic identification appears to be mediated by environmental factors, such as family structure, community, or ethnic groups [52–55]. The "biculturally competent" individual[6] has a strong sense of ethnic identity and functions adequately in two cultures without feeling compelled to choose between the two [56, 57].

Personal self-esteem and group identification must be distinguished. A child may have a strong sense of self-worth but be unprepared to establish a relationship with a dominant culture as a person of a different color [58]. For minority youth, ethnic identification and pride can be an important contribution to their self-esteem and psychic adjustment [59].

Transethnic and transcultural international adoptees do not differ in their self-esteem and adjustment from domestic adoptees, especially if they were adopted in infancy, as an investigation concludes [60]. In fact, many international adoptees have better self-awareness and self-confidence than non-adoptees or domestic adoptees Thus, internationally early adopted children show positive feelings towards their ethnic identity, while older adopted children and children with traumatic experiences in the country of origin often suffer greater troubles in adjusting

---

[6]"…an individual would have to possess a strong personal identity, have knowledge of and facility with the beliefs and values of the culture, display sensitivity to the affective processes of the culture, communicate clearly in the language of the given cultural group, perform socially sanctioned behavior, maintain active social relations within the cultural group, and negotiate the institutional structures of that culture" ([56]: p. 396)

Fig. 7.3 A 9-year-old boy, a monster

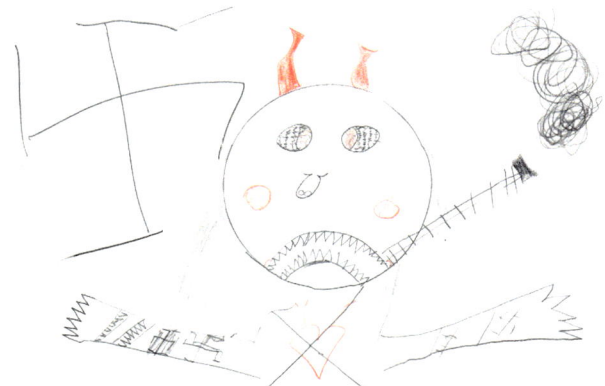

emotionally, linguistically, and socially and have negative attitudes towards their ethnic identity [61].

Ethnic self-identification depends on the attitude of the adoptive parents and the contact with the culture of origin. Many adoptees feel uncomfortable with their physical appearance and are additionally burdened by racist discrimination [62]. Adoptees are assimilated into their adoptive family's culture when adoptive parents create a caring environment, acknowledge their adopted child's physical difference, while emphasizing psychological similarities, and expose their children to persons of the same ethnicity of their country of origin, what facilitates positive identification.

Many studies indicate that for most adoptees the new identity, the one of their adoptive family, is more important than their original one [60]. International adoptees adopt the culture of their adoptive parents; bicultural identification rarely takes place.

A longitudinal study focuses on the identity process, i.e., ethnic identity, national identity, bicultural identity integration, and psychological well-being of adolescents and young adults, who were internationally adopted by Italian families: Bicultural persons may feel divided with regard to their cultural identity and feel dissociated with respect to their cultural orientation. Yet identification with the two cultural systems, that is bicultural integration, leads to better psychosocial adjustment and furthers psychic well-being, such as self-acceptance, autonomy, and the ability to face life challenges [63].

Adopted children are obliged to create their own autobiography about their ethnic and genetic origin, pregnancy, and birth. Phantasms can only come to rest, when they succeed integrating their biological roots and their growing up in the adoptive family. The formation of a unified identity is a highly complex process. Phantasms concerning the biological parents serve the development of identity but represent also potential identity conflicts. Adoptees have a hard time tolerating their internal ambivalence and reconciling positive and negative aspects of their self-image [64].

You think adoption is a story which has an end. But the point about it is that it has no end. It keeps changing its ending. *Red Dust Road*, Jackie Kay.

Confrontation with and Search for the Origin

Adopted children develop an inner relationship with their biological parents [45]. With increasing age - especially during puberty and adolescence - and with a better understanding of the adoption with all its implications [65], a confrontation with their origins takes place for most adoptees [66–68].

If biological roots of a child are erased, his biography will be eliminated. This means a psychic amputation of a child's personal history and of his biological origin. Adoptees, adoptive parents, and society replace what has been amputated with wishful thinking. This may begin with the falsification of the birth certificate and determine the whole life of adoptees. The only characteristic of the adopted child is that he does not really know who he is. The desire to know his biological origin stems from a deep inner psychic urge for essential continuity and wholeness. One of the most important messages communicated to the adoptee is to repress his desire for knowing his roots. It is not uncommon for adoptees, from childhood to adulthood, to search the streets for faces that might be those of their mother, father, or siblings. If the adoptee looks for concrete information, he may be perceived as ungrateful and disloyal. "Every family has secrets, but the adoptee is unique in the extent to which his quest for the most fundamental details of his existence is a direct source of guilt. He has no choice but to adapt to a pervasive sense of separateness and half-life" (Lifton[7] [69]: p. 2–3).

Search for Origins

During adolescence or even later, adopted teenager and young adults - in their search for identity - strive to obtain information about their biological parents and their personal early childhood history.

However, adopted children receive very often only scant information about their origins. In international adoptions, there is generally little known of the prospective adoptive children. It may occur also that adoptive parents "forget" certain information, if - in their eyes - the origin of their adopted child is associated with feelings of shame; this is the case for a child of an incestuous relationships or of the prostitution milieu. The adoption topic is then tabooed, and interest in the origin denied. But the secret about the origin has psychic effects [70, 71]. Due to the lack of information, adopted children create even more phantasms about their origins and personal history.

Marriage, pregnancy, the birth of an own child, or the death of an adoptive parent are cited as triggers for adoptees search. Women search more often for their origins than men. A connection with the central preoccupation of young women with motherhood, maternal role and function, is postulated. Identification and communication

---

[7] Betty Lifton is an adoptee herself; she has written numerous books and was an adoption counselor.

with biological parents about their experience of the transition to parenthood is usually not possible and with adoptive parents too difficult or too painful in case of their infertility. Young adopted women in particular express fears of giving birth to a sick or disabled child, if they have no information regarding genetic hereditary risks. Adoptees also wish and need to tell own children their personal biographical story - where they come from, who they are - and are afraid of transmitting their own identity gaps, caused by the disruption in their generational line.

Vignettes

A young, adopted mother suffers from a depressive anxiety state after the birth of her first child (20 years after her integration into her adoptive family). She tells her psychotherapist that during her pregnancy she lived with anxieties of giving birth to a disabled child, and since the birth of her son she has been flooded with fears of being abandoned or losing someone close to her. She recounts a dream: " I meet my birth mother and my sister in my dream !" and exclaims: "But I had not a single contact in the last twenty years with neither of them." The young mother desires to tell once her son about her biological parents, but she does not even know, whether they are still alive or have already died.

An adopted father in his fifties is reminded violently by questions concerning his birth mother at the moment he is confronted with the loss of one of his children. He seeks psychotherapeutic help and, hoping to find answers, decides to search for his biological mother.

An adopted mother in her forties suffers a breakdown at the death of her child, being desperately forlorn, overwhelmed by feelings of having been abandoned again with intense longing and doubts in her relationships.

Comment

Mourning the death of a child is considered as one of the most painful grief for parents, which often takes several years. Parents, who are confronted with the loss of a child, generally maintain an inner relationship with their deceased child, sometimes during their entire lifetime.

In the above situations, the traumatic experience of the adoptees' losses in their past is reactivated, and the associated emotions of fear, annihilation, and confusion felt again. Their lifelong questioning about her birth mother is awakened once more with a yearning desire of knowing and understanding her. How is a birth mother, who carried and felt her child growing during 9 months in her womb, ever able not to keep it? What happens in her mind?

Studies on Search for Origins

The review of twelve studies of adult adoptees, wishing to search for their biological parents [72], concludes that searching patterns range from unconscious phantasms and associations to conscious ideas and representations up to active searching with the aim to reunite with biological parents [68, 73, 74]. Most of the searchers were young white adult women belonging to the middle class. After a successful search, they felt significant positive psychic changes, not only for themselves but also in their relationship with the adoptive parents [75–78]. Out of fear of hurting or losing the adoptive parents, the search was sometimes postponed or did not take place. The assessment of their adoptive family by adoptees and their phantasms concerning biological parents were quite different [68, 73, 75, 79–81]. Information collected through questionnaires showed that most adoptees had been early integrated into the adoptive family, without multiple previous placements. Almost half of the adoptees cited childhood problems, mainly of emotional nature, e.g., anxiety and confusion, behavioral disorders, depression and learning difficulties. From childhood to adulthood, there was a definite and consistent increase in conscious and preconscious representations of their adoptive status, leading to the desire to obtain specific information about their biological parents. 54% of responders signaled significant health problems (alcoholism, chronic physical or mental illness) in one or both adoptive parents, a traumatic experience for almost a third of the adoptees. For 60%, the lack of physical resemblance with adoptive parents represented a major problem, associated with frustration, embarrassment, confusion, envy, and loneliness. Regardless of how they viewed their adoptive parents - positively or negatively - adoptees cited common themes of forlornness, lack of belonging, incompleteness, and intense anxiety. After successfully finishing their search, the adoptees perceived distinct psychic changes: a better self-esteem and body image, improved interpersonal relationships, and reduced vulnerability in anxiety situations. As the group of non-searching adoptees is hardly accessible to research, the assessment and comprehension of their subjective psychic experiences and their adaptation performance are impossible.

Other studies with adopted adults show similar results [82–86]. Some adoptees advocated for open adoption and for better preparation of prospective adoptive families to meet adopted children' and adolescents' needs for being in touch with their biological parents. However, encounters of adoptees with their birth mother were also experienced as disappointing and stressful for both parts. In contrast, the finding of siblings was often a rewarding experience.

The adoptees interest in their origin usually leads to searching for the biological mother, eventually and usually later also for the father or siblings. In a Swiss study, almost half of the 42 adopted adolescents were interested in searching their biological parents [87]. 70% of the 50 interviewed adoptees, aged 15–18, confirmed to harbor phantasms concerning their origins [88].

According to several studies, adoptees with a rather poor relationship with their adoptive parents are overrepresented among the searchers [89, 90]. Studies by seeking and non-seeking adopted adults conclude that more seekers than non-seekers describe the relationship with their adoptive family and their overall experience of adoption with mixed or, in a few cases, negative feelings. This suggests that ambivalent or negative feelings about one's adoption may be a factor motivating certain adoptees to search. However, as 53% of searchers rated their adoption as a positive experience, negative feelings may not be the only reason for searching. Half of the non-searchers said they were not curious to know their origin or family background and did not feel the need to search for their biological parents or relatives. The other half of the non-searchers showed some interest and curiosity, but worried that their search would severely distress their adoptive parents or themselves [91, 92]. There seem to be differences between adoptees who search and those who do not search, and differences in the group of searchers with regard to their motivations and reasons. If adoptees initiate a search, it does not mean that they are unhappy with their adoption experience or feel negatively towards their adoptive parents. Some only search for background information about their biological heritage [93].

The decision to seek is a complex interaction of various factors. One difference is between those seekers who are dissatisfied with the adoption experience (they seek not only a more complete sense of self, but in addition a relationship with their biological parents) and those seekers who described their adoption as very positive and were mainly interested in issues such as gaining a better sense of self and identity but did not feel the need to develop an alternative filiation relationship with a biological parent.

Adoptees seek answers to questions about their identity (who I am, what do I look like, whom do I resemble) and their self-worth (why I was given up for adoption, why I was rejected, where do I belong). They search for meaning and significance in relation to their origins. Experiences of contact and rediscovery - whether actively achieved in the case of the seekers, or passively in the case of the non-seekers - proved to be extraordinarily helpful in answering questions about identity and self-worth. This did not necessarily imply a desire for a second or alternative family relationship.

Challenges in Meeting Biological Parents

During the search - often lasting for years - the affective investment of adopted children is deeply centered on their birth parents; they sense an intense detachment from their adoptive parents, which may be even accompanied by very painful feelings of alienation. Their true relationships with the adoptive parents, siblings, but also with the extended family seem unreal and inauthentic. In addition, they feel guilty and fear to hurt their adoptive parents, whom they owe so much [94].

While the adolescent adoptees have affectively invested their biological parents with a longing love, boundless hope, and infinite expectations, they also know that they are strangers. A meeting with the birth parents - in response to an emotional longing - is fantasized as a fulfilment of the existential void of identity [95]. Therefore, the encounter with a biological parent may represent a psychic shock. The birth mother or father is a stranger, any woman or man, − despair and disappointment can be immense.

Some adolescents feel that the family "castle" - they did build up in their imagination - falls into ruin, and their inner mental world will be destroyed. They suffer a seemingly endless loss and feel like orphans, saying it would be easier to really be an orphan. The confrontation of the idealized intrapsychic images of the birth parents with the real biological parents is an event, which requires an intense process of cognitive realization and awareness. Adoptees may receive information about a childhood they do not remember, hear stories they often do not trust and are unable to integrate in a biographical narrative. They can suffer from severe depression, multiple psychosomatic symptoms, present with regressive or unbearable revolting behaviors. Some adoptees show unusual and anxiety-provoking behavior and adoptive parents complain of no more recognizing their child.

Grieving is unavoidable, a complex and painful process. But the young adoptees usually do not regret their search and their meeting with birth parents. They feel having acquired something they were missing, often not easily to describe: "We are connected, bound by nothing, we have something common in nothing". The "rope" through which they were entangled with their past and "which held me captive like a slave", as an adopted youth said, "seems finally to unknot" and releases psychic energy, permitting to envision the future.

Vignette

Lionel, 10 years old, "imperatively" wishes to meet his birth mother. In a psychotherapeutic session, he draws the town where - according to his adoptive parents - she lived and probably still lives. "Where does she live? - She could also live here on the same floor as you", he says. To see his biological mother is his "greatest goal"; he wants to know what she looks like, how she lives, if she is being well, and desires to be alone with her, to live with her. He has many questions to ask her. He wants to know, how he was like as a small child, why did she give him away and where does his brother live. In a squiggle game, he draws a spiral: "This will take me to my destination"; he draws the path he must take, the stops where he will rest and calculates that it will take months until he reaches his destination, which is the center of the spiral, i.e., until he will see his mother. In the following squiggle, a face emerges, "a happy face, a woman, my mother", who will happily look at him when he meets her.

Many adoptees are content to receive information. "Knowing that I could know, was allowed to know, was enough for me", said one adopted teenager. Our society ascribes a special significance to genetic origins, as evidenced by the statements "the apple doesn't fall far from the tree", or "as is the father so is the son". Adolescent adoptees lack this "safety net of genetic expectations". One wonders whether the search for birth parents reflects more the need for a connection with the cultural and biological heritage than for establishing an actual relationship with the biological parent [96].

In a study [97], the experiences of 21 couples of adoptive parents - during the meeting of their adopted children with their biological parents - were explored by semi-structured interviews. Adoptive parents often felt neglected, desperate, and confused in their emotions and needs throughout their adopted daughter's or son's encounter. They expressed anxieties of losing their child and feared a deterioration of the parent-child relationship. They questioned their right to parenthood vis-à-vis their child. Sadness and painful feelings about their infertility awoke again.

The so-called heritage journey, birth-country travel, adoption return trips, enable adoptive families with their internationally adopted child to get in touch with ethnic, linguistic, cultural roots and initiate a sense of continuity about the life history of their adoptee(s). Preparation of the journey as well as the integration of the family's shared experiences may represent a stressful episode, having lasting impacts on the child and his family. Returning to the country of origin, where future adoptive parents received their child, has different meanings for them as for their adopted children, who may have no conscious memories at all, or who live their childhood memories differently as their parents [98, 99].

Summary

The need to know one's origin seems to arise from multiple sources, such as the genetically predetermined aspects of personality development and the subjective response to loss, attachment, and cognitive perplexities. The affective confrontation with the perception of being different is very often lived as a disadvantage and associated with the event of having been abandoned.

These issues are of course deeply influenced by the adoptive parents' personality, their individual and family histories. Finally, societal attitudes towards adoption as an "auxiliary solution" and the perception of the adopted child as different, mysterious, also play a crucial role. These attitudes are reinforced by the legislation aiming to "protect" all those involved in the adoption triangle. The search represents the adoptees' attempt to elaborate meaning and significance for the losses experienced, to free themselves from a sense of disadvantage, to consolidate identity concerns (including body image and sexual identity), to clarify cognitive dissonances, to internalize a sense of control, and finally to satisfy the most fundamental need of experiencing human connectedness [100].

> Your children are not your children.
> They are the sons and daughters of life's longing for themselves.
> They come through you, but not from you.
> And even if they are with you, they are not yours.
> You may give your love, but not your thoughts.
> You may prepare a dwelling place for their bodies, but not for their souls.
> For their souls reside in the house of the future, and that remains closed to you, even in your dreams.
> You may strive to be like them, but do not try to make them resemble you.
> For life does not go back, nor does it dwell on yesterday.
> Khalil Gibran ([101]: p. 22).

Family Dynamics

The adoption process is inscribed within the continually changing needs and goal aspirations of each developing individual throughout the various life phases of the family members and the family [102].

The event of adoption modifies the family dynamics. The specific challenges of adoption consist in integrating this event into the individual's biography and the family history. Even if the adoptive parents *are* the true parents for the child, the absent biological parents are not to be considered merely as strangers, as Goldstein et al. [103] describe in their book *Beyond the best interest of the child.*

The significance of the biological parents must be taken seriously by the adoptive family, in order to prevent that wishful thinking and unnamed phantasms about the biological parents arise in the shared family life and are all the more powerful the more they are ignored. The special conditions of adoption create neither new interaction models in the parent-child relationship nor specific communication structures. The significance attributed to adoption, the importance of the child's biological parents in the adoptive family is determined by the family members as individuals, by their biographies and by the family constellation [104].

The integration of the child's origins and past requires that parents and child try, throughout the child's development, to understand these realities together, but also endure the lack of knowledge. This process calls for sincere communication and the recognition of differences between adoptive parents and biological parents as well as between adopted child and biological child [105]. Restitution of what the child has experienced and what is known about him may contribute to his sense of continuity and identity. Thanks to the supportive and emotionally meaningful relationship with both adoptive parents, the child will be capable of coming to term with the losses in his personal history. With mutual significant exchanges, the adoptive parent-child relationship gains a very special quality. Ultimately, only the child alone "knows" - even only unconsciously - his own story, which he begins to recount in fantasizing about his lived experiences, together with his adoptive parents, over the course of his development.

Vignette

Lyo, of Asian origin, came to Switzerland for adoption at the age of four and a half years. Six years later, at the time of the child psychiatric consultation, she has still not been adopted. According to the prospective adoptive parents, Lyo presents behavioral problems (running away, lying, and stealing) and relationship difficulties in the family. In the first meeting with the child psychiatrist, Lyo, ten and a half years old, shares her fear having to return to her country of origin, something her future adoptive parents always threaten her with.

In a squiggle game [106],[8] Lyo draws a telephone - symbol of communication – and bursts into tears and cries in many subsequent sessions, in which she recounts her personal story and memories of her country of origin.

---

[8] The Squiggle Game was described by D. W. Winnicott (1896–1971) pediatrician and psychoanalyst.

It corresponds to a modality of diagnostic and therapeutic dialogue and is a way of maintaining contact with the conscious and unconscious personality interests of a patient. Winnicott conceived his game as interactive, as a form of therapeutic communication with children.

What saddens her most is that her father, a soldier, who was sick and died of an illness she ignores but from which he might have been saved. Lyo does not know if her mother, who had abandoned her when she was 2 years old, is still alive. Her father had entrusted her to a foster mother, whom Lyo remembers very clearly. She lived there with eight other children, and as the youngest she had a privileged place next to her foster mother, both at the table for meals and when sleeping. Life took place in a room, which served as a lounge and dining room during the day and as a bedroom (mattress dormitory) at night. She was subsequently placed in an orphanage, not knowing why. When she arrived in Switzerland, no one was expecting her. Eventually, her future adoptive parents, whose expected child had not arrived, took her in. Lyo would have preferred to stay with her foster mother.

Later, Lyo speaks of her uncertainty if her father was still alive. In times of sadness and loneliness, but especially in conflictual situations with her prospective adoptive parents, she imagines that her father searches for her or that she returns to her country of origin finding him. The most beautiful image of her phantasms is that they both set off to search at the same moment and meet on their way.

Lyo intends to return to her country to look for traces of her family and draws the emblem of her country of origin: for her it represents a symbol of peace—a peace that she wished so much for her country and that would have spared her uprooting.

Comment

The family romance Lyo fantasizes expresses her desire to be reunited with her father and denies his death. It shows the so much longed-for reconciliation with the biological parents and her need to be relieved of her guilt feelings—stemming from fears of being responsible for the abandonment and the suffered rejection—what would greatly improve her self-confidence and self-esteem.

Lyo wishes to be a nurse, who is taking care of small children and also her father. In the narratives she invented during her psychotherapy, she is always caring as a mother for her own children, conceived without a father.

Comment

Lyo's desire to nurse infants as a mother may be understood as an intense need to nurture and heal her intrapsychic abandoned child, a wish to be able to repair her inner self. Her loyalty tie to her father forbids her to fantasize a procreation through a heterosexual relationship; did Lyo unconsciously desired or fantasized to have a child from her father?

The prospective adoptive parents (the mother is 12 years older than the father) informed the psychotherapist in a first meeting that the pregnancy with their biological son led to their marriage, with which their extended families disagreed. After the mother endured several miscarriages, the father wished adopting a girl as a playmate for his son. A first proposed child by the placement agency failed, because—according to the parents—his release for adoption was revoked.

In a next interview, the mother explained that Lyo presented problems since her arrival in the family, the reason why she has not been adopted. For her, the adoption must take place in joy. In a later session, the father speaks in favor for the adoption, the mother remains ambivalent. She believes it is better for Lyo to keep her name.

Even if she is not adopted, she will always remain their child. Behind the parents' disagreement about adoption lay a serious marital conflict.

Comment

Lyo was—in her subjective experience—abandoned in her country of origin by her mother at the age of two, then by her father and finally by the foster mother. Her fears and lack of self-confidence associated with these experiences were continuously reinforced by the hostile attitude of the future adoptive parents, who refused a legal adoption and threatened sending Lyo back to her country of origin.

Adopted children ward off their fears of being again rejected by behaving aggressively: it is as if they provoke a new rejection. The prospective adoptive parents had never been able to accomplish a mourning process of their incapacity to have a second biological child. The reason for adopting Lyo was the father's desire to have a playmate for their biological son. In addition, other motivations—more or less conscious—and expectations regarding the future child were revealed: the parents hoped not only for an improvement of their marital and intra-family relations and communications, but also for a compensation of their narcissistic hurt, due to their incapacity of having a second biological child; they wished to demonstrate their parental and family competence outside, especially towards their families of origin. Since Lyo did not live up to the fantasized expectations, the parents were no longer interested in adopting her. Lyo was never adopted but placed in an institution.

What matters in life is not what happens to you but what you remember and how you remember it. Gabriel Garcia Márquez.

Narratives

Introduction

Narratives belong to the oldest tradition in human history. This is illustrated by the epic poems Iliad and Odyssey of the ancient Greek poet Homer or the Old and New Testaments of the Bible. They are the carriers and transmitters of individual and cultural heritage of previous to future generations. In all cultures, there is a tendency to create stories about human diversity and to share tradition-based meanings: the soul of the people is reflected in their legends [107].

Narrating one's life has a constructive quality; the impoverishment to tell personal narratives or the loss of the ability to turn life events into transmissible stories corresponds to a personal, familial, or sociocultural historical tragedy because the symbolic communication of human experiences is interrupted.

Damasio [108] distinguishes preverbal from verbal narratives. The preverbal narratives are built up in the earliest relationships with primary caregivers through nonverbal communications and contain perception and awareness of emotions and bodily sensations; they can be viewed as fundamental building blocks in the development of self, self-concept, and self-esteem. The preverbal narratives are transformed with the acquisition of language and translated into verbal narratives.

Already infants attempt to grasp storylines and children configure personal experiences into a biographical history. The significance of these experiences is expressed in nonverbal (e.g., gestures, facial expressions, tone of voice, body tone and—posture) and verbal forms (e.g., narrative representation). Verbal narratives correspond to conscious fantasy formations. At the same time, narratives reveal un- and preconscious ideas and fantasies of individual intrapsychic experiences and testify of children's great imagination and creativity. Narratives may also represent defense mechanisms against unacceptable or painful psychic contents. This defensive part of the phantasms often arises due to narcissistic hurts, loyalty conflicts or oedipal problems; it is especially evident in the therapeutic process and will not be elaborated here.

Singer [109] summarizes the research on narrative identity and meaning attribution across the adult lifespan: "Our ability to construct narratives evolves and changes over all phases of the lifespan, as does our capacity for autobiographical reasoning and the ability to make meaning of the stories we tell" (p. 443). New life experiences may change the personal narrative identity, which is related to memory, time, individual features, and critical circumstances. Personal narratives help a subject to be connected to the past, live in the present and anticipate the future.

Emotional experiences can best be represented by describing specific images and episodes in verbal systems. Storytelling offers the possibility of triggering a symbolic process, i.e., emotions will be evoked through associated memories and images and thanks to language linked to verbal systems [110]. Narrative telling serves mainly to ascribe meaning and significance to life events that have interrupted the continuity of experience. During developmental phases and transition periods, personal identity may change, and the corresponding narrative may present the so-called turning points, which change the significance of past experiences and have an impact on a subject's identity [111, 112].

Memories

Childhood memories of the first years of life are modified or constructed at later developmental periods by the process of Nachträglichkeit,[9] that is, by means of "retrospective attribution" ([113]: p. 36). Events and intrapsychic experiences of the past, which the small child was not able to accommodate, find only later meaning and interpretation, what Freud [114, 115] called retranscription of memory. A traumatic life event in childhood may retroactively (nachträglich) lead to symptoms or

---

[9] Nachträglichkeit, retrospective attribution or retranscription of memory according to Modell [111] or deferred action, in French après-coup, is a concept that refers to Freud's original term Nachträglichkeit, conceived as early as 1895 in the Project for a Scientific Psychology ([114]) "Childhood traumas operate in a deferred fashion as though they were fresh experiences; but they do so unconsciously" ([112]: p. 167).

a psychic breakdown. For Freud [116], "impressions from the pre-sexual period, which have had no effect on the child, attain traumatic power at a later date as memories" (p.133). Likewise, threats endured in childhood can have pathogenic effects afterward [117]. At a very young age, a child cannot react adequately to an event, which will only later be understandable [118]. Earliest experiences are not stored in the form of retrievable memories. The missing engrams are often only reconstructed, sometimes starting from "recurrent acting". Unassimilated past affective experiences are brought into the present, and the compulsion to repeat represents the urge to seek re-transcription of a memory in a new context and within a meaningful relationship. Freud [119] considered repetition as a form of memory.

Eickhoff [120] describes the phenomenon of "Nachträglichkeit" as a constant recontextualization of events from earlier developmental phases into later stages. The processing of events later on, introduces a special dimension to temporality: it does not influence the sequence of time but the significance of the event.

Experiences that are not inscribed in a time sequence (past–present–future) tend to repeat themselves. They appear as an everlasting presence. "… The past is not the passive container of things bygone. The past, indeed, is our very being, and it can stay alive and evolve; the present is the passage where the re-transcription and recontextualization of our past continually occur …" ([121]: p. 814). "… for any significant mental event, there is an après-coup effect (Nachträglichkeit), a re-organizing of the mind that lets new forms show up or, conversely, that may bury ideas and affects that had emerged" ([122]: p. 759).

Historical Truth

The notion of "historical truth" is highly complex as the earliest experiences are not encoded as retrievable memories. "His (the analyst's) work of construction, or, if it is preferred, of reconstruction, resembles to a great extent an archaeologist's excavation of some dwelling place that has been destroyed and buried …" ([116]: p. 259). Where Freud speaks of "the probable historical truth" (p. 261), today the terms "subjective truth" ([123]) or "authenticity" [124] are used.

The historical truth is the result of biological, cultural, and individual (preverbal and verbal) influences and does not correspond to the truth of the (re)constructed story, but includes the currently valid, often rapidly-again-modified "truth", which in a psychotherapeutic treatment is elaborated by patient and therapist. Enclosed are the reflections of the intrapsychic dialogue of the patient with himself and—in the exchange of patient and therapist—the emerging and shared current truth, which is constantly modified by conscious and unconscious contributions of both participants, leading to new insights. During a psychoanalytical therapeutic process, the history of a patient is constantly created anew. The patient attempts to establish emotional self-continuity in connecting his past without interruptions with his self-experience in the present.

The past is never dead. It's not even past. William Faulkner.

Narratives of Adoptees

Storytelling allows adopted children to build internal representations of their birth parents, an attempt to compensate for the loss of biological parents. Adoptive parents can replace biological parents in their roles and functions, but it is left to the adopted child, to build up internal coherent parental representations. This seems to be particularly difficult for older adopted children; the older child has to start all over again, because the ongoing process of engaging and interacting with parents or other caregivers has been interrupted. Sooner or later, the adopted child will, in a trustful relationship, begin to narrate—in fantasizing—his past experience. The narratives contain the child's desire to elaborate what has happened to him and is a basic need to ward off feelings of despair, helplessness, fear, shame, and guilt. They also represent wishes to repair what the child—in his phantasms—believes to have destroyed. Finally, these fantasies provide narcissistic gratification, which the child depends on, because of the unbearable injury he has suffered. The narratives contain elements of reality, but represent to a large extent phantasmatic constructions, which the child sometimes tells as if they were real experiences of his past. The stories can also exclude facts of reality that are too painful or too shameful. Children who have suffered physical or sexual violence, for example, often deny having been abused, even when they bear visible marks on their bodies of the suffered abuse. A maltreated adopted boy, whose scars were caused by burns from an iron, said that an iron fell on him.

Children often tell confusing, seemingly incoherent stories that give the impression that they might not correspond to reality. Adults sometimes accuse them of lying. Conversely, the child may highly idealize his past, so that his narrative may be grotesquely at odds with reality. The often far too painful reality must be fought off unless the child represses it. Often, however, children are far too afraid to talk about their past as they imagine revealing secrets, which could have disastrous consequences. Retreating into the inner fantasy world represents a way to endure the traumatic situation, i.e., pushing the traumatic event out of consciousness by investing a counter-world, keeping the memory of the event away or splitting off the original feelings of fear, helplessness, and despair.

According to Wilkinson and Hough [125], children strive to create memories from affective impressions, to control the effects of such memories, and to establish a continuous sense of self in their relationship with others.

Adoptive parents sometimes consider such narratives of memories to be lies, since they can indeed not be verified; however, they are not lies, but a connection—albeit illusory in nature—with the past and thus a way to neutralize the experienced traumatic separation.

Narratives resemble fairy tales or myths. The phantasms of adopted children contain the theme of abandonment. According to Moro [126], the abandoned and exposed child is confronted with an experience of extraordinary danger; he preserves the memory of this endangerment in the form of interactive phantasms between himself and his environment. These phantasmatic productions oscillate between two poles: an extreme psychic vulnerability and the development of an extraordinarily creative potential.

Adoptees confirm often both evolutive tendencies as the example of a highly vulnerable, yet extremely talented adopted adolescent teenager shows, who plays various musical instruments and creates musical compositions, drawings, comic strips, and theatrical performances.

Any aggression, which is not denied and for which personal responsibility is assumed, will be used for repair and restoration; at the core of all play, work, and art lies unconscious remorse for destructive phantasms and a desire to make things right again [127, 128].

Adoptees are preoccupied in their fantasies with their abandonment, lived as a threatening experience, and harbor anxious feelings and fantasies of being at risk of further injuries. The adopted child grows up in a new environment, which very often shares his strong sense of strangeness. The exposure and abandonment can have the significance of a hidden, potential infanticide. In his phantasms, the adopted child asks himself the existential question to whom he owes his survival. Did the child survive thanks to a miracle, a fairy godmother, an angel, a protective animal or because of his personal omnipotence? The narratives try to give answers to such questions.

Vignette

Elia, a ten and a half-year-old boy, adopted from South America, draws—in the presence of his adoptive mother—during an initial interview with the child psychiatrist a whale and comments: "A whale in the sea finds a little boy who has fallen in the water and brings him to the shore; the whale is caught by fishermen, but they let him go because he has saved a little boy". Questions by the child psychiatrist clarify that the little boy is three years old, a lost child and that no one knows what happened to his parents.

Comment

Elia seems to tell his fantasized story of his abandonment; the narrative evokes the biblical heroic tale of Jonah's rebirth after staying in the belly of the whale.

Adoptees' narratives of their past contain numerous questions about guilt and responsibility. Unconscious phantasms of having killed the biological parents, or of having been stolen by the adoptive parents are revealed. But the phantasms also contain the desire for reunification with the biological parents and for reparation. Fears of death or even suicide attempts are based on fantasied wishes to reunite with the lost parent but can also express a need for punishment.

In identifying with the aggressor—the persons responsible for the abandonment—these phantasms are acted out against the adoptive parents or significant other persons, as they cannot be directed against absent birth- or foster parents. The wish for reunion with the biological parents is often expressed in phantasms that the parents are searching for their child, thus confirming the child's narcissistic worth.

Vignette

Cecilia, eight-year-old, is an adopted girl with a physical disability; she brings a "sad parrot" (a stuffed animal) to the first meeting with the child psychiatrist. Its sadness is a secret known only to her. Then she tells her "big dream": "A baby bird has flown away and lost itself. The father of the little bird finds it again and brings it back as a surprise to the mother who is waiting for her baby".

Comment

The dream contains Cecilia's phantasm to be responsible for losing her birth parents and at the same time her wish to be reunited with them [129].

Vignette

The eight-year-old, severely traumatized Alice (she was hospitalized at the age of 18 months in a pronounced state of neglect and with severe developmental delays) draws a girl who is five years old and takes her one-and-a-half-year-old doll for a walk, who—like herself—is called Alice. Alice wishes to be the five-year-old girl. She draws two hearts as an expression of their love, and two flowers and a watering can because the two flowers need water (Fig. 7.4).

Comment

Alice wishes in a regressive movement to take care of herself as a one-and-a-half-year-old baby; she expresses her need to "heal" her intrapsychic infant.

Fig. 7.4 Alice, 8-year-old, a girl taking her doll for a walk

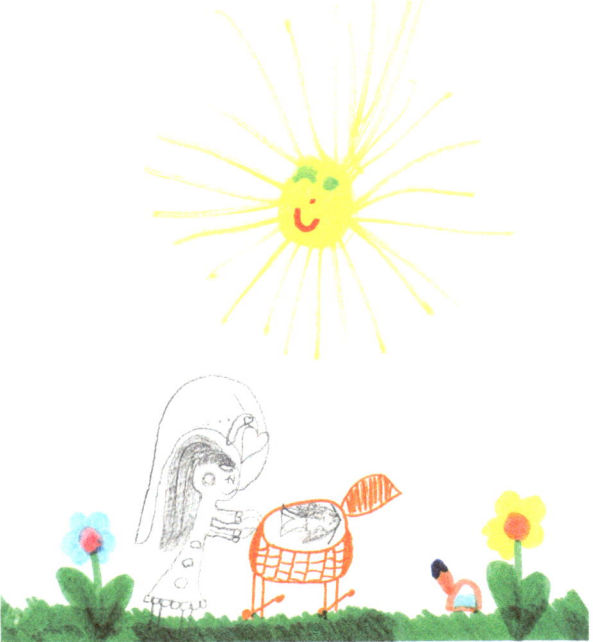

Vignette

A seven-year-old girl is brought to the child psychiatrist because of her jealousy, sadness, and temper tantrums since the arrival of her adoptive sister nine months ago. The adoptive parents inform that Lisa—in her tantrums – did bite the adoptive mother, from whom she cannot tolerate to be separated and in whose bed she sleeps. Lisa had said to be very sad, because she could not live with her birthmother—like her best friend—and to dream about her own birth. According to the adoptive parents, Lisa was separated from her biological mother immediately after birth and treated in a hospital for a serious infection. At the age of two to three years, Lisa wanted to play repeatedly "giving birth" and, in her favorite game, she asked her adoptive mother to choose the dog Lisa among lost dogs.

Comment

In her "giving birth" play scenes, Lisa expresses her wish to know about her birth and her need to be unique, desired, and chosen by her adoptive mother.

In the first child psychiatric interview with Lisa and her adoptive parents, Lisa draws her birth (Fig. 7.5): her adoptive mother gives birth to Lisa with the help of the doctor, in the delivery room, which is equipped with a large lamp.

Comment

Through her rebirth, Lisa tries to undo the adoption and the associated great insecurity in her attachment to the adoptive mother. She seems to reexperience the psychic trauma she suffered at birth (separation from her biological mother, hospitalization

Fig. 7.5 Lisa, 7-year-old, draws being born from her adoptive mother

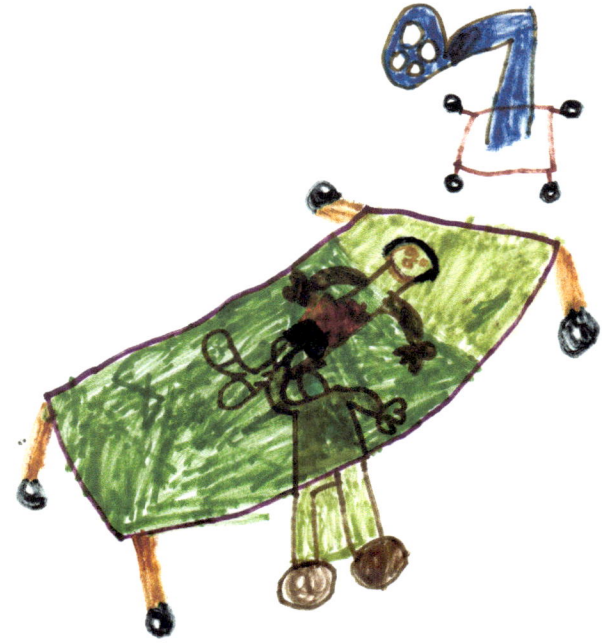

due to serious illness) with the associated emotions such as anger, sadness and above all fear of being abandoned again. Lisa experiences the arrival of her sister as a rejection, as the sister requires the availability of the adoptive parents, who until now have cared solely and exclusively for Lisa.

Vignette

Jonathan, six years old, is addressed for psychotherapy by the school authorities because of his dangerous, suicidal behavior. For the last three years he has been living with his adoptive parents.

While participating in a psychoanalytically oriented group therapy, Jonathan repeatedly tries to hurt himself; he has constantly to be held physically. He accuses the therapists of being thieves of treasures and of children. Finally, he exclaims, "I want to kill myself" and later asks the question "why can't I kill myself?"

Comment

This example shows the frequent phantasms among adopted children of having been stolen by the adoptive parents. Jonathan feels rejected and believes having been snatched and thieved from his birth parents.

He maintains his affective ties to his biological parents and accuses his adoptive parents (in the transference the therapists) of having captured and stolen him. In the role of a helpless and hopeless victim in the traumatic situation of the past, he expresses his pain and despair in auto-aggressive behavior, carried by the phantasm that death could "save" him.

Infantile pain occurs when the basic needs of an infant are not met and is linked with an absence of emotional communication at a stage of the infant's absolute dependence. This experience leads to a distorted development process and is accompanied by unimaginable and unbearable fears of falling, disintegration, and depersonalization. Infantile pain is present before an autonomous self is established and is often warded off by panic and sometimes by suicide attempts rather than by remembering [128].

Narratives also reveal phantasms of narcissistic murderous rage. These phantasms are denied, but expressed in symbolic forms, e.g., in plays and drawings or acted out in aggressiveness, representing in most cases the dramatization of an inner reality, too painful to be tolerated. For their murderous fantasies, adopted children often feel the need to be punished.

Vignette

In the first session after a two-month therapeutic interruption, Mia, a five-year-old adopted girl tells: "I killed my girlfriend's mother". The girl asks her psychotherapist to build a prison and lock her up in it, chained by hands, feet, as well as by her whole body.

Comment

Being held by shackles in prison reduces the unbearable feelings of fear associated with the fury of having been abandoned and rejected. The imprisonment represents a protection against the dread that phantasms of murderous rage might be realized, leading to the relationship breakup, as it happened in the past with the birth parents.

The necessity to be safeguarded is expressed be seven-year-old Maurice, who draws a dog, which is also 7 years old and, as Maurice says, loves his fence, behind which he feels secured.

Comment

Maurice is identifying himself with the dog and discloses his feelings of vulnerability, which reflects adoptees' often extreme need of containment and protection.

Vignette

The future adoptive parents request a child psychiatric consultation for eight-year-old Carlos who presents aggressive behavior at school and in the family. Carlos originates from South America and has been living in the adoptive family for 9 months.

Carlos draws a submarine in a whale and says: "This is a (male) submarine that causes the (female) whale to explode; it perishes and dies".

Comment

The submarine, representing the boy, seems to be—in Carlos' phantasm—responsible for the death of the whale, representing his pregnant birth mother.

The loss of the biological parents appears to the adopted child often as a confirmation of his fear having "carried out" his murderous fantasies, i.e., having killed his birth parents.

Antisocial tendency arises from loss or deprivation and is an emergency signal. One could say the acting out is an alternative to despair. At the root of any antisocial tendency [127, 128] there is a lived experience of loss. The resulting aggression represents almost always a dramatic acting out of a despairing inner reality, impossible to endure.

Vignette

In a psychoanalytical psychodrama group therapy, the boys (aged between ten and thirteen, three of them adopted) play their imagined story of an orphan girl who is locked up in prison. She must be punished because she has no parents. A queen wants to adopt the girl; however, the girl refuses.

In the discussion that follows the play, the boys explain that the girl killed her birth parents and must therefore be punished. The boys agree that it is nonviable to have two sets of parents.

Comment

The phantasms of the family romance, namely, to descend from nobler, i.e., royal parents, emerge in the story, but cannot be "realized" in the play. It is as if the real existence of biological parents renders the intrapsychic elaboration of the family romance unimaginable. An adoption is rejected in the play. The girl behaves loyally to her birth parents.

Vignette

Prospective adoptive parents request a child psychiatric evaluation for their eight-year-old boy who has been rejected by the first adoptive family. Philip repeats a play scene, in which an evil infant, who has sickened and killed his parents, must be punished. The house, where the infant lives, is burning. The authorities, the police, and the fire department, called for help, are unable to control the evil infant. Finally, the evil infant transports the sick and dead parents to the hospital and the authorities to the prison.

Comment

Philip's phantasms demonstrate his feelings of being an evil and destructive infant who is responsible for the relationship ruptures with his former caregivers. He seems to have lost all trust in any authority, which could restore law, order, and safety. He, who has destroyed his loved ones and his home in a murderous way, must try to restore order and heal the injured or dead.

Where parents do not provide a protective and supportive environment, the child creates a different reality, which maintains the illusion that he will be able to satisfy his own needs and help himself thanks to his belief in his own omnipotence [127].

Adopted children may express their belief to be an unwanted child through psychosomatic or behavioral symptoms. Children bear fantasies of having been bad, dirty, or monstrous. "I am not desired" appears in the self-representation as being rejected. Therefore, the adopted child's unconscious hope is that, for instance, his regressive or psychosomatic manifestations will not be dismissed, but accepted by his adoptive parents. He expects that the adoptive parents recognize his past identity and help him to preserve it.

Vignette

Adoptive parents report that their eight-year-old boy, who suffers from hemophilia, is constantly pulling at the collar of his clothes as if he were trying to hold on to them, tearing his shirt or sweater. Ricardo either shows very regressive behavior, e.g., wets at night, or extremely dangerous acting out (suicidal tendency). He never tells anything about his past, answers questions only with "I don't know", repeatedly plays birth scenes and comments: "My (birth)mother is afraid that I am dead".

Comment

Ricardo, in holding on his clothes, seems to try a kind of self-holding, wishing to regress to the time of his birth (play of birth scenes). Is Ricardo so desperate that he would prefer to be dead or is he preoccupied by anxieties that his birth mother might already be dead or that he may die?

The antisocial tendency, emanating from deprivation, represents the child's claim to return to the satisfactory condition before his deprivation and is always a call for help and accompanied by hopefulness [127]. Manifestations are stealing, lying, aggressive and destructive activities; these acting-out behaviors are signals of distress and alternatives to despair.

If the adopted child is hopeless in terms of being able to repair the original trauma, he lives in a state of relative depression or dissociation, which conceals the constantly threatening chaotic state. However, when the child begins to invest a person, engages in a significant relationship, then the antisocial tendency begins to manifest itself, as a compulsive need to either make unrealizable demands, followed by e.g., to steal the significant person, or to initiate—through destructive behavior— a severe or even punishing answer as the following vignette illustrates.

Vignette

A first child psychiatric evaluation of Frederick takes place at the age of ten for his behavioral disorders (stealing, lying, running away) and auto—aggressive acting out (physical injuries). At the age of five, Frederick was placed with a foster family for adoption; however, a legal adoption did not take place because of Friedrich's psychosocial problems. The foster parents informed that Frederick, at the time when he was welcomed into his future adoptive family, had asked to change his name; since then, he called himself by their family's last name and by a first name he had given himself.

In the first interview with the child psychiatrist, Frederick establishes contact very cautiously; initially he appears suspicious, observant and controls the relationship.

In a squiggle game [106] he draws half a fir tree (Fig. 7.6) and comments: "It will soon be winter. The fir tree will be a Christmas tree, it will be cut down; it will be sold; it will be decorated, but then it will be thrown away."

Comment

Frederick seems to be telling his own story, namely that of a half-child (deprived of his birth parents) who cherishes the hope of growing up in the new foster family into a beautiful Christmas tree that will never be given away.

Frederick associates that he has seen a photo of his birth father on which only half of him is depicted. To the question concerning his biological parents, Frederick replies that he knows nothing about his birth parents, does not want to know anything because this involves too disturbing thoughts, which he prefers to block out.

To the following squiggle, Frederick tells the story of two robbers whose main concern is to steal. The next squiggle is about a parrot who flew all the way to America. Friedrich adds that he has had no contact with his birth mother, who has left him forever for America when he was 4 years old.

He addresses—in his story about the parrot—his mother: "Hello, how are you, many greetings from your son", and continues that the mother greets him back but closes the door again immediately. The parrot flies through the window, but the mother is already gone. He tries to reach her by phone, but she unplugs the phone. Then the parrot pokes a hole in the glass window and pecks his mother with his beak.

Comment

Friedrich's narrative tells his wish to be able to contact his birth mother, his longing to know her, as well as his rage having been abandoned and rejected by her. A mourning process over the loss of his biological parents and his past, marked by relationship ruptures and milieu changes, has until now not taken place. Friedrich is overwhelmed by violent aggressive impulses which he tries to fight off and control

Fig. 7.6 Frederick,
10-year-old, half a fir tree

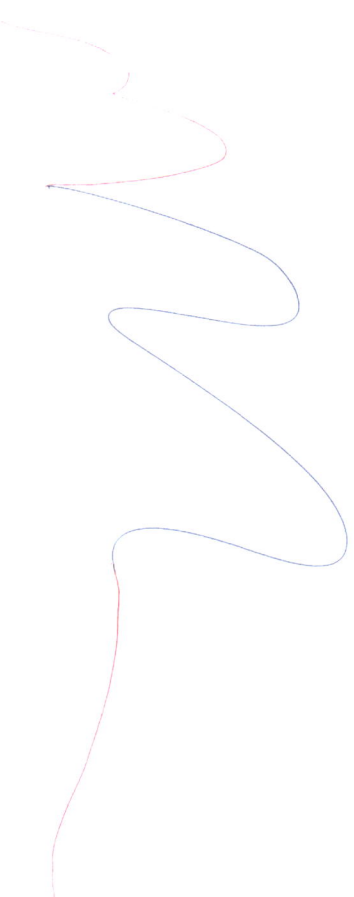

and which find expression in his physical injuries and his antisocial and dangerous behavior.

Friedrich uses partially maniform defenses, which can be considered as an inability to give full meaning to his psychic realities. Embarrassing, painful memories, especially losses, must be denied. A child or adolescent behaves as if cut off from his memories of the past and finds himself in a kind of enduring present, in which there is neither loss nor death [130]. Adoptive parents observe again and again that their adopted child lives into the day, unable to project himself into the future, or if he does, then only in the form of omnipotent, unrealizable projects, an escape from a too painful intrapsychic reality.

If a child begins to fantasize about his experienced past, it is of little importance whether these narratives represent elements of reality or not. It is above all essential that the child communicates his inner psychic reality in his own way and a trusted and emotionally available adult person listens attentively to his story. This significant adult must be able to identify himself with the child, to empathize with the child's suffering and pain without being flooded by similar feelings himself. The adult has to avoid making a judgment about the child or the persons who did not take care of the child or whose victim he became. Listening corresponds to enduring the horror and the unbearable feelings the child suffered.

When adopted children are not able expressing in words what they experienced, they may show through their symptomatic behavior what happened to them. If adoptive parents listen attentively to their child's narratives during his development, a very important process of awareness and symbolization of unconscious and pre-verbal contents and emotions takes place. The narratives change as the child can only gradually perceive, feel, and express the so far unconscious emotions associated with his phantasms. This process depends on the child's ego development and his ability to endure his emerging emotions. A child needs an adult who is emotionally tuned in and available to empathize with his despair, to help him understand his lived past and ascribe meaning and coherence to it. This process allows the child to slowly admit the feelings of grief about his painful losses and the linked injuries. Grieving enables the child to find and build up his own identity vis-à-vis the dual parents and eventually the dual cultures, what contributes to the restoration of the child's narcissistic equilibrium.

Summary

Narratives told by the child to a significant caregiver promote a grieving process and the working through of loss and psychic trauma. Thanks to the narration, the phantasms and lived emotions of the traumatic experience can be perceived, felt, and expressed, and thus the traumatic experience be transformed. However, if the traumatic event remains unspoken, i.e., withdrawn from verbal discourse, secrets emerge from the unimaginable or unspeakable events. The presence of a secret disrupts any meaningful relationship, including the parent-child relationship. An adopted child's affective history is updated in the hope that the significant caregiver will be able to help him process and make sense of his experienced events. Only words make experiences nameable and communicable [131]. The unhindered emotional dialogue between adoptive parents and adopted child is so important as otherwise unnamed fantasies, desires, fears, and feelings about the biological parents, the origin, and personal history of the child lead to additional intrafamilial secrets. The revelation of the fantasized and/or real past allows for a shared experience, based on the narrated story told, and strengthens the affective bond between adoptive parents and child [132]. The narratives, which adopted children tell, allow for an integration of split-off mental content, consisting mainly of "translating" unconscious and preconscious processes into metaphorical language.

The most difficult and undoubtedly most important task for adopted children is to be able to bring together in their intrapsychic world the representations of their birth parents and other significant attachment figures—if such existed—with those of their adoptive parents [133]. Thanks to this phantasmatic convergence, a sense of genetic ancestry and belonging, and thus a true parent-child bond and relationship will evolve. "The adopted child must include two separate sets of parents within his representational world. He must also integrate into his representation of himself the fact that he was born to one set of parents but has been raised by another set of parents". ([134], p.108).

References

1. Guyotat J. Mort/naissance et filiation. Etudes de psychopathologie sur le lien de filiation: Masson; 1980.
2. Lévy-Soussan P. Travail de filiation et adoption. Rev Franç Psychanal. 2002;1:41–9.
3. Julien P. Tu quitteras ton père et ta mère. Paris: Aubier; 2000.
4. Juillerat B. L'atome de parenté est-il soluble dans la psychanalyse? Topique, no. 75, Psychanalyse et anthropologie, p. 81–103, et dans Penser l'imaginaire, essais d'anthropologie psychanalytique, p. 11–133. Lausanne: Payot. 2001.
5. Toshio T. Characteristics of children in substitutive and adoptive care. Washington: American Public Welfare Association; 1985.
6. Boszormenyi-Nagy I, Spark G. Invisible loyalities. New York: Harper and Row; 1973.
7. Boszormenyi-Nagy I. Trust-based therapy: a contextual approach. Am J Psychiatry. 1980;137(7):767–75.
8. Freud S. The psychogenesis of a case of homosexuality in a woman, vol. XVIII. London: SE Hogarth Press; 1920b.
9. Blos P Jr. Psychic and somatic expressions of preverbal loss: analysis of a child adopted at thirteen months of age. In: von Klitzing K, Tyson P, Bürgin D, editors. Psychoanalysis in childhood and adolescence. Basel: Karger AG; 2000. p. 59–70.
10. Colon F. The family and child placement practices. Fam Process. 1978;17(3)
11. Farber S. Sex differences in the expression of adoption ideas: observations of adoptees from birth through latency. Am J Orthopsychiatry. 1977;47(4):639–50.
12. Lawton J. Review of psychiatric literature on adopted children. Arch Gen Psychiat. 1964;11:635–44.
13. Nickman SL. The adoption experience: losses in adoption. Psychoanal Study Child. 1985;40:365–98.
14. Wiener H. On being told of adoption. Psychoanal Q. 1977;46
15. Anthony EJ, Brinich P, Bradzinsky D, Goodman W, Hajal F, Schechter M. Problems of adoption: familial, developmental and biological findings as guides to treatment. In: Symposium presented at the 36th annual meeting. Amer. Acad. New York: Child Adolescent Psychiatry; 1989.
16. Macintyre JC. Resolved: children should be told of their adoption before they ask. J Amer Acad Child Adolesc Psychiatry. 1990;29:828–9.
17. Brodzinsky DM, Schechter MD, Brodzinsky AB. Children's knowledge of adoption: developmental changes and implications for adjustment. In: Ashmore RD, Brodzinsky DM, editors. Thinking about the family. Views of parents and children. Hillsdale: Erlbaum; 1986. p. 205–32.
18. Newman JL, Roberts LR, Syré CR. Concepts of family among children and adolescents: effects of cognitive level, gender, and family structure. Dev Psychol. 1993;29(6):951–62.
19. Borduin CM, Mann BJ, Cone L, Borduin BJ. Development of the concept of family in elementary school-children. J Genetic Psychology. 1990;151:33–43.

20. Jordan VB. Conserving kinship concepts: a developmental study in social cognition. Child Dev. 1980;51:146–55.
21. Belsky J, Steinberg L, Draper P. Childhood experience, interpersonal development and reproductive strategy: an evolutionary theory of socialization. Child Dev. 1991;61:647–70.
22. Maccoby EE. Different reproductive strategies in males and females. Child Dev. 1991;62:676–81.
23. Freeark K, Rosenberg E, Bornstein J, Jozefowicz-Simbeni D, Linkevich M, Lohnes K. Gender differences and dynamics shaping the adoption life cycle: review of the literature and recommendations. Am J Orthopsychiatry. 2005;75(1):86–101.
24. Brodzinsky DM, Schechter MD, Braff AM, Singer LM. Psychological and academic adjustment in adopted children. J Consulting and Clinical Psychology. 1984;52:582–90.
25. Baethge G. Aengste und unbewusste Phantasien in Adoptivfamilien. Prax. Kinderpsychol. Kinderpsychiat. 1993;42:49–55.
26. Brunet M (1989). L'Amour adopté. Ed. Renaudot.
27. Brinich PM. Psychoanalytic perspectives on adoption and ambivalence. Psychoanal Psychol. 1995;12:181–99.
28. Freud S. Family romances, vol. IX. London: SE. Hogarth Press; 1909a.
29. Robert M. Roman des origines et origines du roman. Paris: Bernard Grasset; 1972.
30. Soulé M. La vie de l'enfant: le nouveau roman familial. Paris: Éditions ESF; 1984.
31. Freud A. Annual report, January 1942. In: The writings of Anna Freud, vol. 3. New York: International Universities Press; 1973.
32. Freud A. Wege und Irrwege in der Kinderentwicklung. Bern/Stuttgart: Huber/Klett; 1968.
33. Rosenberg EB, Horner TM. Birthparent romances and identity formation in adopted children. Amer J Orthopsychiatry. 1991;6(11):70–7.
34. Fullerton CS, Goodrich W, Beth Bermann L. Adoption predicts psychiatric treatment resistances in hospitalized adolescents. J Amer Acad Child Psychiatry. 1986;25(4):542–51.
35. Priel B, Kantor B, Besser A. Two maternal representations: a study of Israeli adopted children. Psychoanal Psychol. 2000;17:128–45.
36. Blum H. Adoptive parent: generative conflict and generational continuity. Psychoanal Study Child. 1983;38:141–63.
37. Bürgin D. Adoption: trauma oder chance? In: Biermann G, editor. Handbuch der Kinderpsychotherapie (pp- 586-600). München: Reinhardt; 1992.
38. Waber-Thevoz H, Waber JP. Le lien d'adoption à l'épreuve du temps. Neuropsychiatrie de l' Enfance et l'Adolescence. 2000;48:179–98.
39. Nietzsche F. Die Geburt der Tragödie oder Griechentum und Pessimismus. Leipzig: Druck und Verlag C.G. Naumann; 1895.
40. Huth W. Adoption und Identität. Wege zum Menschen. 1980;32:49ff.
41. Breccia M. Destini delle Identità [Fates of Identities]. Int J Psychoanal. 2010;91(6):1550–7.
42. Erikson EH. The problem of ego identity. J Am Psychoanal Assoc. 1956;4:56–121.
43. Erikson EH. Identity: youth and crisis. New York, W.W: Norton; 1968.
44. Erikson EH. Life history and the historical moment. New York, W.W: Norton; 1975.
45. Hoksbergen R, Juffer F, Textor MR. Attachment und Identität von Adoptivkindern. Prax Kinderpsychol Kinderpsychiat. 1994;43:339–44.
46. Brodzinsky DM. Adjustment to adoption: a psychosocial perspective. Clin Psychol Rev. 1987;7:25–47.
47. Kohler JK, Grotevant HD, McRoy RG. Adopted Adolescents' preoccupation with adoption: the impact on adoptive family relationships. J Marriage Fam. 2002;64(1):93–104.
48. Pinderhughes EE, Rosnati R. Introduction to special issue: adoptees' ethnic identity within family and social contexts. In: Pinderhughes EE, Rosnati R, editors. Adoptees' ethnic identity within family and social contexts. New directions for child and adolescent development, vol. 150; 2015. p. 1–3.
49. Manzi C, Ferrari C, Rosnati R, Benet-Martinez V. Bicultural identity integration of transracial adolescent adoptees: antecedents and outcomes. Journal of Cross Cultural Psychology. 2014;45:888–904.

50. Friedlander ML. Ethnic identity development of internationally adopted children and adolescents: implication for family therapists. J Marital Fam Ther. 1999;25(1):43–60.
51. Richards B. What is identity? In: Graber I, Aldrige J, editors. Culture, identity and transracial adoption. London: Free Association Books; 1994.
52. Feigelman W, Silverman AT. The long-term effects of transracial adoption. Soc Serv Rev. 1984;8:588–602.
53. Grotevant HD. Assigned and chosen identity components: a process perspective on their integration. In: Adams G, Gullotta T, Montemayor R, editors. Adolescents identity formation. Newbury Park, CA: Aage; 1992. p. 73–90.
54. Phinney JS. Ethnic identity and self-esteem: a review and integration. Hispanic Journal of Behavioral Science. 1991;13:193–208.
55. Rotheram MJ, Phinney JS. Introduction: definitions and perspectives in the study of children's ethnic socialization. In: Phinney JS, Rotheram M, editors. Children's ethnic socialization: pluralism and development. Beverly Hills, CA: Sage; 1987. p. 10–28.
56. LaFramboise T, Coleman HLK, Gerton J. Psychological impact of biculturalism: evidence and theory. Psychol Bull. 1993;114:395–412.
57. Scherman R. A theoretical look at biculturalism in intercountry adoption. J Ethn Cult Divers Soc Work. 2010;19(2):127–42.
58. Taylor RJ, Thornton MC. Child welfare and transracial adoption. J Black Psychol. 1996;22:282–91.
59. Phinney JS, Rosenthal DA. Ethnic identity in adolescence: process, context, and outcome. In: Adams G, Gullotta T, Montemayor R, editors. Adolescent identity formation. Newbury Park, CA: Sage; 1992. p. 145–72.
60. Textor MR. Auslandsadoptionen. Forschungsstand und Folgerungen Praxis Kinderpsychol Kinderpsychiat. 1991;40:42–9.
61. Simon RJ, Alstein H. Adoption race, and identity: from infancy through adolescence. New York: Praeger; 1992.
62. Benson PL, Sharma AR, Roehlkepartain EC. Growing up adopted: a portrait of adolescents and their families. Minneapolis, MN: Search Institute; 1994.
63. Ferrari L, Rosnati R, Manzi C, Benet-Martinez V. Ethnic identity, bicultural identity integration, and psychological Well-being among transracial adoptees: a longitudinal study. In EE Pinderhughes and R Rosnati (eds.). Adoptees' Ethnic Identity Within Family and Social Contexts. 2015;150:63–76.
64. Swientek C. Wer sagt mir, wessen Kind ich bin? Von der Adoption Betroffene auf der Suche. Freiburg/Basel/Wien: Herder; 1993.
65. Textor MR. Inlandsadoptionen: Herkunft, Familienverhältnisse und Entwicklung der Adoptivkinder. In: RAC H, Textor MR, editors. Adoption: Grundlagen, Vermittlung, Nachbetreuung, Beratung. Freiburg: Lambertus; 1993. p. 41–63.
66. Ebertz B. Adoption als Identitätsproblem. Zur Bewältigung der Trennung von biologischer Herkunft und sozialer Zugehörigkeit. Freiburg: Lambertus; 1987.
67. Sorosky AD, Baran A, Pannor R. Adoption. Zueinanderkommen – miteinander leben. Eltern und Kinder erzählen. Reinbek: Rowohlt; 1982.
68. Trisiliotis J. In search of origins: the experiences of adopted people. London, Boston: Routledge and Kegan Paul; 1973.
69. Lifton BJ. Twice born, memoirs of an adopted daughter. New York: Penguin; 1976.
70. Delaisi G, Verdier P. Enfant de personne. Paris: Ed. Odile Jacob; 1994.
71. Verdier P, Soulé M. Le secret sur les origines. Paris: ESF; 1986.
72. Bertocci D, Schechter MD. Adopted adults' perception of their need to search: implications for clinical practice. Smith College Studies in Social Work. 1991;61:179–96.
73. Day C, Leeding A. Access to birth records: the impact of section 26 of the children act 1975. London: The Association of British Adoption and Fostering Agencies; 1980.
74. Webber J, Thompson J, Stoneman L. Adoption Reunion: a struggle in uncharted relationship. Unpublished study for the Children's Aid Society of Metropolitan Canada; 1980.

75. Bertocci D, Schechter MD. Adopted adults' perception of their need to search: an informal survey. Unpublished Study; 1987.
76. Depp CH. After Reunion: perceptions of adult adoptees, adoptive parents, and birth parents. Child Welfare. 1982;61:115–9.
77. Lion A. A survey of 50 adult adoptees who used the right of the Israeli'open file' adoption law. In: Paper presented at the annual meeting of the international forum on adolescence. Jerusalem; 1976.
78. Slaytor P. Reunion and resolution: the adoption triangle. Austalian Social Work. 1986;39(2):15–20.
79. Kowal K, Schilling KM. Adoption through the eyes of adult adoptees. Amer. J. Orthopsychiatry. 1985;55(3):354–62.
80. Sorosky AD, Baran A, Pannor R. The adoption triangle. Anchor Books, Anchor Press, Garden City, New York; 1984.
81. Thompson J, Stoneman L, Webber J, Harrison D (1978) The adoption rectangle: a study of adult adoptees search for birth family history and implications, Toronto (unpubl).
82. Campbell LH, Silverman PS, Patti PB. Reunions between adoptees and birth parents: the adoptees' experience. Soc Work. 1991;36(4):329–35.
83. Humphrey H, Humphrey M. Damaged identity and the search for kinship in adult adoptees. Brit J Medical Psychology. 1989;62:301–9.
84. Rushbrooke R. The proportion adoptees who have received their birth records in England and Wales. In: National Statistics. Population Trends; 2001. p. 104.
85. Schechter MD, Bertocci D (1990) The meaning of search. In: Brodzinsky DM, Schechter MD (Eds): The psychology of adoption (pp. 62–90). New, Oxford: Oxford University Press.
86. Swientek C. Auf der Suche nach den Eltern – auf der Suche nach Identitä. Adoption – die unendliche Geschichte. In: Hoksbergen RAC, Textor MR, editors. Adoption. Grundlagen, Vermittlung, Nachbetreuung, Beratung. Freiburg i.Br.: Lambertus; 1993b.
87. Keller-Thoma P. Adoption aus der Sicht des Adoptiv"kindes". Zürich: Schweiz. Gemeinnütziger Frauenverein/Adoptivkinder-Vermittlung; 1987.
88. Stein LM, Hoopes JL. Identity formation in the adopted adolescent. In: the delaware family study. New York: Child Welfare League of America; 1985.
89. Aumend SA, Barrett MC. Self-concept and attitudes toward adoption: a comparison of searching and nonsearching adult adoptees. Child Welfare. 1984;63:251–9.
90. Textor MR. Die unbekannten Eltern. Adoptierte auf der Suche nach ihren Wurzeln. Zentralblatt für Jugendrecht. 1990;77:10–4.
91. Howe D, Feast J. Adoption, search and Reunion: the long term experience of adopted adults. London: The Children's Society; 2000.
92. Howe D. Age at placement, adoption experience and adult adopted people's contact with their adoptive and birth mothers: an attachment perpective. Attach Hum Dev. 2001;3:222–37.
93. Passmore NL, Feeney JA, Peterson CC, Shimmaki K. Depression, emotional Arousability, and perceptions of parenting in adult adoptees and non-adoptees. Adopt Q. 2006;9(2–3):23–35. https://doi.org/10.1300/J145v09n02_02.
94. Jardin F. Réflexions sur l'adoption d'enfants âgés: les difficultés de l'i¬dentité. Neuropsychiatrie de l'enfance. 1981;29(6):297–304.
95. Steck B. L'adoption: une aventure semée d'embûches. Patient Care. 1992;8:12–24.
96. Dickman GE. Adoptees among students with disabilities. J Learn Disabil. 1992;25(8):529-531, 543.
97. Petta GA, Steed LG. The experience of adoptive parents in adoption Reunion relationships: a qualitative study. AmerJ Orthopsychiatry. 2005;75(2):230–41.
98. Gustafsson J, Lind J, Sparrman A. Family memory trips – children's and parents' planning of adoption return trips. J Heritage Tourism. 2019; https://doi.org/10.108 0/1743873X.2019.1702666.
99. Wilson SL, Summerhill-Coleman L. Exploring birth countries: the mental health implications of heritage travel for children/adolescents adopted internationally. Adopt Q. 2013;16(3–4):262–78. https://doi.org/10.1080/10926755.2013.790865.

100. Brinich PM. Adoption from the inside out: a psychoanalytic perspective. In: Brodinsky MD, Schechter MD, editors. The psychology of adoption. New York: Oxford Press; 1990. p. 42–61.
101. Khali G. Der Prophet, 7. Aufl., S. 22. München: Deutscher Taschenbuch Verlag; 2002.
102. Hajal F, Rosenberg EB. The family life cycle in adoptive families. Amer J Orthopsychiat. 1991;61(1):78–85.
103. Goldstein J, Freud A, Solnit A. Beyond the best interests of the child. 2nd ed. New York: Free Press; 1973.
104. Huth W. Psychoanalytische Reflexion und therapeutische Verfahren in Adoption und Familiendynamik. Band 11: Pädagogik; 1982.
105. Steck B. Aspects psychologiques de l'adoption. Rev. méd. Romand. 1987;107:1025–35.
106. Winnicott DW. Therapeutic consultations in child psychiatry. London: Hogarth; 1971.
107. Murray HA. Explorations in personality. New York: Oxford University Press; 1938.
108. Damasio AR. Descartes error. Emotion, reason, and the human brain, a Grosset/Putnam book. New York: G.P. Putnam's Sons; 1994.
109. Singer JA. Narrative identity and meaning making across the adult lifespan: an introduction. J Pers. 2004;72(3):438–59.
110. Bucci W. The power of the narrative: a multiple code account. American Psychological Ass., 1994.
111. Riessman C. Strategic uses of narrative in the presentation of self and illness: a research note. SocSci Med. 1990;30:1195–200.
112. Riessman C. Analysis of personal narratives. In: Fortune AE, Reid WJ, Miller RL, editors. Handbook of interviewing. New York: Columbia University Press; 2013.
113. Modell AH. Other times, other realities. Toward a theory of psychoanalytic treatment. Cambridge: Harvard University Press; 1990.
114. Freud S. Further remarks on the neuro-psychoses of defence, vol. III. London: Hogarth Press; 1896.
115. Freud S. In: Masson JM, editor. The complete letters of Sigmund Freud to Wilhelm Fliess,1896. Cambridge: Harvard University Press; 1985.
116. Freud S. Project for a scientific psychology, vol. I. SE London: Hogarth Press; 1895.
117. Freud S. Two case histories, vol. X. London: SE Hogarth Press; 1909b.
118. Freud S. An infantile neurosis and other works, vol. XVII. London: SE Hogarth Press; 1917–1919.
119. Freud S. Beyond the pleasure principle, vol. XVIII. London: SE Hogarth Press; 1920.
120. Eickhoff FW. (1956) on nachträglichkeit: the modernity of an old concept. Int J Psychoanal. 2006;87:1453–69.
121. Scarfone DA. Matter of time: actual time and the production of the past. Psychoanal Q. 2006;75:807–34.
122. Scarfone D. The analyst at work. Live wires: when is the analyst at work? Int J Psychoanal. 2011;92:755–9.
123. Frey J (2006) in Collins S (2011).
124. Collins S. On authenticity: the question of truth in construction and autobiography. Int J Psychoanal. 2011;92:1391–409. https://doi.org/10.1111/j.1745-8315.2011.00455.x.
125. Wilkinson S, Hough G. Lie as narrative truth in abused adopted adolescents. Psychoanal Study Child. 1996;51:580–97.
126. Moro MR. L'enfant exposé. Grenoble: Editions La Pensee sauvage; 1989.
127. Winnicott DW. The maturational processes and the facilitating environment: studies in the theory of emotional development. In: The international psycho-analytical library, vol. 64. London: The Hogarth Press and the Institute of Psychoanalysis; 1965. p. 1–276.
128. Winnicott DW. Home is where we start from. New York London: WW Norton & Company; 1986.
129. Steck B. Narrative von adoptierten Kindern und Jugendlichen über ihren Beziehungs- und Herkunftsabbruch. Analytische Kinder- und Jugendlichenpsychotherapie. 1997;95(3):335–50.

130. Winnicott DW. Collected papers: through pediatrics to psychoanalysis. 1st ed. London: Tavistock; 1958.
131. Tisseron S. Tintin et les secrets de famille. Aubier; 1992.
132. Steck B. Eltern-Kind-Beziehungsproblematik bei der Adoption. Praxis der Kinderpsychol Kinderpsychiatrie. 1998;4:240–62.
133. Ferrari P. La filiation en psychopathologie de l'enfant. Ann Pédiatr. 1986;33(8):713–8.
134. Brinich PM. Some potential effects of adoption on self and object representations. Psychoanal St Child. 1980;35:107–33.

Chapter 8
Clinical Vignettes

"Who are You? You who exposed me out of cowardice? Out of necessity?
    You, ghost of my childhood, you haunt my childhood dreams.
    You were my comforter in moments of despair.
    To you I turned, you I implored in my weeping, in my suffering as a child.
    You were always my ghost, who had no name, who had no face, how often I fell asleep
calling you, stretching out my arms to you, hoping each time that you would appear.
    You never came, you never told me in my sleep the reasons for my mother's flight.
    My mother! No words are possible to describe the hatred that I bore her as a child,
    I cursed her. Basically, is it you or is it her, that I must condemn?
    Which of you two is the more guilty? Yes, in my eyes you will always be guilty, even if
the circumstances prove you right.
    I have suffered too much, and I am still suffering.
    Your exposure has affected my emotional life.
    As if I have brought misfortune and hurts to the persons who love me and who are not
responsible for it.
    I wish so much, one day in the future, to see you with my own eyes, caress your faces
with my hands, just for a moment, to be your child.
    But to be the child of a love union and not only of a sensual one.
    Adopted young women

Vignettes of psychoanalytical psychotherapies give insight into how creatively and often surprisingly adoptees deal with critical life events. Psychic injury and grief in children, adolescent and young adults are closely related to their developmental age and to their caregivers. Adoptees try to understand and process traumatic experiences by building a fantasy world explaining what happened to them. They also tell their phantasms in stories. The attribution of meaning to the experienced event is constantly re-vised by the adoptee in the course of his development. Within the safe and reliable framework of a psychotherapeutic process, the creative imagination of the adoptee unfolds. In listening to the adoptees voice, to the language of trauma and to the silence of its mute repetition, therapists bear witness to the adoptees' suffering. With the help of the therapist, the adoptee learns to consciously experience fears and feelings related to the trauma and to verbalize them in symbolic language.

© The Author(s), under exclusive license to Springer Nature   207
Switzerland AG 2023
B. Steck, *Adoption as a Lifelong Process*,
https://doi.org/10.1007/978-3-031-33038-4_8

This process allows to understand and integrate memories and emotions associated with the traumatic experience.

Preschool Age

Vignette

Anna, four and a half years old, is brought to the child psychiatrist by her adoptive father who informs, that his daughter is haunted by death, speaking in a confused way, and presents a general developmental delay. Anna was brought to Switzerland for adoption by the prospective adoptive parents from an orphanage in South America when she was one and a half months old. Anna lost her adoptive mother to sudden cardiac death when she was two and a half; her developmental process came then to a standstill. Anna has only begun to speak 6 months after the death of her adoptive mother, i.e., at the age of three. She then screamed desperately, crying that she wanted to be reunited with her mother in heaven. After the death of the adoptive mother, a governess and the maternal grandmother took care of Anna and her 3 years older, also adopted brother. According to the adoptive father, the maternal grandmother maintains a real cult around the death of her daughter. Six months ago, the adoptive father remarried. Anna expresses her ambivalent feelings towards her stepmother in saying to her: "This is not your home", and in asking her: "You are not going to kill yourself ?"

In individual child psychiatric sessions, Anna plays the story of a sick grandmother and a sick girl and comments: "The sick girl does not know her illness but has caused it herself. The girl cries because she has lost her mother and wants to be reunited with her. Therefore, the doctor burns the girl (cremation) in order to cure her." Annas comments reveal her wish to be reunited with her mother.

In the following play with the scenotest,[1] Anna says that she lights a fire to tree toys and explains: "You die, when you are burned". She narrates, that the four-and-a-half-year-old baby is not afraid of being burnt, as she wants to find her mother again who will recognize her child. In another scene, Anna comments that she is an infant and carries a baby from her father and therefore (for this "stupidity" as she says) must leave her home.

Comment

The play scenes demonstrate Anna's intense efforts to resolve conflicts and make amends. She expresses her feelings of being sick and of having caused her illness herself. She wishes to be healed by the doctor (in the transference the psychotherapist) who will burn her and thus enabling her to find her mother again. In Annas phantasms, she must die to be reunited with her mother. In a regressive movement as an infant, Anna deals with her guilt feelings. She is punished and has to leave her

---

[1] The scenotest of von Staabs is used as a play and communication aid in a diagnostic-therapeutic interview.

home for her oedipal[2] desire, which she expresses by her saying to carry a baby from her father. Is Anna in her unconscious phantasms asking herself, if she is responsible for the death of her mother, as a consequence of her oedipal rivalry, and must therefore be punished, by falling ill and dying? Her anger and fear of her aggressiveness towards the stepmother, who takes her mother's place at father's side, Anna expresses by saying "this is not your home" and "you will not kill yourself". In the second phrase, Anna denies her preconscious wish for her stepmother to die, as her anxiety is too great to endure a new loss, which would represent a repetition of her earlier losses of her birth and adoptive mothers, her care persons in the orphanage and the governess.

As Anna resumed her developmental process after these sessions, psychotherapy seemed not indicated, as priority was given to her affective engagement in the relationship with her stepmother.

One year later, the adoptive father returned with the question of Anna's upcoming integration into school and informed the child psychiatrist, that Anna presents herself in kindergarten as a silly girl, speaking confused and having problems with time orientation. Her development is still delayed and her integration in kindergarten difficult, as she apparently tends to show off, behaves like a boy and jumps into everyone's arms.

Anna remembers the past psychotherapeutic intervention. At the beginning of the new individual sessions, Anna surprises by her appearance and behavior of a mentally deficient child, presenting a confused speech. Then – after the first contact – she resumes an adequate relation and recounts her recurring nightmares, from which she awakens in horror, not being able to fall asleep again. In these dreams she is beaten by men and, in self-defense, kills them. She also dreams of her father's death. In other nightmares she dies by "child-eaters". She speaks of her constant pains in her throat and back and her intense weeping when an animal dies.

Comment

Anna is overwhelmed by unbearable feelings, which she manifests in psychosomatic symptoms; in identification with a dying animal, she expresses her mourning and shares her great sadness. She is haunted by her multiple fears, especially the fear that her father might die.

Anna wishes to be no longer afraid and to be free from her nightmares. She confides that she never speaks of her greatest sorrow, which is that her mother died, but the death of her mother is the reason for her fear that she is going to be killed. Anna's fear of revenge is obvious. To be afraid, Anna says, is stupid and evil, and she is stupid and evil, because she is afraid and therefore nobody loves her.

---

[2] Already the baby is able to establish triadic exchanges and build triadic relationship structures. Yet the infant has not a clear representation of the sexuality and the relationship between his parents. In the course of development, between about 2 and 5 years, children perceive the sexual differences of their parents. The conflicts associated with this development are called *oedipal*, a child's feelings of desire for the opposite-sex parent and jealousy and anger toward the same-sex parent.

Fig. 8.1 Anna, 5
½-year-old, a mare and its
adopted small baby

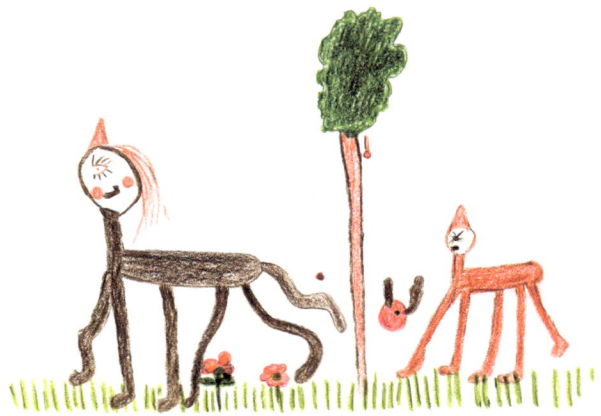

Annas incapacity to speak about the death of her adoptive mother and to find out its cause seems to be synonymous in Anna's mind with not being allowed to know, i.e., being stupid.

Anna draws a mare that will soon be 6 years old; next to it there is a tree and an apple, poisoned by men (Fig. 8.1). The worm who is eating the apple dies. The mare has adopted a small baby (a foal) because she wishes to have a child but is too afraid of a husband. A misfortune is going to happen: the foal will eat the poisoned apple and fall sick but will not die.

In Anna's imagination, the apple of the tree of knowledge is poisoned. In a double identification with the mare, representing herself as a soon-to-be 6-year-old, and her foal, representing her baby self, Anna's desire to know the cause of her adoptive mother's death, to be informed about her adoption situation (the foal is adopted); her associated fears are evident. The foal will get sick but does not die.

The adoptive father reports that Anna—after this third session—suffered a breakdown and wept for hours in her father's arms. Sobbing, she said: "When I was born, I killed my mama"; "my mama could never be a grandmama"; "I never want to be a mama, I never want to have children, as I will die like my mama".

The adoptive father compared this event to a "rope with knots"; during Annas emotional outburst, one knot after another was undone. Thereafter and for the first time, affective ties between Anna, her adoptive father, and also her stepmother were built up. Subsequently the adoptive parents experienced Anna as deeply changed and felt that she was "quite a different child".

Comment

At the beginning of this second encounter, Anna indeed presented herself as a dumb and quite confused girl. However, she was very soon able to express her phantasms, feelings, and fears in coherent stories through play scenes and drawings, which allowed to gain awareness and comprehension of her fears of dying like her adoptive mother, losing her father, or being killed, as well as of her guilt feelings out of her belief having caused the death of her adoptive mother and her need to be punished for it.

The question arises whether Anna partially succeeded in distancing herself from the past and the fate of her adoptive mother, respectively in starting a mourning process and giving up her identification with her adoptive mother.

The adopted foal falls ill but does not die with the poisoned knowledge, which might signify: "No, I did not kill my adoptive mother, and—when I allow myself to know—I will fall ill, but not die."

Mourning the loss of a mother or father improves with increasing age and a more advanced, harmonious development stage. Coping with the death of a parent is aggravated by pre-existing critical life events, as is the case in the adoption situation. Children have great difficulties to accept a loss when their psychic pain is too intense for the affect tolerance of the developing self or the disruption of the narcissistic balance, i.e., the loss of being loved is experienced as too threatening. Wishing to undo what happened, aggressiveness towards or idealization of the lost parent serve to avoid the perception of ambivalent and guilt feelings towards the deceased person. The child has to give up the identification with phantasms about the cause of death, but also with unconscious phantasms of death wishes, as these unconscious phantasms hold aggressive impulses and cause feelings of guilt. The kind of rational understanding and conceptual integration of the loss of a meaningful loved one within the globality of a child's conscious and preconscious phantasmas is of central significance for grief work and resuming psychic development.

School Age

Vignette

Joël came from India to Switzerland for adoption at the age of six. He accuses his adoptive parents having stolen him; he got lost, he said, and his birth parents could not have found him again, because his adoptive parents took him with them. He thinks that his mother did not take care of him because he was an ugly infant. Joël feels responsible and guilty of having been abandoned, maintaining the innocence of his birth parents.

He comments his drawing, which has symbolic meaning, as follows: "I'm towing myself; this is a new red car, which doesn't run and needs to be repaired. The sky and the sun know what happened to me" (Fig. 8.2).

Comment

Joël presents himself as a new car, which probably corresponds to his perception that he no longer lacks anything materially. The car is red, the color of love; Joël knows that he is loved by his adoptive parents. But the car is not moving, not functioning, like Joël who presents severe learning and relationship disorders. He says the car must be repaired, what suggests Joel's awareness of his problems and of his needs for help. Joel's personal history is unknown, except of the fact that he lived in a men's prison in India before he came to Switzerland for adoption. The sky and the sun are the same in India and in Switzerland; they alone know his past, Joel seems to say.

Fig. 8.2 Joël, 6-year-old, a
new red car, which
doesn't run

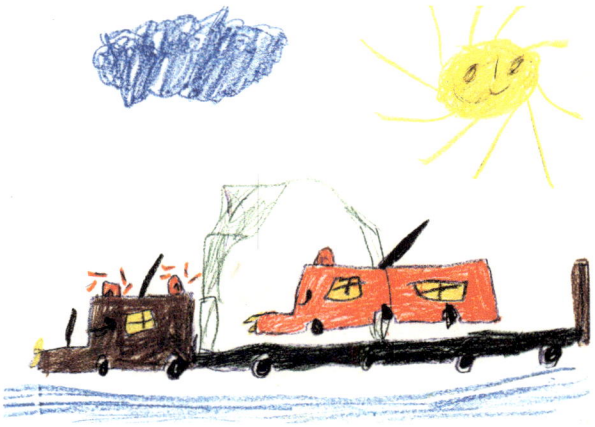

On the arrival of his two-year-old sister from India for adoption, Joël, now 8 years old, reacts with violent jealousy. He proposes to his adoptive parents to leave home for a boarding school, so that they can enjoy being together with his sister without him. Joël experiences his sister's arrival as a rejection and prefers to leave his home, thus fleeing from enduring again unbearable feelings of abandonment.

Adopted children tend to anticipate and act out potential separation situations, by running away, escaping. In this way painful feelings associated with previous separations, which may be re-actualized in separation situations, can be avoided. Aggressive emotions associated with having been abandoned cannot be directed against the absent biological parents and are often expressed towards the adoptive parents in form of behavioral disorders, such as lying, stealing and aggressiveness. In a certain sense, the adopted child "uses" his adoptive parents for processing his past lived injuries.

Transition from Childhood to Adolescence

Vignette

Pascal, originally from South America, was integrated into a Swiss family for adoption at the age of eight and a half years. The child psychiatrist received the following information about Pascal's personal history: The biological mother died when Pascal was 3 years old, the biological father placed his son for a very short time with the maternal grandfather, then in an orphanage of his country of origin; as this house burned down, Pascal was transferred to a second orphanage.

At the age of 9 years, having spent 6 months in his future adoptive family, the adoptive parents were no longer capable to deal with Pascal's severe behavioral disorders (running away, stealing, lying, aggressiveness and destructiveness). The adoptive father suffered a mental breakdown; both prospective adoptive parents felt unable to care for Pascal and keep him in their family, all the more as he allegedly had asked that their own biological son should leave the house. The parents considered Pascal as mentally ill and required his treatment in a psychiatric hospital.

In the individual child psychiatric interview, Pascal draws and tells his recurring nightmare: "A man from my country (of origin) comes to pick me up and to take me back there". Pascal is afraid of this man, afraid of the dark and cannot sleep. The man carries a pistol, has evil eyes, and wants to kill him. Pascal erases—in his drawing—the person who represents him. The police come to put the man in prison, but the man kills the policemen. Pascal continues with his drawing and says: "I have grown up". He draws himself and comments: "I have a sword, I defend myself, I now kill this man; he is dead, can no longer move and I sleep peacefully".

Comment

The integration of Pascal into the future adoptive family led to a mental breakdown of the adoptive father, the rejection of the child and his expulsion from the family.

Pascal's nightmare contains the phantasms of infanticide and parricide, the law of "either I or the other", i.e., of a fundamental violence [1]. Did the rejection of the future adoptive parents remind Pascal of his previous painful experienced losses of significant persons? Does he carry unconscious murderous feelings related to the lived relationship breakups and must be punished and killed for these unconscious phantasms, as he recounts in his story about his drawing? Or is it a reactivation of his Oedipus complex, in which Pascal desires an intimate relationship with the adoptive mother, demands the expulsion of the brother (a rival) and fears the revenge of his adoptive father? Already now Pascal announces that, armed with a phallic potency, he will avenge the "crime" of having been—in his subjective lived experience—rejected, expulsed, abandoned.

Subsequently, Pascal was integrated into a first institution, then into a second, where he set a fire. Did Pascal reenact his experience of the burned orphanage, an event associated with his relationship ruptures? Pascal is finally integrated into a second adoptive family, which—although confronted with his massive difficulties—legalizes his adoption. The adoptive parents desire a psychotherapy for Pascal, who is now 11 years old. According to their account, Pascal seeks refuge in his past, which he glorifies; he wants to return to his country of origin, although he has suffered so many painful experiences there. Pascal also tends to present himself as a victim, e.g., he denies to outsiders that he has been adopted and complains that his adoptive parents make no effort to adopt him.

In the individual child psychiatric interview, Pascal recounts the following dream:

> I visited C. (name of the village where he had lived with his first prospective adoptive family). I knocked on my parents' door, but no one answered, the inhabitants had left the village. I woke up with great fear.

He then draws "a crooked house that will soon fall" and comments: "The house will fall into the water: A ship, an airplane and a crane try to save the house. But the house cannot be saved, the house is dangerous, it will destroy everything in its fall" (Fig. 8.3).

Fig. 8.3 Pascal, 11-year-old, a crooked house that will soon fall

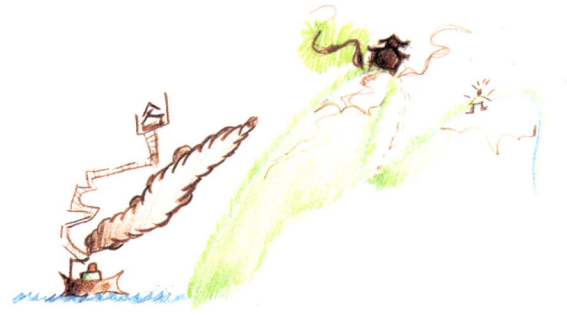

Comment

The house seems to represent Pascal, who expresses his auto-aggressiveness in saying "the house will fall" and his hetero-aggressiveness, "the house will destroy everything".

He then draws the orphanage where he lived in his country of origin and speaks of all the children he has known and his longings. He tells of multiple fears that haunt him in bed at night: fear of suffocating, fear that a monster will open the door and tear his face, fear that someone will operate on him.

Pascal does not know, how to explain his great dissatisfaction since he loves his adoptive mother and the whole family and is loved by all family members. He tells—while drawing—the story of a thief who lives on the street and owns nothing, but who enjoys stealing so that he does not have to work: "The thief will go to prison; he will escape, but he will be put back into prison, what he likes. His family is dead; he is all alone and does not know what to do. He can't be helped because he doesn't want to be helped; he wants to stay alone as always, but he doesn't like being alone". Pascal refuses psychotherapeutic help.

Comment

Pascal states that he is inhabited by a murderous rage, which is so dangerous that it is better to destroy himself (the fall of his house cannot be prevented). His fear of his own rage and of further rejection leads to his inability to form meaningful relationships. He is the perpetual thief who owns nothing, who is alone but does not like it. His losses of significant relationships have added up. Pascal was never really offered an opportunity to grief his multiple losses in his personal history—within the context of a significant relationship with an adult—resulting in his persistent depression.

Legally adopted at the age of eleven, Pascal denies his adoption. Although he testifies loving and being loved by his adoptive family, his unprocessed personal history with its associated and split-off emotions seems to suffocate him. Fears of punishment in the form of castration (surgery) or depersonalization (tearing his face) seem to haunt him. Pascal's defense mechanism is to seek a personal non-existence, thus avoiding responsibility and escape persecution [2].

Pascal's drawing of a tree (Fig. 8.4) and his comment illustrate Pascal's life experience in the most impressive way. "This is my life tree". To the tree on the left,

Fig. 8.4 Pascal, 11-year-
old, my life tree: at the
beginning (left) and now
(right)

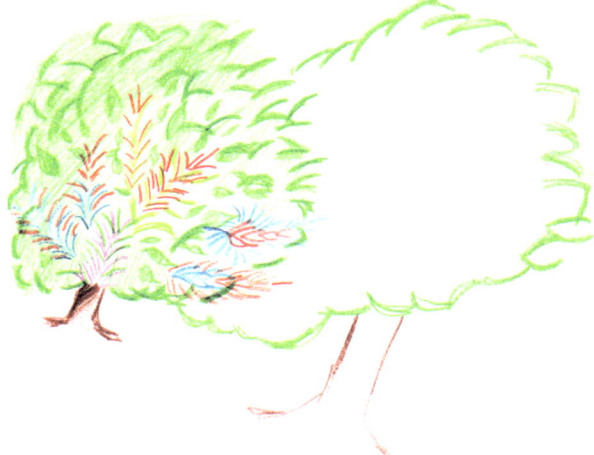

Pascal says: "This is the tree at the beginning of my life". It is richly filled out and drawn in all its detailed dimensions. To the right tree: "This is the tree now"—an empty tree that has only preserved its outer form.

At the age of eight and a half years, when Pascal was integrated into the first adoptive family, he expressed with his behavioral disorders a cry for help, hoping to be able to resume his development and to cope with and process his personal history with the help of his future adoptive parents, but he was again rejected.

According to Winnicott [3, 4], the antisocial tendency is usually a sign of emotional deprivation suffered in infancy or toddlerhood and is linked with the child's hope for a supportive environment, provided by trusting caregivers. At a moment of hope, the child perceives a situation, in which he believes being able to rely on and begin to invest a new relationship with caregivers. The environment, the adoptive family, is thereby constantly tested by the child who wants to make sure that his adoptive parents are capable of enduring his aggressive behavior, of preventing his destructiveness or of helping him making amends for it. Adoptive parents need to recognize the positive elements in the child's antisocial tendency and make themselves continuously emotionally available for their child.

Pascal's nightmare at the age of eight and a half years reflects first his victim position (he is killed), then his identification with the aggressor: "I will be the one who kills". At the age of 11, Pascal seems to have given up all hope. The thief can only express his needs in a repetitive way, but each time he is punished and recaptured. The "crooked house", despite efforts to save it, will fall. Pascal denies having been adopted by his second adoptive parents and wants to return to his country of origin, as if hoping to find help there. Pascal's psychic defense organization (splitting, denial, identification with the aggressor, projective identification[3]) allows him

---

[3] Projective identification is a process, in which, in a close relationship, an unconscious fantasy of aspects of the self or of an internal relation representation is attributed to an external person.

not to feel his much too painful emotions. He creates an intrapsychic emptiness and thus avoids unbearable affects. His rejection of psychotherapeutic help might indicate his tremendous fear that far too painful emotions would erupt and overwhelm him in an individual psychotherapy.

Vignette

Jan, an adopted, early pubertal boy, was presented to the child psychiatrist by his adoptive parents because of non-acceptance of his adoptive filiation and behavioral disorders.

Already in the first hours of his psychoanalytic psychotherapy, Jan speaks of the difficulty of having four parents as well as of his boundless rage, a state in which he could kill someone. He calls himself being a hero.

Comment

Jan gives expression to his immense fear that he could act out his murderous fantasies. Simultaneously, he speaks of a problematic identity development, which may be related to the continuity break in his generational lineage.

At the time when Jan, in the beginning of puberty, should complete an age-appropriate individuation and separation process from his adoptive parents, he is confronted with highly painful and unprocessed experiences of loss from his childhood.

Growing up has—in unconscious and preconscious phantasms—obviously to do with murder and manslaughter. In order to take the place of the father, the father must seemingly be killed. "We…find at this point the origin of the idea of hero, of the hero, who, after all, always, rebels against the father and kills him in some way" (Freud 1939, p. 193).

In the psychotherapeutic sessions, Jan's infantile needs erupt as boundless desires and violent outbursts of rage, manifesting his difficulties in controlling aggressive impulses, as well as his immense regression tendency, both amplified by intensive drive impulses. Themes of Jan's pretend play enactments and drawings are struggles for life and death, with only two positions, the one of a perpetrator or the one of a victim. Jan identifies predominantly with the perpetrator role. In identification with an omnipotent aggressor, an active position, he manages to ward off feelings of helplessness and powerlessness, but also of pain and grief, and thus avoids a passive victim role. Denial, splitting, and projective identification serve as protective defense mechanisms against painful mortification and narcissistic injury.

The psychotherapist addresses Jan's feelings of pain, sadness, and despair and the resulting unspeakable rage he may have felt when he was abandoned as an infant; she tells Jan that he seems harboring the idea to be entitled to inflict on others what he himself experienced as so painful.

In various pretend role-scenarios Jan plays an omnipotent, omniscient emperor or king—an identification with an idealized part of his self-representation—who possesses a murderous destructiveness and who tortures and devalues the therapist in the role of a miserable, stupid, help- and hopeless slave—a projection of a part of his self-representation, which he perceives as worthless. Jan enjoys these role-playing scenarios greatly and with time, he succeeds to give his sadistic boundless-ness, his grandiose omnipotence, and his megalomaniac phallicity a certain form and structure. In her slave role, the therapist expresses her feelings—perceived by projective identification—of pain, helplessness, powerlessness, anger, and sadness. Jan accepts more and more that the therapist relates his play scenes to his personal history.

Separations are for Jan associated with high vulnerability. They represent anni-hilation, humiliation, and devaluation. He experiences each separation as extremely painful because the emotions, Jan lived in past relationship breakups, are reacti-vated. These most intense feelings of pain and sadness occurred most likely during the loss of the infant's omnipotently controlled attachment to the primary object, his birth mother. The confrontation of traumatic experiences in infancy with his present reality activates Jan's most violent, painful, and angry feelings of disappointment, when the injuries in the "continuity of his being" are reawakened.

Comment

Several years of therapy allowed Jan to come to terms with the loss of his biological parents and the associated painful traumatizing experiences of his past. In his manic defense, Jan maintained the omnipotence fantasy of being able to dominate situa-tions that could evoke fear or pain and thus to keep away feelings of fear, sadness, and pain. Careful interpretations of the unspeakable pain and narcissistic "rage", resulting from the losses Jan experienced in his early childhood, allowed him to begin a mourning process. Gradually, the integration of the dissociated mental con-tents took place. The integration process consisted in translating unconscious and preconscious parts of experience, which were characterized by primary processes, into the metaphorical language of secondary processes, i.e., in transferring the memory fragments stored in implicit memory into symbolized and narrative memo-ries of explicit memory. A change in the quality of Jan's relationship helped him to gain a better understanding and attributing a more coherent meaning of his experi-enced past. A selective identification process within the four parental representa-tions allowed Jan to build a personal identity.

It is quite conceivable that Jan will be confronted again with his adoption situa-tion during a life transition phase or critical life experiences and will then continue a mourning process, which is not yet completed; the representations of the biologi-cal parents, especially of abandoning their child, as part of the child's self-representation may remain a source of vulnerability, unless Jan succeeds in attributing to his four parental representations a specific richness.

Heredity is according to Guyotat [5] an absolute necessity. If transmission fails, inheritance is replaced by chronology. The rupture of emotional bonds between mother and child is a loss of what the mother could have transmitted to her child. The traumatic moment of this situation is then incorporated and reappears at a cru-cial moment, as a re-traumatization, for example at the arrival of a sister or brother for adoption, which was the case for Jan, who wanted to kill his sibling.

Adolescence

Normal intrapsychic development in adolescence involves a grieving process over the loss of childhood and the transformation of mental representations, the primary significant relationship representations of the internalized parental figures. According to their development, adolescents have to abandon their internalized primary love relationships and give up the familiar experience and functioning of their childhood. This process is associated with an increased investment of the self, a narcissistic retreat, and often accompanied by a depressive mood and insecurity in self-perception and feelings. In this transition period infantile conflictual or critical experiences reemerge and need to be elaborated again. If adolescents are not capable of containing their emotional distress resulting from personal intrapsychic conflicts or critical events, they depend even more on the attention from caregiver. Yet at the same time adolescents fear the dependence of adults, often lived as a submission to others or as an intrusion.

Specific Features of the Adolescent Period for Adoptees

Adolescence represents a critical phase for adopted adolescents, as their curiosity and interest in their genealogical history are intensified. The preoccupation with existential questions and the associated feelings of loneliness and strangeness may be accentuated in adopted adolescents as a result of the transgenerational rupture in their personal history due to adoption. The testimonies of adopted adolescents show how their past—their experience of loss of relationship with biological parents as well as loss of cultural ties—complicates the process of their identity development. The adoptees' losses are real experiences, as opposed to the symbolic loss that all adolescents live during their separation process from their parents. The physical changes occurring during pubertal development can lead to an intense preoccupation with the origins of their bodily characteristics. The bodily transmission shaped by the biological parents is neither modifiable nor erasable [6]. Anxieties and feelings of deficiency and insufficiency, which concern the entire body, but especially the sexual organs, find expression in phantasms such as not being able to procreate or giving birth to a malformed baby—"a monster", said one adopted adolescent. There is also a fear of an incestuous relationship with an unknown family member, as the following vignette demonstrates.

Vignette
A nine-year-old adopted girl, who has been in psychotherapy for one year, repeatedly enacts play scenes in which she presents herself as a young woman falling in love. The young woman wonders whether the man courting her might not be her brother, whom she has not seen for such a long time that she would no longer recognize him. According to the adoptive parents, her daughter does not have a brother.

The relationship breakup with biological parents can—especially during puberty—lead to an unconscious or preconscious rejection of the sexual body, to hatred of one's own body or to a distorted self-image.

Infertile adoptive parents may perceive the awakening of sexuality in their adolescents as a personal threat. The procreative adoptees may trigger feelings of jealousy, rivalry, and inferiority in their adoptive parents. The prohibition of incest for adoptees is not based on a biological reality but established by law. In adoptive families, the oedipal situation may be intensified by the absence of the usual incest taboo.

Adopted adolescents who have been exposed to environmental failures or assaults are at increased risk of reacting to adverse environmental situations by developing a false self. " ...a true self hidden, protected by a false self. This false self is no doubt an aspect of the true self. It hides and protects it, and it reacts to the adaptation failures and develops a pattern corresponding to the pattern of environmental failure. In this way the true self is not involved in the reacting, and so preserves a continuity of being. However, this hidden true self suffers an impoverishment that derives from lack of experience" [7].

> I always have to make a constant effort to maintain the image other person's see of me, an image, I think, they like. I am afraid they will discover that it is only an image and then, when I drop my mask, they will no more love me.

This adopted teenage girl's statement corresponds to her perception of a lack of personal authenticity. The formation of a false self is built up to protect the vulnerable core self. The function of a false self prevents the development of individuation and autonomy processes but allows to submit unconditionally to the real or fantasied demands of the environment and to eliminate the threat of a potential disaster in the external reality. At the time of adolescence, which is a complex developmental phase, the maintaining of a false self, which enables some children to appear as if they are promising, is very often no longer possible; the adolescent's breakdown reveals that a true self is barely developed or hardly exists [3].

In adolescence, crisis situations in adoptive families are frequent, often severe, even violent, and lead to child psychiatric consultations. The adoptive parents say that they had no problems with their adopted child during the infancy or latency period. They describe "model" children of whom they were proud. At the same time, however, they often noted that their child had difficulty making a decision or a choice and preferred to let the parents decide for him. The child, thanks to his efforts to adapt, seems to be integrated into his adoptive family in such a way that his parents perceived his false self-personality as his true person. The false self can fit effortlessly into the family structure and be easily mistaken as healthy. In adolescence, the adoptive parents are unexpectedly confronted with strange behaviors of their son or daughter, which often makes them feel highly insecure and fills them with apprehension.

The adolescent crisis can take various forms and manifest itself in different ways: the crisis may be linked to the adolescent's physical development and lead to psychosomatic symptoms; violent forms can be expressed in delinquent behavior, in escape or in self-aggression (drug abuse, suicide attempt, multiple accidents). Another pathological form of the personality of a false self at the time of adolescence does not manifest itself in external appearances, but seems to take place internally, for example in depressive states. This situation may be accompanied by a refusal of any professional or social realization or integration, as well as an inability to form meaningful relationships outside the family. Some teenagers or young adults focus their efforts and affective preoccupations on the search for their origins, driven by the hope of "discovering their true selves". In most cases, adopted adolescents who exhibit a false self-pathology hardly ever realized a mourning of the losses suffered in their personal biography. Until the age of adolescence, their personality structure enabled them to continuously adapt to the wishes and expectations of the adoptive family—at the expense of their own individual development. A kind of unconscious, "tacit contract" of ignorance and misjudgment existed between adoptive parents and adopted child, which abruptly broke with the onset of adolescence. In this agonizing despair, neither parents nor adoptees find points of orientation.

Vignette

Bernard, a 17-year-old teenager, was adopted at the age of 3 years. He wants to move out of his adoptive family and live in a youth home. In the first family meeting with the psychiatrist, intra-family communications turn out to be extremely difficult. Bernard excludes himself from his family and does not participate in the conversation. According to the adoptive parents, Bernard was found on the street in an Asian country; as a little boy, he often said, wishing to live with his true mother.

In individual interviews, Bernard speaks openly about his adoption, which he does not consider a positive measure. He does not feel like a member of his adoptive family, but of his country of origin. He wants to help his country of birth and return there to seek out the traces of his origins, but without his adoptive parents, since his country of origin belongs to him alone.

Bernard tells having suffered from a depressive state for months, the last episode because of a love disappointment, which led to his first suicide attempt with medication. He describes himself as very sensitive in affective relationships and wishes to have a serious love relationship. He admits having been smoking excessively and drinking a lot of alcohol for a long time. His appearance—long hair, always dressed in black—is much criticized by his adoptive parents, for whom it is important how he presents himself outside their family. "I am their (his adoptive parents') extension". For his adoptive parents, "he is not himself". Bernard thinks, he was adopted to show an image of his adoptive parents' righteousness. "I lived up to that image when I was a kid. Everyone thought I was adorable. My parents were proud, now it's the opposite."

Three weeks later, Bernard shows up for his therapy session with a dislocation of his right arm, which causes him severe pain, but he laughs about it. He talks about his parents' marital problems and his mother's loneliness and depression.

The adoptive parents are deeply hurt and disappointed by the behavior of their son, and reject him, saying: "We have raised a child, but he is not our son." The father depreciates his son's therapeutic communications with the psychiatrist as gossip and puts an end to his son's treatment.

Three months later, Bernard takes part in a burglary and disregards—in the eyes of his adoptive parents—his status as an adopted son. The father asks for information about the possibilities of relinquishing his custody. The mother's depressive condition worsens, she needs medical treatment. Bernard is allowed to resume his psychotherapy.

Comment

Antisocial tendencies are clinical signs, often signifying a cry for help as well as hopeful expectation. The antisocial manifestations may mask a significant loss or an experience of a meaningful relationship breakup, i.e., a psychic trauma in the past, having impacted the affective development of the person concerned. As soon as a child lives in an environment offering some hope for a secure containment, he will resume his development, which has come to a standstill because of a traumatic event [2, 4]. Until adolescence, Bernard maintained the unconscious contract of an ideal child who fulfills the parents' expectations and confirms them narcissistically in the outside world.

Bernard's adoptive parents had applied for adoption after the stillbirth of a baby with congenital malformation. As long as Bernard represented a substitute for the lost idealized child, the adoptive parents could avoid grieving the loss of their dead born infant. Their incapacity to carry out a mourning process has hindered Bernard to work through the grief of the losses he suffered in his own personal history, A child is not able to fulfill a mourning process alone; for this task he needs the help of a meaningful adult person who offers a dialog in a continuous relationship. The rigidity of the family structure, the considerable communication difficulties within the family, as well as the expectation that Bernard remedies the narcissistic injuries of his parents, impaired Bernard's own personal emotional development. The adoptive parents were not only burdened by the traumatic event of having lost their biological child but had based their unconscious motivations to adopt a child on the hope that this "replacement or substitute" child will help them overcome their personal hurts. The risk of disappointment and unfortunate evolution in such an encounter of mutual emotionally stressful expectations is high.

When parents are unable to accomplish a mourning process over the loss of their child, then a sibling often assumes the grief work of the parents. The surviving or adopted child may unconsciously be designated to alleviate the parents' feeling of guilt or may be compared with the lost idealized child and never be able to fulfill the parents' expectations. The replacement or substitute child must build up a myth and identity around a "foreign body", which the parents have deposited in him, because of their attachment to another child, whose loss they deny and whose aliveness they maintain in their intrapsychic world (in "crypts" through incorporation fantasies, according to [8]). The substitute child tries to identify himself with the lost love object, his parents were unable to mourn, and to internalize it, even if the child did not know the lost sibling. This conduct is motivated by the child's desire to understand the parents yet is often accompanied by uncanny feelings [9]. A substitute child may have a serious disadvantage for his own identity development, as he is constantly compared to the idealized dead sibling. Thus, the replacement child faces a lifelong search for a personal identity.

Bernard concludes his psychotherapy a year after the first consultation, by saying with a laughter: "Next time my parents will order a child from a catalogue". He tells his psychotherapist, that he imagines to be the father of a child, who will be unlike him and whose psychic and physical differences he will accept. Bernard expresses his desire to make up in a child of his own what he missed, namely, to be recognized and accepted in his psychic and physical otherness.

Vignette

Fanny, 18 years old, of Asian descent, came to Switzerland at the age of six and a half years for her adoption. During the first interview with the psychiatrist, Fanny expresses her tremendous fear of going crazy. She has the impression that she has been dismembered, her body being split off—an uncanny feeling of alienation. She says no longer sensing anything in her body; even if it is true that her body is here, it should be in her country of origin. She speaks of her nightmares, in which she is rejected, despised, ignored by everyone; waking up in tears, she wishes to die. When she perceives rejection, she is running away, fleeing. For years she has been obsessed with thoughts and feelings of persecution and is haunted by existential questions to which she cannot find answers. She remembers the words of her mother, kneeling in front of her: "You will come back when you have grown up". Why did precisely she had to leave her biological family?

Fanny seems to suffer from psychotic symptoms and fears a disintegration of her personality. She agrees to regular psychotherapeutic sessions.

Three months before starting psychotherapy, Fanny had attempted suicide with medication after a love disappointment. She describes how she had been highly dependent in this symbiotic relationship, which she repeatedly broke off but always resumed. She thinks she sought paternal protection, which she had never known.

"I am destroying myself". She regards the sexual aspect of the relationship with her boyfriend as "ridiculous" as she never enjoyed it. Memories of her childhood emerge, and she says that at the age of five, she had been sexually abused by an older boy.

Six months later, Fanny successfully passes her intermediate exams at the art academy. However, she decides to give up her education and to quit everything she had ever done at the request of others. "I had a trigger inside me; the trigger is called: I Fanny". She leaves her apartment and breaks off the relationship with her adoptive mother, telling her: "If I'm hurting you so much, it's because I've never really been your daughter and never will be." She feels like "a larva" in need of attention, nourishment, and maturation.

Comment

Fanny becomes aware of her true self when she says, "I had a trigger inside me, I Fanny". She feels that the development of her true self has come to a standstill in a larval stage. Her suicide attempt can be understood as the destruction of her false self and her wish to preserve her true self. "When suicide is the only defense left against betrayal of the true self, then it becomes the lot of the false self to organize the suicide. This, of course, involves its own destruction, but at the same time eliminates the need for its continued existence, since its function is the protection of the true self from insult." ([3]: p. 143).

The poverty of the true self is accompanied by emotions of futility and despair. Fanny feels an increasing impoverishment of feelings in her relationships and social contacts.

She shows a need to continuously expose herself to injuries; her individual existence is thus filled by responding to these wounds.

> Instead of cultural pursuits one observes ...extreme restlessness, an inability to concentrate, and a need to collect impingements from external reality so that the living-time of the individual can be filled by reactions to these impingements (Winnicott [3], p. 150).

In Fanny's appreciation, her adoptive parents failed her adoption. They told her, the reason to adopt a child was to give their bedridden biological son, who suffers from a hereditary disease, a sister and playmate. It was also her brother who chose her name. "It is as if a child wishes to have a dog; it is bought, and the child gives it a name and plays with it." Her adoptive father had left the family, her mother worked full time and—always tired—never had time for her, Fanny said. "I raised myself". She thinks her adoptive parents didn't really wish to have an additional child. Her adoptive father, whom she would prefer to forget, had promised her many things but never kept them, including a visit to her country of origin.

Fanny complains being tired, empty, without passion, without energy, without desire, but not daring to kill herself, because the souls of those who commit suicide must wander forever. As she could no longer read or enjoy anything, she had tried alcohol, smoking and drugs to help herself. Then she speaks of her past years, in which she has neither been able to be interested in others nor to realize anything of her own. Therefore, she absolutely needs to return to her country of origin; she fears much more to find her family, than to know that members of her family are already dead. Fanny is convinced that her mother has already died. She recounts having lost the only two photos she possessed of her family, one of her parents and one of her younger sister. She wonders if she could finally realize something by fulfilling her mother's mission, "You'll come back when you have grown up."

Comment
The adoptive parents had suffered severe narcissistic wounds because of their son's serious hereditary illness, followed by their renouncing to have another biological child. Their motivation to adopt a child was based on the phantasm of reparation, namely, replacing the missing sibling for their son. On the one hand, Fanny reminds the narcissistic injuries of her adoptive parents, who—for this reason—had difficulties to emotionally invest her; on the other hand, she stood for the adoptive parents' need for reparation, resulting from their guilt feelings towards their disabled son. In this context, Fanny was not able to fulfill a grieving process over her own losses. In the relationship with her partner, she reenacted repetitively the traumatic experienced breakup of her attachment to her biological family and her country of origin.

Vignette

Martina, a 17-year-old Asian teenager, was adopted at the age of five. In the interview with her adoptive parents, they complain about her daughter's instability on a professional and relational level and especially about her love adventures. They fear that Martina could end up a drug addict or being pregnant. The adoptive mother informs the child psychiatrist that Martina's birth mother was a prostitute, an information she had always kept secret from Martina. She herself was never able to overcome her shame- and anxiety feelings about the potential hereditary burden of her adopted daughter.

In the individual psychiatric interview, Martina presents a severe depressive state, she cries during the whole interview and recounts that her adoptive mother had told her: "You can earn your money on the streets at night".

Comment

The adoptive mother and the adopted daughter seem to share a common phantasm concerning the biological mother. Through her behavior, Martina keeps reminding the information regarding her birth mother, shameful for her adoptive mother and kept secret by her. But with her message to Martina: "You can earn your money on the street at night", the adoptive mother points to the secret of Martina's origin. The ambivalence of the adoptive mother is evident: on one hand she wishes to keep the secret, on the other to reveal it. Martina seems to enact the phantasms of the secret's content, unknown to her. Obviously, through all these years the adoptive mother did not achieve a positive attitude towards the birth mother. She upheld the prostitution myth (a sinful sexuality in her eyes), which allowed her to disgrace the biological mother and to feel confirmed in her own self-esteem.

The secret was shared and maintained in the mother-daughter relationship over all these years; Martina expressed her fantasies—of what her parents could not name—through her behavior and by her severe depression; the secret inhibited a mourning process of her losses and hindered her ability to engage herself professionally and relationally.

A secret always arises in a meaningful relationship and is a shared experience [8]. The formation of a secret seems to be comparable to the creation of a "void," a hidden space in the psyche of an individual, which is subsequently often filled with bizarre fantasies.

All children with filiation problems will sooner or later question their environment out of their curiosity [10]. If they remain without an answer, they will express their need to know with their behavior, i.e., with their symptoms. "The event, which cannot be expressed by the parents, often produces behavioral and affective manifestations in the child" ([11]: p. 144).

Martina's acting-out can be understood as escaping her anxious feelings of inner emptiness and meaninglessness. Cognition urges and sexual drives are interconnected. Desiring to learn to know his origin, a child will try to transcend the prohibition of knowing his true filiation. Sexual curiosity concerns not only the difference of the sexes, but also the genealogical dimensions of origin and filiation. A too powerful interdiction or a contradictory discourse in this respect burdens the child and leads to an inhibition of his drive for knowledge and finally—by forbidding him to think his origin—to a real developmental inhibition of any school learning (Ferrari 1986). Martina had great learning difficulties and memory problems.

Vignette

The child and youth protection service asks for a psychiatric evaluation of Natacha, an incest child of the mother-grandfather relationship. Natascha was admitted into the future adoptive family when she was a few months old. The adoptive parents, informed about the incest, declare 15 years later that they forgot this fact.

Natascha, 15 years old, reveals—in her first interview with the child psychiatrist—that she is pregnant. She believes to be pregnant, because she wishes to belong to someone, namely to her future baby. This desire—or perhaps it is the desire to know her birth origin—is so absolute that Natascha is convinced of her parthenogenetic pregnancy. It seems inconceivable for Natascha to integrate—on a mental level—a father into the procreation process.

The question arises, if Natascha, who is in reality not pregnant, is trying to enact the elements of her biological mother's life that are shameful for and kept secret by the adoptive parents; or does she attempt to "realize" a secret wish of her sterile adoptive mother?

The following years of Natascha's life proved to be devastating; she entered into violent relationships with foreign men, which she repeatedly broke off, and she showed herself incapable of pursuing an apprenticeship or a job. She committed several suicide attempts and was victim of multiple accidents.

Comment

Adopted adolescents or young women harbor (pre)conscious phantasms of pregnancy and having a baby to "fill" a painful inner void, to satisfy their longing for a biological connection, to gain feelings of belonging and an experience of completeness, as well as to encounter the physical image of their biological parents.

The sexual acting out of adopted adolescent girls can have the meaning of an unconscious identification with the biological mother. What phantasms are acted out or realized by adopted teenagers who are the offspring of single mothers and adopted by infertile mothers? Like their biological mothers, they may conceive being single, or like their adoptive mothers, they may suffer from infertility.

Vignette

Vera, an 18-year-old European-born teenager adopted at 10 months—she is an only child—and her adoptive mother request a psychiatric consultation for Vera, who presents the following symptoms: multiple accidents, school performance problems and relationship difficulties. The dialogue in the first interview between adoptive mother and daughter is characterized by mutual hostile attacks; mother and daughter tell that at home they reciprocally act out their aggressive behavior. Vera threatens to run away and commit suicide.

Subsequently, the daughter's primary amenorrhea is casually mentioned, for which she is undergoing gynecological treatment. Later the adoptive mother reveals that the adoptive father is sterile, but that she has declared herself infertile to her and her husband's families. Does the symptomatology of amenorrhea indicate the paternal sterility that was kept secret, or does it represent the daughter's identification with her adoptive mother?

Vignette
Cecilia, adopted at the age of some months from an institution in an East Asian country, is informed about her adoption at the age of four, when her adoptive parents separate. As a young adult, she tried in vain to find her biological parents. She seeks psychotherapeutic help for her multiple anxieties such as to be abandoned, to take false decisions, to disappoint her adoptive parents or to lose her adoptive mother with whom she lives. Engaged in a relationship with a man of her age, she is haunted by feelings to be abandoned or betrayed by her friend, dreading that he will leave her for another women. She verbalizes doubts about her appearance and compares her looks with other women. Obsessed by these thoughts, she has difficulties to concentrate and suffers from insomnia. After some months of psychotherapy, she announces—to the surprise of her therapist—that she has never dared to tell her friend that she is adopted. The psychotherapeutic process reveals how overwhelmed with shame and guilt feelings the patient is about her adoptive affiliation.

Summary

These examples of adopted adolescents or young adults of various ages show different symptoms but have in common a childhood history that is largely unknown. Their psychopathological behavior indicates a break in their developmental line. The actual psychological developmental tasks in adolescence are impaired. Individuation, disengagement, and separation processes from the adoptive parents are complicated by the inability to grieve losses of birth parents, as well as of ethnic, linguistic, and cultural losses. The anxiety to engage a process of coping and coming to term with these losses is too overwhelming, as it may trigger existential fears of annihilation and death. The "threat of annihilation"' is a primitive fear that precedes all fear and includes the fear of death.

The severity and chronicity of these adoptees' symptomatology reflect their enormous suffering. They are particularly vulnerable to compulsively reenacting traumatic experiences, as they have no conscious memory of the traumatic event(s), leading to repeated suffering either for themselves as victims or for others as perpetrators. The acting out can manifest itself in delinquency, drug addiction, love adventures, promiscuity and serves to avoid intolerable fear feelings, inner emptiness, meaninglessness, and insignificance and are accompanied by broad inhibition of the ability to think. The adolescents remain dependent on external reality and the presence of a reference person to feel their existence. The question is, if these are reenactments of traumatic experiences out of an unconscious need for punishment, e.g., self-healing attempts, which however fail.

The clinical vignettes show the adoptees inability to integrate contradictory aspects of relationship investment[4] and to differentiate between their internalized self- and object representations. The persistence of their psychic defense organization (splitting, dissociation, denial, projective identification) hinders an individuation process and impairs the integration of an autonomous self-image. According to Laufer [12], the psychopathological manifestations result from the breakdown of developmental functions in adolescence. An integration of the sexualized adult body into the body-self-image does not take place. The developmental stillstand is a potential pathology since the differentiation of male and female identification processes (a specific task of adolescence) has been interrupted. This rupture in the developmental line severely affects the relationship with oneself as a sexual individual, the relationship with other persons, and the relationship with external reality. For adopted adolescents, the rupture can also be understood as a repetition of previous interruptions in the adolescent's personal history.

Therapeutic interventions in these situations are demanding and complex. Frequently, the need for a psychotherapeutic treatment has first to be worked out with the adopted adolescent and his adoptive parents. Adopted youth often refuse psychotherapeutic help, or the adoptive parents devalue the therapeutic proposition; all they wish is that her son or daughter behaves as he or she used to before puberty. A new "as if" adjustment may occur, leaving the psychopathology unchanged.

The central theme of the therapy is concerned with understanding the meaning for the adolescent's developmental breakdown and thereby his experienced brutal loss of significant persons in his individual history. In a therapeutic transference relationship, the adoptee will learn to comprehend the signification of his breakdown and subsequently be able to better cope with his lived experiences, to which as a child he was helplessly exposed. A mourning process begins gradually: transformation and integration of the losses in the adoptee's personal history take place progressively and lead to the consolidation of his authentic personality.

Young Adulthood

Vignette

In the initial psychiatric interview, a 21-year-old adopted young man, Leander, complains of being in a persistent state of depression, having no job and not knowing what to do with his life. He tells having always been a bad student, and although he has good intellectual capabilities, he has never passed any exams.

Leander was adopted at the age of 5 months from South America. At age 20, he returned to his country of origin in search of his mother, he unfortunately did not find. He describes his birth mother as a "shadow without a face, a God, my lifesaver

---

[4] In psychoanalytic theory, the investment of psychic energy in an object of any kind, such as a wish, fantasy, person, goal, idea, social group, or the self, such objects are said to be cathected when an individual attaches emotional significance (positive or negative affect) to them.

for all my feelings in any conflictual situation." He is living in a state of expectation: either he wants to find his birthmother or to know that she is dead. He thinks that the catastrophe happened during his conception. He says having constantly lived in a bubble, allowing him to always keep distance. If a person establishes a close relation with him, he is immediately afraid of losing her. He keeps himself and his state of adoption secret. Of his past he has forgotten everything, also what happened in his adoptive family. For Leander forgetting is an automatic process. He recently re-read what he had written a year ago about his stay in his country of origin; he read this text as if someone else had written it.

In a psychotherapeutic session he says about himself:

> I always got everything. I never lacked anything. I have always granted myself everything immediately, if not realizable, I no longer desire it, thus I do not feel any deprivation or sadness. I never get angry; I never cry, I feel nothing. I am empty inside, the reason why I collect and keep things, so that the outside is filled with objects. Like objects, people must be present and available when I need them, if not, then they shall not disturb me. I love myself; it flatters me when someone loves me, but I do not love him, I only use him. I always managed to give an image of myself, to appear instead of to be. In all my relationships, I succeeded each time that the other person leaves me. When someone begins to love me, I withdraw, I will become more and more intolerable, until the other person abandons me. I could never break off a relationship; I cannot admit making a mistake and I am incapable of taking responsibility. I would like to lay in my girlfriend's arms for hours like an infant, but I cannot ask her to be my mother all the time.

Leander wished to change his last name, replacing it by the name of his birth mother. At Christmas—the most difficult time of the year—Leander feels alien, not belonging to his adoptive family, an orphan. During this period, he awaits the return of his biological mother, hoping for a rebirth. Leander thinks he has suffered enough and is entitled to everything.

Comment

Leander seems to fear his inner emptiness, resulting from his splitting off his painful emotions. He tries to control his feelings of void and meaninglessness in accumulating numerous objects, a sort of a compensation. The psychic emptiness—the consequence of his pronounced defensive strategies—blocks Leander's ability to carry out learning processes and lets him forget everything. Leander seems never to have processed the psychic traumatization he suffered from the breakups in his past history. Not knowing if his birth mother is still alive, he seems incapable to grieve her. He presents a pathological grief disorder.

In complicated grief, the affective investment of the psychic representation of the lost beloved person is crystallized forever, as if the sufferer is trying in vain to bring the lost person back to life. His love is frozen around an image and accompanied by intense longing and pain [13]. For Leander, the loss of his biological mother remains present, and he wishes to resurrect her each Christmas.

Leander has apparently never been able to mourn the traumatic moments of losing his biological mother, a catastrophe, which happened 21 years ago when he was 5 months old and probably not at his conception, as he thinks.

Leander's breakdown took place at a stage of development when he was dependent on maternal or parental support. According to Winnicott [2], such an experience of primitive agony[5] must be re-experienced by the subject and processed at a later development stage; only then it can be integrated and memorized. In a kind of repetition compulsion, Leander seems to avoid establishing a meaningful relationship, for not having to re-experience painful feelings of loss. By means of intense phantasms, he maintains the bond with his biological mother. Such fantasy activity may reinforce the organization of a false self. Painful experiences are split off and/or repressed for self-protection. The individual behaves as if cut off from the memories of his past, giving the impression of being in a kind of eternal present, where there are neither losses nor death. This (hypo)manic defense mechanism allows avoiding a confrontation and coping with psychic reality; a mental elaboration and meaning attribution of the lived events do not take place. Arduous memories, painful losses can thus be denied.

Leander believes he must remain hidden; the fact of his adoption must never be revealed. The secret of the adoption hides a much greater mystery, that of his origins and of his biological mother's motivation for having given him up for adoption. Leander refers to his birth mother as a god (goddess) who will return at Christmas for his rebirth, thus maintaining the phantasm of being the son of God. This status of a son of God seems on the one hand to be analogous to the Christian religion of a spiritual procreation, and on the other hand to relate to omnipotent phantasms of a primary mother-child-unity [4], from which the biological father is excluded.

Leander lives in a world of "abundance", supposedly without frustrations, without effort, a passive life without creativity and meaning, where everything is futile and useless. The question arises whether the phantasm of being the son of God was nourished by his adoptive parents? Leander has—"like a god"—generated life in his adoptive parents: a biological sister was born one year after his integration into his adoptive family.

Thanks to Leander, his adoptive parents were able to overcome their sterility; they became mother and father of a biological child, Leander's sister. Is it their gratitude and/or their guilt that prevented them from confronting Leander with reality, i.e., setting limits and encouraging him to take developmental steps appropriate to his age? Leander, for his part, lives in the belief that he can dispose of the world as he pleases. Is he considered a sacred, holy child because he created life?

---

[5] The primitive agonies and the defenses against them are:

    1. A return to an unintegrated state. (Defence: disintegration.)

    2. Falling forever. (Defence: self-holding.)

    3. Loss of psychosomatic collusion, failure of indwelling. (Defence: depersonalization.)

    4. Loss of sense of real. (Defence: exploitation of primary narcissism, etc.)

    5. Loss of capacity to relate to objects. (Defence: autistic states, relating only to self-phenomena.) (Winnicott [2]: pp. 89–90)

References

1. Bergeret J. La violence fondamentale. Paris: Dunod; 1984.
2. Winnicott DW. Fear of breakdown Int R Psychoanal. 1974;1:103–7.
3. Winnicott DW. Ego distortion in terms of true and false self. In: The maturational processes and the facilitating environment: studies in the theory of emotional development. The international psychoanalytical library, vol. 64. London: The Hogarth Press and the Institute of Psychoanalysis; 1965. p. 1–276.
4. Winnicott DW. Home is where we start from. New York London: WW Norton & Company; 1986.
5. Guyotat J. Mort/naissance et filiation. Etudes de psychopathologie sur le lien de filiation. Paris: Masson; 1980.
6. Berger M. L'enfant et la souffrance de la séparation. Paris: Dunod; 1997.
7. Winnicott DW. Clinical varieties of transference. In: Collected papers. Through pediatrics to psychoanalysis. London: Tavistock; 1955–1966.
8. Abraham N, Torok M. L'écorce et le noyau. Paris: Flammarion; 1987.
9. Hirsch M. Psychodynamik und Identitätsschicksal des Ersatzkindes. In: Sohni H, editor. Geschwisterlichkeit— Horizontale Beziehungen in Psychotherapie und Gesellschaft. Göttingen; 1999.
10. Bourdier P. Famille et connaissance des liens de parenté. Psychologie Médicale. 1982;14(10):1541–9.
11. Tisseron S. Tintin et les secrets de famille. Paris: Aubier; 1992.
12. Laufer M. Psychopathologie de l'adolescence et objectifs thérapeutques. In: Ladame F, editor. Jeammet P La Psychiatrie de l'adolescence aujourd'hui. Paris: Presse universitaires de France; 1986. p. 61–86.
13. Nasio JD. Le livre de la douleur et de l'amour. Paris: Editions Payot & Rivages; 1996.

Chapter 9
Professional Help

Suffering and pain are always the prerequisite of comprehensive knowledge and a deep heart. It seems to me that truly great people must feel great sorrow on earth — Fyodor Mikhailovich Dostoevsky

Introduction

The integration of an adoptive child into his new family is a complex and often turbulent process that requires a lot of time, strength, and emotional commitment from the adoptive parents. The adoption situation represents a special challenge that adoptive parents believe they must be able to meet, since they desired to have a child and opted for adoption. Difficulties and problems are therefore often denied or repressed for a long time, since they are associated with adoptive parents' feelings of incompetence and insufficiency. Seeking help is perceived by many adoptive parents as a kind of confirmation of a fantasized failure or as an attribution of blame and guilt. It is not surprising, then, that adoptive parents often "put forward" the child first and relate his problems to his heredity.

Therapeutic interventions [1–5] include family counseling as well as individual psychotherapies [6–8] or psychodrama group therapy for the child, with accompanying interviews with his parents [9–11], or counseling with adoptive parents alone. Self-help groups for adoptive families [12], adoptive parents or adoptees may also be a great source of support.

It is often not easy to make the "right" therapeutic choice. Usually, adoptive families sense best how and when to begin with accepting and receiving help. Sometimes the intervention aims first to work out with the family the willingness for a therapeutic process. The treatment of adopted children cannot be separated from the one of their adoptive parents. Clinical experience proves favorable, if the same therapist is available for therapeutic interventions with the child and his family

B. Steck, *Adoption as a Lifelong Process*,
https://doi.org/10.1007/978-3-031-33038-4_9

to meet the complex triangular situation of biological parents, adoptive parents and adopted child.

"The treatment of an adoptive child will necessarily include analysis of transference manifestations deriving from both the adoptive parent and the (unknown) biological parents, about whom the child will have constructed elaborate fantasies in order to make sense of his adoption" (Brinich [13], p. 126).

Therapeutic Interventions with Families

"The adopted child is always accompanied by the ghost of the child he might have been had he stayed with his birth mother and by the ghost of the fantasy child his adoptive parents might have had. He is also accompanied by the ghost of the birth mother, from whom he has never completely disconnected, and the ghost of the birth father, hidden behind her. The adoptive mother and father are accompanied by the ghost of the perfect biological child they might have had, who walks beside the adopted child who is taking its place. The birth mother (and father, to a lesser extent) is accompanied by a retinue of ghosts. The ghost of the baby she gave up. The ghost of her lost lover, whom she connects with the baby. The ghost of the mother she might have been. And the ghosts of the baby's adoptive parents" (Lifton [14] p. 11). "To help all members of the adoption triad, therapists must be able to see the ghosts that accompany them. These ghosts spring from the depths of the unresolved grief, loss, and trauma that everyone has experienced. They represent the lost babies, the parents who lost them, and the parents who found them. Too dangerous to be allowed into consciousness, they are consigned to a spectral place I call the *Ghost Kingdom*" (Lifton [15] p. 1).

In psychotherapeutic processes with adoptive families, it is important to bring up the biological parents and to help adoptive parents and adopted children to reveal their (un)conscious fantasies concerning the biological parents [9]. This will encourage the child to ask questions about his origins and the reasons for his release for adoption. Adoptive parents will address their fears about the adopted child's heredity and past and raise questions about rights and responsibilities of their parenthood. The link between the family romance fantasy of the parents with the one of the adopted child needs to be elaborated, while keeping in mind the significance of the birth parents. What role does the child in his phantasms ascribe to his adoptive parents and what position do the adoptive parents wish to assume in the eyes of their adopted child? Are they the idealized parents of the child's fantasy romance or foster parents raising a child? Should the adopted child correspond to the idealized imaginary child of the adoptive parents? Or is he respected as the real child with his origins, his past and his difficulties? The expression and reflection of these phantasms lead inevitably into the biographical past of both the adoptive parents and the adopted child.

What adoptive parents, adopted child, and biological parents have experienced in common are losses. For the *child*, it is the loss of his birthparents, grandparents and possibly siblings, his cultural, ethnic, and linguistic roots; for the *biological parents*, it is the loss of their child; for the *adoptive parents*, it is usually the loss of their reproductive capacity, sometimes the loss of a biological child, of a parent or a sibling. Working through the feelings associated with losses leads to an affectively shared togetherness and strengthens the emotional bonds between adoptive parents and adopted children. Revealing the fantasized and/or real past of adoptive parents and adopted child creates a narrative history shared together. The past needs no longer to be denied and the common future can be envisaged with greater freedom. The inclusion of biological or adopted siblings, at least on a mental basis, is important in therapeutic processes with adoptive parents and children. Information about past events and circumstances is certainly highly significant for adopted children; however, if too much importance is attributed to these information, difficulties or problems connected with the adoption will remain attached to unknown events or circumstances. The knowledge of real facts does not magically improve the parent-child relationship; the goal is rather to communicate in non-hurting words, to recognize and share conscious and unconscious phantasms, feelings and fears associated with not-knowing. A psychotherapeutic process with adoptive parents and adopted child is associated with painful mourning of experienced losses.

Continuity Interruption

Adoptive parents and adopted children as well as biological parents' continuity in their life stories has been interrupted by losses or critical life events. Carried by the hope of finally being able to overcome and integrate these experiences into the personal and family history, they very often expose themselves to situation, in which they re-experience traumatic events and thus repeat painful past situations. The interruption of temporal continuity in their personal histories may represent a breakdown for the adopted child and the adopting parents.

For the child, the breakdown is the void of origin, a non-experience of his genesis, the absence of a mirror image, which includes the self. For the adopting couple, the procreative incapacity prevents them from projecting themselves into the future, from inserting themselves in the biological cycle of birth - procreation - death and from making the generational leap from the role of son - daughter to the one of parents.

Adoption too often takes the form of repetition of this traumatic situation, the unconscious hope being to succeed in mastering this event at last and to reestablish a continuity in one's self- representation; then only the experience can be remembered and become "history" [16].

Special Therapeutic Attention for Transracial Adoptive Families

Approximately half of adoptions are transracial and consist of predominantly white parents and children of color from diverse ethnic or racial backgrounds, according to the US children's bureau.[1] The task for adoptive parents in this situation and for their adopted children represents a complex and lifelong process and depends on multiple child-, parent-, and family variables. Even if adoptive parents have the very best knowledge of the culture of their child's origin, help him in his ethnic–racial socialization process and prepare him for possible discrimination, it is finally up to the adopted child to cope with his singular situation: to develop his specific identity, to accept his difference and learn to deal with discrimination. This working through process and overcoming wrongful events is an arduous challenge for adopted youth [17].

Psychotherapeutic Processes with Adoptive Parents

> The treatment of adopted children usually cannot be divorced from the treatment of the adoptive parents because adoption is almost always linked in the parents with powerful affects and conflicts related to the issues of infertility, illegitimacy, and parenthood. Beyond these, the adoptive parents need to be able to deal with the ambivalence of their children without resorting to externalization and projection. … While the child is loved, he is also representative of the parental failure to conceive (Brinich [13], p. 125–126).

In a study to explore the impact of the child's traumatic past on parental representations and subsequent parent-child interactions, over forty French parents who adopted one or more children internationally, participated in a semi-structured interview [18]. The results of the qualitative analyzed interviews showed the difficulties of the parents to identify emotionally with their child's pre-adoptive traumatic experience, as well as their tendency to deny its significance. Denial and affect absence may indicate defensive mechanisms for own protection and is associated with insufficient reflecting and elaboration of the child's personal past history. If remembering their own past is too overwhelming for adoptive parents, they are hardly able to be confronted with the past of their adopted child.

Additional themes of the narratives revealed parents' perception of their child's otherness and strangeness, sometimes accompanied by cultural depreciation of the child's country of origin, as well as their anticipated anxiety for their child's repeating painful situations of his past. These results demonstrate the importance of psychotherapeutic interventions to help parents with regard to their representations of their child and their interactions with him.

The goal of psychotherapeutic treatments with adoptive parents is to improve parents' sense of competency and to support parents' processing of critical

---

[1] The Children's Bureau supports programs, research, and monitoring to help eliminate barriers to adoption and find permanent families for children.

experiences in their personal biography. Preventive and therapeutic interventions aim at allowing parents to discover and strengthen their parental role and functions, while at the same time expressing their conflictual burdens. Adoptive parents need to recognize their implications and meaning in the histories of their own parents and to understand the personal life story of their own intrapsychic child. It is essential to consider the inner child in the adult person and the intergenerational dynamics, as well as the parents' creative anticipation for their children [19].

Psychoanalytic therapy with a child, whose parents experienced psychic trauma in their own childhood/adolescence, represents - in the presence of transgenerational legacies - a specific challenge for therapists. When forming a viable alliance with the parents, which is necessary for the psychotherapy with their child, it is important to approach the existing parental pain with cautiousness and diligence. The unprocessed personal life stories of the parents, their unresolved grief or painful secrets are usually associated with an insufficient identity formation. Parents often seek a reparation of their own traumatic experiences, which affects their ability to recognize their child as a separate, autonomous, and different person.

Fraiberg et al. [20] in *Ghosts in the Nursery*, describes the repetitions of unprocessed, often traumatic past experiences of parents and their inner representations in the attachment and relationship with their child, who, with his birth, becomes a tacit partner in the tragedy of his parents. Parents - who remember the pain and suffering they endured in childhood - are usually protected from blind repetition with their own child. By reflecting back, they identify with their injured self of their childhood. This is not the case for parents who repressed their painful emotions and stayed in an unconscious alliance and identification with the feared figures (the aggressors and the betrayers) of their personal life history. The parental past is then imposed on the child. In the psychotherapeutic accompaniment of parents, it is essential for parents being capable to remember their childhood experiences and thus to be relieved of their associated painful emotions. As Fraiberg writes: "The key to our ghost story appears to lie in the fate of affects in childhood" (p: 420).

The transgenerational transmission of traumatic experiences from parents to their children takes place, mostly non-verbally and unconsciously, through body language (e.g., facial expressions or gestures), through the parent's emotional state of mind and its affective expression, and through the regulation of closeness and distance. The lack of symbolization of elements, transmitted nonverbally, leaves the affected child without speech for relevant experiences, what may impair his development of self- and object relations.

Children often perceive the emotions associated with their parents' traumatic experiences (such as fear, pain, anger, despair, shame, or helplessness) only diffusely or in a distorted way and are therefore unable to sense the parental feelings in a differentiated way. They not infrequently feel obliged to take over the parent's unaccomplished mourning and - sympathizing with the parent's unresolved grief and concerned for the parent's well-being - burden themselves with feelings of guilt [21].

A child perceives the injuries and neediness of his parent and tries to support him with a caring relationship. Out of his needs for love and care, the child unconsciously makes himself available, identifies with the parents' unprocessed traumatic experiences, and adopts also "cryptic" elements, which he is unable to integrate into a coherent world of representation. Parents rarely register the parentified role-taking and the associated often severe stress for their child, who is overburdened with the task of processing transgenerational transmitted pain, guilt, silences, and conflicts of loyalty from their parents [22]. Parents burdened by the reactivation of their traumatic experiences and associated affects may not succeed in alleviating their child's anxiety [23]. Psychoanalytic work must deal with the parents' repressed emotional pain and/or projections onto their child. The combination and condensation of traumatic experiences and the constantly varying and changing nature of the transference make such treatments particularly complex.

Processing Intrapsychic Conflicts and Critical Experiences in the Parents' Personal Biography

Adoptive parents feel frequently obliged to engage in an inner confrontation and psychic processing, sometimes already upon arrival of their child, or later during his development steps or developmental transitions. They sense that their parenting skills are questioned by the relational constellation with their adopted child, or they may even feel rejected as mother or father. They have second thoughts about their decision to adopt a child and doubt their motivation.

Psychotherapeutic work with adoptive parents usually leads to their personal history. Individual critical life events are often related to the (unconscious) motivation to adopt a child. Conflicting, psychic stressful experiences in the adoptive parents' biography are worked through in psychotherapeutic processes with the adoptive couple, or with the adoptive mother or father alone.

In psychoanalytical sessions, the transference relationship facilitates communication of the patient's unconscious formations and permits the search for sense and signification of unconscious phenomena in a context of containment [24]. The unconscious includes thoughts, memories, affects, motivations, dreams, creating meaning and influencing behavior. It is constantly working in sleep as well as in waking state. Conscious and unconscious processes are considered more and more as representations of mental phenomena emerging in a continuous form. Breuer and Freud [25] already postulated that the unconscious had a function in sustaining "psychic continuity", when there was discontinuity in consciousness.

Improving Parents' Sense of Competency and Enhancing Adoptive Parenting

Adoptive parents are sometimes bewildered by their adopted child's unknown, unusual, strange behavior. As they did not live with and care for their child in his early years, they perceive their adopted child as foreign. Their incompetence feelings may be associated with anxiety or depressive symptoms. Therapeutic interventions aim to support and help parents to better understand the meaning of their child's behavior, which often represents a reenacting of his lived adverse experiences in the past. With greater knowledge, parents' confidence increases and their skills in responding to the child's behavior improve. The resulting feelings of compassion and empathy for their child enables him to build up trust in the relation to his adoptive parents [26, 27].

Specific Interventions

Specialized psychological interventions with adoptive parents alone or with their adopted children, which use video-feedback, allow parents to reflect on their interactions with their child and to induce changes in his behavior [28, 29]. In a systematic review of psychological therapeutic interventions, involving only adoptive parents or with adoptive parents and their children, the effectiveness of these therapeutic interventions was explored, mainly if they succeed in enhancing the adoption experience and improving parent and child outcomes. Findings reveal generally positive results: adoptive parents accept the interventions, however - due to the multiple and various patterns of interventions - no specific recommendation can be made [30].

Over 200 child psychotherapists in the UK were interrogated in an online survey about their working practices with children in care and adopted children. Findings revealed that the majority conducted assessments, psychotherapies and worked with foster care persons and adoptive parents. They emphasized the need for a long-term psychotherapeutic treatment with these children and the significance for working with the professional network of the child [31].

Psychoanalytical Psychotherapy

One of the goals of psychoanalytical treatment is to understand the inner world of a patient, which unfolds in the significant relationship between patient and therapist. The patient's personal experiences and the meaning he attributes to his experiences are at the core of psychoanalytical investigation, with the aim to favor the patient's specific processes to understand the affective and cognitive contents of his mind. The intention of the therapist is to try to understand the patient's unconscious emotional experiences and to achieve, together with the patient, a careful common understanding of what is "true" for the patient in his unconscious emotional experience ([32]).

In psychoanalysis, transference refers to the process in which a patient's unconscious feelings are actualized and projected onto the analyst. Transference contains the patient's communications, his verbal expressions such as dreams and narrations, and his nonverbal communication such as posture, bodily movements, facial expressions, gesticulations, and his voice, the "musical dimension" of the transference [33]. The relationship between patient and analyst represents in part a shared "musical experience," allowing the affective and emotional world to be expressed. This musical dimension is an essential means in the analytical work as it facilitates the affective and emotional, often traumatic experiences, stored in the patient's implicit memory, which cannot consciously be remembered, to be relived in the transferential encounter. Often the understanding of a patient's personal history has to be elaborated from his enactments, by working on transference and countertransference elements; then recollections come to mind, and psychic continuity is being created.

The psychotherapist has to offer a continuous containment and relatedness for the patient's emotional engagement in the therapeutic process; the patient will then be able to reveal his lived affects of endured traumatic events, by simultaneously keeping a certain control and thus gradually decrease his feelings of fear, confusion, and helplessness. The patient will be able to "comprehend" the lived traumatic experience, even if not able to remember what exactly happened to him in reality [34].

The communicative exchange between patient and therapist takes place on verbal and preverbal levels. There are always at least two levels to be listened to: what a patient tells or shows both at the infant- or young child age and at the real age of the subject. The self of the infant or young child is the one that presents his suffering in various forms, whereas the self of the real age patient is often present with different contributions and functions such as "helping" or "guiding" the therapist and supporting the therapeutic process. Therefore, the therapist has to continuously adjust his listening according to the different "selves" of his patient: at the infant stage for example, the patient requires a caring and affectionate presence of his therapist. He has to be able to wait, yet never leave a patient on an emotional level alone. He must record any communication (whether nonverbal, enforced by means of projective identification or verbal), preserve, and transform it into language and give it back to the patient. "Being found" by spoken words is often the secret hope of patients with subjective experiences of having felt lost or abandoned when their inner emotions were not met by a caregiver's affectionate engagement and attuned speech. The analyst attempts to perceive, sense, and comprehend the intrapsychic lived experience of the patient and returns in words the meaning of the patient's experiences.

Individual Psychotherapy with Traumatized Adoptees

Treatment with adoptees having experienced traumatic events in infancy or early childhood is a demanding task, which must be accomplished by a reliable therapist who establishes a secure, protective, and continuous relationship with his patient. The therapeutic work aims to help a patient, who compulsively repeats his traumatic experiences in actions, somatic states, or emotional distress, by analyzing and understanding with him the unconscious dynamics, underlying his reenactments. Through an appropriate containment and a careful transformation into words, there is the possibility of new relational experiences in the dialogue between patient and therapist with partial transformations of disabling representations.

Patients need to be reassured that expressing the overwhelming feelings associated with the trauma will not bring the trauma back. The goal of working through traumatic experiences is to enable the patient to gradually decrease his highly intense emotional charge and at the same time create meaning of his lived events. It is the responsibility of the therapist to guarantee that re-traumatization does not happen during trauma processing work.

The therapeutic process with traumatized adoptees can be particularly complicated because the traces left by trauma exert a continuous influence on their psychic functioning. The attempt to get rid of this burdening element may be carried out by a repetitive ejection into conscious experiences or by means of encapsulation, i.e., by transforming it into a kind of psychic crypt. The compulsion to repeat has the character of an enactment, in which the traumatic potential of the external reality is revived, often to satisfy an unconscious need for punishment. However, the core of the trauma - the non-mentalized and non-metabolized - remains. These reenactments of traumatic events can be considered as repetitive self-healing attempts, which however fail.

During the movements of the therapeutic process, the intrapsychic conflict configurations (e.g., between self- and object representations) are - as transference phenomena - transformed into interpersonal disturbances between adoptee and therapist. These enactments and repetitions are not exact copies of earlier ones, but recurrent attempts to find more favorable coping options, more appropriate expressions, and adequate solutions [35].

The more destructive tensions in an adoptee's environment exist, the more demanding is the processing of personal and intrapersonal relationship conflicts in the therapy; the distinction between internal and external problems is often not easy to recognize for both the adoptee and the therapist.

Against destructive attacks of a patient, it is essential that psychotherapists demonstrate their capacity to contain the aggression and "survive", what designates at the same time their separate existence from the patient. Adoptees need help to begin mourning. Children have no model of grieving because a true mourning process only takes place in adolescence, with the ongoing movements of detachment, disengagement, and separation from primary caregivers. It lies in the therapist's responsibility to assure that pathological grief does not occur during trauma processing.

Adoptees, who have experienced continuity interruptions in their development, will create continuity in their psychotherapy. Separation means loss for adoptees and is very often equated with death. The intense anger over loss may cause pathological grief. If patients succeed to bring their anger gradually into the therapeutic relationship and ensure that the relationship remains alive, the emergence of pathological grief can be avoided. Bringing aggressive, destructive affects into the therapeutic relationship is critical for adoptees because they fear that the vehemence of their affects could destroy the therapist on whose availability they depend. The murderous rage must be brought progressively into the relationship. In this way intrapsychic processes find partial expression on an interpersonal level. In identification with the adoptee, therapists enter into the adoptee's world of loss. A patient needs his therapist as a symbolic substitute figure with whom the rage over the loss can be processed.

The end of a therapy session is frequently experienced by adoptees as an expulsion or rejection, which reactivate their pain of separation and is therefore felt as an aggressive act. At the same time, it indicates the limited nature of the relationship with the psychotherapist. When a patient is overwhelmed by the re-enactment of the traumatic loss, the therapist has to be the container of the unwanted feelings of loss and separation. Through the therapist's ability to hold externalized fear or anger within himself and to transform these emotions into words, he also assumes a certain auxiliary ego function for the child. The therapist's containment corresponds to a complex empathic taking over of an unbearable part of the adoptee's inner world by the mechanism of projective identification.[2] It represents for the patient a psychic attitude with which he will increasingly be capable to identify, namely how the alive-part in the therapist prevails over the death-bringing-part. Psychic processing means mentally representing a highly vulnerable area, keeping the associated affects under control and distinguishing intrapsychic from external events, the latter especially on the emotional level. This process takes place gradually in a secure therapeutic relationship.

The excess of trauma is accompanied by its shadow, the silence of the inexpressible (Barrois [36] p: 195).

The earlier children who have suffered psychic trauma receive help, the greater their chance of not becoming "shadow children". Chronically traumatized children do indeed give the impression of shadow figures. They are also described as automatons or robots. Having cut off their memories of the past, they live joylessly into the day, apparently in a kind of perpetual present, which strives to exclude any absence, be it through separation, loss, or death, and without any wishes for the future.

Play in the Psychotherapeutic Process with Children

"In the case of children's play we seemed to see that children repeat unpleasurable experiences for the additional reason that they can master a powerful impression far more thoroughly by being active than they could by merely experiencing it passively" (Freud [37] p: 35).

---

[2] Projective identification is a process, in which - in a close relationship, such as between parent and child or psychotherapist and patient - an unconscious fantasy of aspects of the self or of an internal relation representation is attributed to an external person. Projective identification is a defense mechanism in which the individual projects qualities that are unacceptable to the self onto another person.

"It is in playing, and only in playing, that the individual child or adult is able to be creative and to use the whole personality, and it is only in being creative that the individual discovers the self" (Winnicott [38] p: 54).

Vignette
Cindy, a seven-year-old girl from India, tells in a psychotherapeutic session the following story of a caterpillar: "The caterpillar was cut by bad people; therefore, it is blind. Birds took the caterpillar to C (first letter of the village's name, where the girl lives with her adoptive parents); there the caterpillar promised never wanting to see again, but to remain blind forever as it loved more than anything else to never see again."

Comment
The caterpillar speaks for Cindy, who expresses her greatest wish to never again perceive and feel the horrible experiences she had lived in her country of origin, before coming to Switzerland for her adoption. Cindy was able to use her psychotherapy and to "transform herself into a seeing butterfly".

Play provides an abundance of creativity. "Within the inner life of the child, play is a mental process which takes its stand along with, intermingles with, builds upon and integrates with many other mental processes in the developing child's mind - thinking, imaging, pretending, planning, wondering, doubting, remembering, guessing, hoping, experimenting, revising, and working through" ([39]; p. 137). In the area of play there is a potential space between an individual and his environment. In this area two persons can create new representations together, offering different solutions and significant meanings, sometimes out of chaotic and senseless elements [38]. Winnicott considered playing as an important feature fostering development. The therapeutic and restorative functions of playing have already been discussed by Anna Freud [40].

The spontaneous play of children in analytic psychotherapy enables the expression of intrapsychic processes by means of an abundance of representations. Without any demands or major restrictions, play offers an infinite number of creative variations of expression and their link with conscious and preconscious processes. In repetitive play enactments, the child attempts to master past painful experiences. In their play and related transference movements, children show their relationship and associated phantasms with their significant caregivers. Play enables the child to experiment - in the outside world - with identifications and solutions of intrapsychic conflict situations, to adapt affects and ideas accordingly and to gain a better self-understanding and self-awareness. "Pretend play" encourages the expression and representation of unconscious desires and conflicts, and their verbalization in play is less anxiety provoking for the child, as it provides simultaneously protection. In a second step, the child's play stories can be related to his difficulties and personal history.

Adopted children's symbolic repetitive play with birth, babies, and their mothers represent often not only their own preoccupation, but also the unresolved grief of the adoptive parent's failure to have a biological child. In the play-scenes of lost and found babies, the child tries to find an explanation for his loss. Children explore their relationship with significant others and show, in their fantasy play, not only their wishes, but also their expectations with regard to their adoptive parents or other meaningful persons, even how these should answer their needs and desires.

Psychoanalytic Therapeutic Process

The psychoanalytic process is based on an intersubjective relationship, involving the creation of a relational space in which latent development resources and resilience perspectives of a patient and mutual expectations of the patient and therapist are recorded. New functional possibilities and opportunities for more suitable integrations are explored and a more profound understanding of a commonly shared narrative is elaborated. The aim of the psychoanalytical process is directed towards working out new scope, open space and freedom and creation of alternatives, as well as more suitable forms of coping with life events [41]. Fostering the adoptee's developmental progression and helping him to experience a sense of coherence and personal continuity over time further the emergence of his self, the awareness of his intrapsychic reality with feelings and fantasies as well as of the boundary to his outer world. The assessment of a working alliance with both adoptive parents and especially with the adoptee has a special meaning. The investigation and diagnostic procedures should allow the patient to experience how the therapeutic process will evolve. With his functional parts, the patient will work together with the therapist on the dysfunctional structures of his inner world.

The indication for individual psychotherapy must consider the child's motivation and interest in therapeutic work. Children and adolescents usually do not seek help on their own but are referred for evaluation by parents, teachers, and physicians. Regardless of the existing disorders, it is necessary to bear in mind the age and the cognitive, affective, and psychosocial development of the child as well as his interpersonal relationship environment, his family and social situation. Age-, gender- and development-specific characteristics of contact and relationship - a child/adolescent creates with a psychotherapist - need to be assessed. Further the patient's ability to express and communicate, i.e., his dialogue, as well as his emotional experiencing and cognitive processing are to be estimated, and also his ego functioning level and defensive qualities. Will the child/adolescent be able to benefit from the therapeutic relationship offer, does an emotional movement and deepening take place? It is necessary to understand the kind of relationship a child engages with the therapist and how transitional spaces between child/adolescent and therapist are formed. These first interviews allow a diagnostic and therapeutic evaluation [42]. In any psychotherapy indication, the therapist is influenced by his or her own references, training, and value systems. In all considerations regarding desirable therapeutic approaches, the psychotherapist has also to evaluate, which therapeutic measure is possible at a specific time.

In *psychoanalytical psychotherapy* the therapist needs to be attentive to the non-verbal expression of emotions emerging in the transference relationship with the patient, as the events of these affects, stored in implicit memory,[3] can neither be recalled nor verbalized. It is the affective resonance of the therapist that the patient needs to hear, to feel understood in his infantile demands, wishes, deprivation, and distress. The therapist must name the affective atmosphere, sensed in the transference. The often very intense and confused emotions of the patient have then to be verbally differentiated in various nuances by the therapist, so that the patient can perceive and consciously experience his feelings and to qualify them with words as for example fear, anger, sadness, pain. Fantasies and images related to the patients' feelings emerge and associations and memories linked to these emotions are then revealed by the patient. Psychotherapists need to listen carefully to how and what a patient hears from their interventions, interpretations, the sound of their voice, or their silence. What a patient recalls and what meaning he attributes by his own associated reflections are essential elements for the therapeutic process ([43]).

The therapeutic relationship allows a patient to elaborate an understanding of his subjective lived experience and to learn to deal with overwhelming feelings, thoughts, ideas, and phantasms. The patient learns that all psychic states can be expressed and contained in the therapeutic relationship. Symbolic and semantic processing of somatosensory, emotional, and sensory implicit memories of lived events enables their translation into explicit memories, their transformation into declarative memory, so that they no longer need to be expressed by the body and/or by acting out. The integration work of split-off mental contents consists in translating unconscious and preconscious parts of experience into metaphorical language i.e., in transferring the memory fragments stored in implicit memory into symbolized and narrative memories of explicit memory.

The patient in his suffering and with his pain can be helped by a meaningful dialogue in a continuous relationship. In the safe and reliable framework of a psychotherapeutic process, a patient's creative imagination will unfold. Trust, sympathy, and the desire to work together constitute the main components of the therapeutic alliance, a kind of bridge, always to be maintained during the therapeutic process, allowing the movements of the transference relationship to proceed. Some patients need repeated recognition of such functional ego performances before they are ready to deal with pathological, i.e., dysfunctional, or disturbed relational aspects. The aim in an analytical psychotherapy is to guarantee the patient sufficient affective security allowing him to experience consciously partly repressed fears and feelings, associated with his lived traumatization into conscious experience. In the transference relationship, these affects can be named and verbalized in symbolic language.

The re-experiencing of former feelings is very painful. But grief work is urgently needed to avoid secondary traumatization through the patient's re-enacting his lived traumatic situations. The work-through process allows to understand and integrate the memories associated with the traumatic experience. Psychotherapeutic

---

[3] Implicit memory refers to the faculty of remembering motor or perceptual skills as well as emotional experiences; implicit nondeclarative memory, is automatized, and is not retrievable. Explicit or declarative memory refers to the conscious, intentional retrieval of past information or events.

interventions thus serve to ascribe meaning and significance to life events that have interrupted the continuity of a patient's personal life history.

Vignette

Helen, an Asian girl, arrived in Switzerland at the age of four-and-a-half and was placed in her prospective adoptive family (parents with two biological sons). After a suicide attempt at age 16, Helen left her adoptive family and lived with her godfather.

From her personal history it is known that her biological mother left her when she was 5 months old, her biological father remarried when she was three and Helen lived with her father and stepmother for one-and-a-half years.

At the age of 18 and a half years, one month before her baccalaureate, Helen began a psychotherapy, which lasted three and a half years. Shortly after her graduation, Helen left Switzerland for a few weeks - as she had planned for a long time - in search of her biological father, who had emigrated to another continent. After reuniting with her father and his family (stepmother and two half-siblings) and returning to Switzerland, Helen suffered from a severe state of depression. She saw various specialists for her multiple somatic symptoms; no organic pathology was diagnosed.

During the following 3 years, at age 19–22, Helen prepared for the entrance exam for psychomotor therapy training, which she failed three times despite great efforts. Simultaneously, she continued the search to find her birthmother in her country of origin. Helen described her many short-lasting heterosexual relationships, which she always broke off, as disappointing and longed for a stable, continuous relationship. She assumed a connection between her emotional relationship difficulties and her inability to start professional training. If she succeeded in a professional career, she believed, she would also be able to engage in a significant emotional relationship.

Helen had her first sexual relationship with her brother (a biological son of her adoptive parents), which was the reason for her suicide attempt at the age of 16 and her wish to leave her family. She had kept this relationship - incestuous in her eyes and against the law - secret from her adoptive parents. To reveal the secret, family therapeutic sessions took place, which helped Helen in her elaboration process of her past history in the adoptive family and led to a greater closeness of all family members.

A few months after these interviews and a short time before the last opportunity for Helen to pass her entrance exam, she said: "If I pass the exam, my success will be related to the death of one of my closely related persons." She knew - she continued - that her birth mother was dead, because she had been unable to find her, and that *she herself* must have caused her death. She thought that it was not her mother, who had abandoned her, when she was 5 months old, but that she had killed her mother.

Comment

Helen's statement was a turning point in the psychoanalytical therapy, a mutative experience, and a point of reference in the narrative history of Helen, representing significant insight for her and her therapist and leading to an intimately profound understanding. These now-moment [44], sacred-moment [45] seconds of eternity [46], shared between patient and therapist enhance the therapeutic relatedness and enrich the therapeutic process. The ancient Greeks called such a moment kairos,[4] a cyclic or mythic time, differentiated from chronos, a linear or sequential notion of time, thus emphasizing how perception and sense of time are influenced by phantasms, memories, and subjective experiences.

One can assume that Helen's fear - a person close to her would die if she allowed herself to successfully pass the exam - represents her own fear to suffer a breakdown. Helen had experienced at the age of 5 months the loss of her birth mother, a breakdown she has never been able to mourn and integrate in her adult personality. The past is "unknowingly" projected into the future and the recollection can only take place by reliving and mastering the traumatic event in the present. The subject must return to the moment when her emotional development was interrupted by the traumatic experience in infancy or early childhood.

Winnicott's concept of the "fear of breakdown" refers to "the fear of a past event that has not yet been experienced" ([16]: p. 107) and tends by compulsive repetition to be reactivated; the emotions associated with the original critical event are repeatedly relived on an interpersonal level and may represent a re-traumatization. An infantile event of "primitive agony", of an original breakdown, remains actual, unrepresented, and can only be inscribed into the past if taken up by the ego in present experiences and having been worked through, integrated, and remembered.

Helen's feared breakdown in the future already happened a long time ago. Her fear of breaking down has its roots in her need to "remember" the original breakdown. Helen's original breakdown took place at a development stage when she has been dependent on maternal or parental support; yet a protective environment was missing in Helen's infancy and childhood. According to Winnicott [47], the original experience of "primitive agony" must first be brought into the present experience of an individual and his coping process before it can belong to the past. To be able to continue his emotional development from where it came to a standstill, a patient must return to his early childhood or infancy.

Helen endured a very critical time in her psychotherapy, her psychic vulnerability being extreme. In her regressive movements, she was overwhelmed by intense emotions of sadness, pain, rage, and terrorizing fears of annihilation, disintegration, and depersonalization. Finally, she was able to recognize that her fantasies originated from feelings of helplessness and guilt. She learned to distance herself from the upsetting fantasied memories and to tell and envisage different meanings for the traumatic events she had been exposed to in early childhood. By (re)constructing her personal history (narration), she reached a turning point and gained a sense of self-continuity with feelings of being connected to the past without disruptions to the present.

---

[4] Kairos (ancient Greek: καιρός) signifies a moment of indeterminate time, a window of opportunity for change, whereas Chronos (ancient Greek: Χρόνος) "time" refers to chronological or sequential time.

The historical truth does not necessarily correspond to the truth of the (re)constructed story, which contains the again and again modified "truth," elaborated by the patient and therapist. During the course of a psychoanalytical therapeutic process, reflections of the intrapsychic dialogue of the patient with himself and the emerging and shared "certainty about the current truth" - continuously modified by conscious and unconscious contributions of the patient and the therapist - lead to new insights and create the history of a patient constantly anew.

Helen passed her exams and subsequently terminated her psychotherapy. At this time, she was almost 22 years old, her biological mother's age, when pregnant with her. Transmission from parents to children - from one generation to another - seems to be an absolute necessity [48]. If such a legacy cannot be realized, the need for transmission of heritance is replaced by chronology as demonstrated in this vignette: Helen was able to begin a mourning process of her losses at the age when her mother was expecting her. Later, Helen established a meaningful relationship with a partner.

Comment

A mourning process can be considered as engaged if the mourner is able to accept that his love for the new chosen person does not threaten to replace the love for the lost person [49]. The image of the lost person must never be erased but maintained up to the moment when the mourning person succeeds to keep the love for the lost person coexisting with the love for a newly chosen person. Pain is alleviated at the moment when the grieving person finally admits that his love for a new person will never erase the one for the disappeared or lost person.

Summary

For each individual adoptee and his family, it is essential to establish a therapeutic concept and to respect the autonomy of the adoptee and in the case of a child or adolescent his parents. Throughout the therapeutic process, the focus must be the adoptee's development, not his symptoms, with regard to his entire personality. Listening to the parents' or family's story intensively and over time creates a containment of their anxiety and guilt and helps them to adjust and accept the changes triggered by the therapeutic process [39]. The psychotherapist has to offer a significant relationship and a meaningful dialogue to the adoptee and his family. The analytical process is never linear and both patient and therapist undergo unconscious processes; the experiences of past events and the associated emotions are reactivated in the current relationship. The psychotherapist needs to be aware that it is the patient who "knows" - at a certain moment of his treatment - what he can assume in order to continue the psychotherapeutic process, what is helping him to transform disabling representations and to progress in his personal development.

Psychoanalytical Psychodrama Group Therapy

Psychodrama therapy was created in the 1920s by Moreno [50, 51]. Psychoanalytic psychodrama provides direct scenic insights into both the inner life of the individual and the functioning of the group. The analytic approach in psychodrama therapy opens a special access to latent personality areas.

In every civilization, individual or private myths provide a fundamental basis for childhood development, serving the social organization, such as the parent–child relationship. In therapeutic psychodrama, the child can explore his individual myths, for example, the Oedipus myth, which Freud used as basis for his concept "oedipal complex".[5]

The dramatic nature of psychodrama can be compared with the classical Greek tragedy: The Greeks have left us poetic and dramatic texts of people and heroes struggling with unpredictable gods. The myth in the tragedies is reinterpreted again and again in manifold versions.

The therapeutic psychodrama obeys the rule on which the classical tragedy is based, namely the unity of time, place, and action. Transgressions of the human order, based on collective faith, and their reparation are displayed In the Greek tragedy. The hero, as well as the spectators perceive the transgression as a fault (Greek: ἁμαρτία = hamartia). Order and rules are expressed in symbols and are reflected in laws and prohibitions, which determine human generations and sexual relationships and vary according to each civilization.

In the psychoanalytical psychodrama sessions, children play as heroes transgression and reparation, thus expressing each child's fundamental situation. Children experience the principles of human reality such as the difference between generations and gender. The child understands more intuitively than rationally the phenomena of birth, incest, death, love, and hate. He learns to adapt his wishes to the order of human reality.

According to Anzieu [52], the effectiveness of the psychodrama lies in its symbolic value. The task of the therapists is to represent the private myths in the play and to portray those myths in word and deed. This allows the child to experiment with relationships pattern, to invent new relationship opportunities, and to free himself, due to his increasing awareness, of unconscious conflictual obsessions.

The attractiveness of the psychodrama is the "realization" of children's phantasms, emotions, and wishes of magic satisfaction. The interindividual relations during the play are in a constant process of development, confront the child with the order of coexistence among persons, which the child over time does no longer deny. The symbolic function of the therapeutic psychodrama is situated between looking for an enjoyment and the necessity of recognizing a given and preexisting order. The

---

[5] Already the baby is able to establish triadic exchanges and build triadic relationship structures. Yet the infant has not a clear representation of the sexuality and the relationship between his parents. In the course of development, between about two and five years, children perceive the sexual differences of their parents. The conflicts associated with this development are called oedipal.

inner drama of the child is shown in the outside world, in a space that is inhabited by persons who sooner or later symbolize the interindividual situation of the original conflicts. The repetitions of the emotional disorders lead to symbolic (re)constructions, unknot conflictual situations, and release emotional energy. Inhibitory or pathogenic affects are revived and appear in the transference relationship.

The participation of the therapists is threefold: physical, emotional, and reflective. Between the two poles of body language on one side and verbalized thoughts on the other, the therapists use opportunities - depending on the situation and moment of the therapeutic process - for therapeutic interventions or interpretations in the hic and nunc. They address their understanding of the child's early psychic trauma, respectively, its consequences, which are expressed in the play, without searching for the biographical facts (this information is told by the child' parents in parallel interviews sessions).

Psychoanalytically oriented psychodrama therapy deals always with the child's personal history. The told stories reveal a child's relationships and his interpersonal situation. Children rarely speak directly of themselves. The symbolic interpretation addresses the mythical story. The identity and similarity of the mythical story with the personal drama of the child are at the root of the spontaneous and effective dramatization taking place in the psychoanalytic therapeutic psychodrama [10, 11].

The spatial and temporal framework and the "pretend play" are basic elements. There are three times units: In the first, group members are asked to tell a story, which may correspond to a real experience, however, invented narratives are generally preferred. The roles for the chosen story are then distributed. The second is the time of playing, while the third is the time of discussion, of retrospective processing, i.e., understanding and meaning attribution to the play scenes for each child and the group.

The playing time: Each child plays his attributed role; the therapists are engaged as well. The scenic-expressive presentation of the imaginary stories, told by the children and worked out together by the group, allows each child's present experience to unfold, with unconscious dimensions emerging and offering insight into the individual child's personal history. The played story comes to light in relationships and interpersonal interactions with the members of the group and the engaged therapists. Suppressed, repressed[6] or split-off feelings emerge and are progressively verbalized; constantly recurring emotional conflicts are being elaborated and eventually resolved.

In psychodrama therapy, the child will try out new relationship patterns, invent alternative relationships and, thanks to his increasing awareness, free himself from unconscious adverse entanglements. The phantasmatic conflict configurations with the original emotional disturbances, repeatedly enacted in scenic representations, need to be gradually processed; the resulting symbolic (re)constructions allow with time to resolve conflictual situations and release emotional energy in a cathartic way.

---

[6] Repression is unconsciously blocking unwanted thoughts or impulses, whereas suppression is voluntary.

Regressive Needs

"It is a sophisticated game of hide-and-seek, in which it is a joy to be hidden but a disaster not to be found" ([53], 186).

Many adopted children desire repeatedly to play hiding; there intensive wish is to be searched and to be found. There joy of having been found seems to symbolize the so much needed reassurance from the therapists' attentive presence and active participation.

In group therapy or psychodrama groups, adopted children express their regressive needs; they want to be carried, to drink at mother's breast, to be cared for like infants; they insist on living a holding experience [54]. Through their nonverbal behavior, adopted children express experienced states of confusion, disorientation, and overwhelming emotions of their past, which they are incapable to communicate with words. Archaic fears of fragmentation, disintegration, annihilation, and death are expressed through bodily manifestations. Children drop or throw themselves to the ground; they are often hypotonic or show poorly coordinated motor hyperactivity. They seem not knowing their own body boundaries, are ignorant of what is outside and what is inside their body, as if having lost contact with their own body. In their motor clumsiness, children often bump into each other or hurt themselves, the bodily pain provides a sense of feeling their existence.

Personalization means a firm relationship between the mind and the body. Depersonalization and disintegration are emergency mechanism, serving the ego[7] as a defense against unbearable sensations, originating from the body. Disintegration is painful and perceived as a threat [55]. In psychoanalytic psychodrama group therapy, emotionally deprived adopted children first learn to perceive and become aware of their feelings, to know their bodies, especially their body boundaries, and to distinguish between the inside and outside of their bodies. As long as children act with their bodies, a mental process will not take place. Parallel to their body investment, children's linguistic and symbolic abilities evolve. With time they learn to integrate archaic aggressive and destructive impulses and to subordinate their feelings and fantasies of magical omnipotence to a reality principle. Only when adopted children no longer enact their suffered psychic traumas in repetitive form and in a hypomanic way, they will be able to represent their lived traumatic experiences in play scenes. A mental process of psychic working through follows, allowing emotional and cognitive development to resume. Phantasmatic conflict configurations of traumatic experiences are being processed through their repeated enactments in play scenes. The efficacy of the psychodrama therapy is achieved by the symbolization process, namely the assimilation and accommodation of all feelings, associated with the traumatic experiences, into a mental elaboration.

---

[7] Ego-integration is the process of the development of an inner world, the capacity to make sense of one's own experience.

Summary

Psychic stressful, highly painful situations represent cumulative psychic traumas leading to different post-traumatic consequences. Offering a meaningful dialogue and a sustainable relationship within the safe and reliable framework of analytical psychotherapy helps the adoptee to unfold his fantasies and to express his pain and suffering. In analytical psychotherapy, the goal of processing traumata is to reduce the high intensity of the emotional distress, to elaborate meaning of the lived experiences and to understand - in working through the trauma - its impact on the adoptee's development. In the transference, psychoanalytic work opens the possibility of a kind of reenactment of conflicts in the present and thus of retrospective attribution.[8] This enables a patient - in the therapeutic relation with the therapist - to feel and understand his emotions, associated with his lived traumatic events. The compulsively repetitive and unchanged experience can be transformed, and dissociated parts integrated. The transformation of psychic pain through the process of symbolization promotes psychic growth. Phantasms, dreams, myths, daydreams, and artistic creations represent mental expressions of lived events and their assimilation. Emotional experiences, which are only present as a void in memory, often appear in the therapeutic relationship in the form of nightmares with feelings of terror, fear, distress, or anxiety; in this situation, communication in words lacks emotional resonance or is impossible, leading to persistent silence. Psychic working through and integrating past affective experiences with the aim of finding one's identity and regaining those psychic functions which were impaired by defenses, such as dissociation and isolation, is an extremely painful process.

Specific Topics in the Therapeutic Process with Adoptees

Loss and Reparation

Loss is a central theme in all therapies. For adoptees, loss is potentially reversible. The effort to regain the lost object - the birth parents - may take an active form when adoptees search for parents or relatives. They try to compensate for the relationship breakup, hoping to gain a sense of wholeness. Adoptees report desperately to feel a painful emptiness and complain to experience their environment as if time and place have been suspended. The adoptees' grief cannot be described as pathological because the birth parents are alive in their consciousness, i.e., they are still present.

---

[8] Retrospective attribution (Modell 2006) or deferred action (in German Nachträglichkeit) implies a complex and reciprocal relationship between a significant event and its later reinvestment with meaning.

Adoptees live different intensities of emotional vulnerability when confronted with additional losses or rejections [56].

The therapist is sometimes fantasized as a long-lost relative, the reason why adoptees often show great curiosity regarding their psychotherapist. He may also be idealized as a birth parent substitute and the adopted child wishes to resemble him. These are attempts and strong wishes to make up for the original loss and to be relieved from associated mysterious representations and phantasms.

Vignette

Johannes, 9 years old, wants to know "everything" about his psychotherapist and constantly presses her with personal questions about her relationships, her life story, her professional motivation, her faith, and wishes to get to know the therapist's family. Johannes rejects any intervention of his therapist, such as his curiosity concerning his birth parents, their biography, and his own life story before the adoption. He threatens to break off the psychotherapy he just started if the therapist does not answer his questions. Johannes says being entitled to know as much about the therapist as she knows about him. He estimates that he is the one to ask questions and not the therapist. After an interview with his adoptive parents, which was prepared with Johannes, he accuses the therapist - who informs him about the conversation she had with his adoptive parents - of not having asked his permission. He insults the therapist for being ignorant and not interested.

Comment

Johannes projects his anger towards his biological parents, which were not interested in him, and his ignorance onto his psychotherapist. He does not know his biological family, his origins, his parents' and his own personal history.

Why he was given up for adoption, why his biological parents were not interested in him, remain unanswered questions for him. He menaces to break off the relationship with the therapist as his biological parents have broken off the relationship with him.

Envy and Jealousy

Adopted children - compared to biological children - lack many personal contents and facts about their family background, such as their biographical and medical history, kinship structures, cultural, linguistic, or ethnic ties, and physical similarities with the adoptive parents. Adoptees consider these privileges to be a necessary condition for their physical and psychic well-being. The lack of these advantages is felt as privation or loss and is accompanied by feelings of envy and jealousy [57]. The adoptees' experience of being not like others (like members of the adoptive family or like others in the peer group), often represents a continuous frustration, with feelings of inauthenticity and nonbelonging. Adoptees try to appropriate these envied favorable attributes, hoping to gain a better psychic well-being.

Body Image and Sexuality

The adoptee's body is the only connection with his birth parents. A child's (un) conscious attempt to be the same or similar corresponds to a process arising from the infantile experience of his undifferentiated self. Subsequently primary parent-child relationship representations are internalized by the child [58]. The more differentiated and structured the world of internal representations and skills acquired by the infant and the young child is, the greater is his autonomy from the caregivers, on both psychological and bodily levels. Imitation and identification processes serve to develop and strengthen feelings of belonging and promote the formation of all subsequent developmental steps. The adoptees' emotions relating to their body image are associated with their unconscious or conscious intense desire to get to know the physical image of their birth parents.

The development of their sexual identity reflects sometimes the adoptees' identification with a fertile (the biological parents) or non-fertile (the adoptive parents) sexual identity. Female adoptees may fantasize themselves sterile like their adoptive mother or impulsive, i.e., promiscuous like the biological mother. The representation of their sexual identity is often associated with loss, punishment, rivalry, and rejection. For female adoptees, reproductive capacity is frequently accompanied by mystery, anxiety, fear, and the need to differentiate themselves from the adoptive sterile mother. Reproductive capacity and its relation to sexuality are issues that can stir up envious resentment (unconscious or conscious) on the part of the adoptive mother towards the female adoptee. Female adoptees harbor fantasies that their release for adoption is due to their gender, the birthmother would not have rejected a boy. For adoptees and their therapists, the working through of the adoptees' phantasms and fears concerning their own body image and sexuality, as well as the one of both sets of parents, is a highly complex process.

Control

In psychotherapies, the question arises whether the control over an event is situated within the adoptees' area of influence, i.e., within his power (internal control), or if the adoptee is convinced having no power of influence, believing that the control lies outside his person (external control). Adoptees often complain that the adoption situation has prevented them in their attempts to actively care for and meet their needs. They adopt a helpless position and regard adoption as the main cause of their personal developmental impairment. They sometimes behave in a particularly passive manner and tend to allow others to take responsibility for them. Since their release for adoption was determined by others, they assume that the source of their decision-making and orientation in life lies outside. Overcoming this characteristic passivity of adoptees, accompanied frequently by a paralysis of ego functions (e.g., an inability to distinguish cause from effect), is one of the most difficult goals of treatment.

Sense of Belonging

Adoptees lack the subjective experience of their self as holistic, truthful, and thus the ability to plan their own personal development, starting from the past into the present and anticipating the future [59]. The discourse of adoptees repeatedly points to themes of disruption, separation, rejection, abandonment, and exclusion. The social environment, lacking understanding and empathy, often does not identify this psychic amputation. Adoptees manifest their sense of mistrust through acting, distancing, or withdrawing their engagement in the therapeutic relationship; they may question the continuity of their therapy. This defensive organization is built up against fears of rejection and repudiation. Overwhelming feelings of dependence and clinging behavior may express the adoptees desire to perceive a sense of belonging.

Conflicts around attachment and separation intensify the longing for a biological connection, i.e., to be really part of a biological family with its past, present, and future. There is a great desire and yearning to belong to the genetic ancestors and to be remembered by the descendants. Internalized parental figures are split in accepting parts (adoptive parents) and in abandoning parts (biological parents). In a psychotherapeutic process it is of central importance that the therapist represents for adoptees an undivided, unified object. Working on the defensive split of the parental figures is essential for enabling the adoptee to integrate into *one* parental image the abandoning, rejecting and the adopting, accepting, partial representations of the parental figures [60]. This helps the adoptee for his part to "adopt" his adoptive parents, i.e., to evolve from a passive position "I was adopted" towards an active and engaged attitude "my adoptive parents are my parents".

The therapeutic work in the adoption situation must deal with aggression [61]. Accepting and understanding the child's destructive movements is not enough. The child must make the experience of the destruction of the object and realize that the object survives and really exists outside himself, outside of the subject's omnipotent control. For Winnicott "use of the object" means its destruction in fantasy and its survival in reality. The working through aggressiveness in the therapeutic transference relationship is demanding, however essential for promoting that adoptees are capable to establish integral object relations and to develop freely according to their wishes [62].

There can be no keener revelation of a society's soul than the way in which it treats its children. Nelson Mandela.

Placement Office

Placement agencies, private or public institutions, vary greatly from country to country, in the USA even from state to state.

The placement agencies are confronted with a variety of tasks and difficulties. Professionals working in the adoption field seek for a better preparation of the applicants for adoption, of the children to be adopted, and for more intensive follow-up support for adoptive families [63, 64].

An interdisciplinary team is required, available for the adopted child, the adoptive parents, and the adoptive family, ensuring continuous care and support by the same contact persons; their positive influences contribute significantly to the relationship formation of adoptees and their families. The task assignment of the intervening third party is to accompany childless couples in their exploration of prospective parenthood, support the building up of the parent-child attachment after the child's admission and recognize the act of the child's adoption, his legal parentage.

Mediatory accompaniments need to be provided during a certain time, to enhance a dialogue with all parties involved in the adoption situation and to promote progressive and mutual psychic processing of all family members, thus contributing to the integration of the child - with his personal history - into the adoptive family and the family's history.

The tasks of placement agencies can be divided into those before the adoption procedure, during the care relationship and after the legal adoption has taken place [65]. Pre-placement and post-placement services must prepare and empower adoptive parents to deal effectively with the emerging difficult adoption situations. This is especially indicated for parents who adopt children with complex or developmental trauma disorders; helping these children to integrate permanently into their new family is a highly demanding, emotionally stressful, and unpredictable task [66].

Before the Adoption Procedure

The referral agency is the place where information is exchanged, providing not only information about the child to be adopted, his social, medical, and genetic history, but also pointing out - to prospective adoptive parents - the specific issues involved in adopting a child and the potential problems and difficulties that may arise.

Prospective parents need to be informed that the first encounter with their future child may represent a stressful, even traumatic event. In international adoption, parents generally travel to meet their child in his country of origin and then return home with him. In the first parent-child interaction, parents are confronted with the child's living conditions and his often-poor health, visible by his bodily presentation. Parents may feel forlorn and fearful, worrying about their or their future child's aggressive or rejecting reactions and the child's health [67].

Literature references on adoption, contacts with other adoptive parents and support groups prove to be helpful for prospective adoptive parents [3, 68]. In France, the evaluation process, before permission is given to adopt a child, usually takes 9 months, which corresponds to a "psychological pregnancy". The discussions with social workers, psychologists, psychiatrists, and child psychiatrists during this time play an extremely important role in preparing the future adoptive parents to accommodate their child [64].

In other words, it lies in the task assignment of the adoption professionals' responsibility to prepare future adoptive parents for the adoption of a child, a highly significant event [69]. Prospective adoptive parents should receive as detailed information as possible about the child to be adopted. This includes information about the child's personal history, his biological parents, social and cultural environment, stage of development, somatic and or psychic disorders, including their severity and associated potential risks. Whenever possible, this information ought to be available before the adoption procedure.

The specific difficulties associated with the adoption situation need to be addressed at the time of the arrival of the child, in the further course of his development, as well as in critical developmental transitions. Relevant literature should be made available to prospective adoptive parents and the opportunity offered to discuss with professionals and to exchange with experienced adoptive families.

During the Care Relationship, before Legal Adoption

This period represents a critical time, in which crisis situations may arise. Simultaneously, the first encounters and contacts between parents and child take place, which are of greatest importance: the child faces a period of high vulnerability, due to the circumstances of his uprooting, and the future adoptive parents are confronted with a period of unpredictability, uncertainty, often associated with fears and disappointments. During this critical period of a child's integration, the family, the adoptive parents, or individual family members benefit to be assisted by professionals.

After Legal Adoption

Specific counselling and therapy sessions by professionals, familiar with adoption, ought to be created and provided to adoptive families [70]. In certain circumstances, family therapy in a variety of settings is recommended, e.g., at home, at school, and in the community, considering the specific differences of each adoptive family [65]. According to adoptive parents, support groups for adoptive families proved to be most helpful. In therapeutic interventions with adoptive families, it is important to understand the perspective of the family context; adoptive parents should not be blamed for their children's difficulties. Understanding the impact that adoption has on each stage of the child's development and acknowledging the child's past are crucial [71, 72]. Therapeutic treatment aims to help adoptive parents find better ways of relating to the inner emotional, phantasmatic, often confused imaginative world of their adopted child. Understanding the child's emotional fantasy world improves adoptive parents' coping with his behavior. Parents need to be reassured that their adopted child's problems arise from the child's pre-adoption experiences and not from the parents' insufficient parenting skills [73].

The results of questionnaires and semi-structured interviews (9 months after the adoptive child's placement) showed that the newly formed adoptive families need support mainly in the domains of promoting children's health and development, strengthening family relationships, and fostering children's identity. Further requests for assistance are how to face contacts with birth parents, relatives, and other significant care persons and how to deal with financial and legal issues [74].

Interventions by the placement agency must be tailored to the adoptive family's living situation. The collaboration of all persons concerned, and all professionals involved in the adoption situation is required and their needs to be supported by objectivity, impartiality, and mutual respect. Adoptive parents, adoptees, and siblings are to be informed about the assistance available and are to express their wishes about possible therapeutic measures and make their own decisions. Professional help is intended to strengthen adoptive parents and their families in their competences, but not to devalue, blame, or patronize them. In particularly difficult adoption situations, joint planning with the adoptive parents and their families, regarding the measures to be taken in a crisis, proves to be advantageous.

In the USA the goal of the National Child Traumatic Stress Network (NCTSN) is to raise the standard of care and improve access to services for traumatized children, their families, and communities throughout the United States. Interventions consist in trauma screenings for all children and youth coming into contact with the child welfare system and address trauma by multiple interveners for children, biological parents, foster and adoptive parents, and caseworkers [75].

Postplacement support must be adapted specifically to the individual needs of each adoptive parent and adoptive family; anticipation and identification of when and what is required, as well as for whom, is a challenging task, demanding of involved practitioners some experience with adoptive families [76].

With regard to treatment measures of traumatized children and adolescents, there is often a painful decision to take, of whether to let a child stay in the care of persons or institutions who are sources of hurt and threat, or whether to expose the child to abandonment and separation distress by taking him away from familiar environments and persons to whom he is attached, but who are likely to cause him further substantial harm [77].

Trauma-informed parenting workshop - by the NCTSN - aims to improve parents' and caregivers' awareness of the impacts of trauma on their children and to reduce their challenging behaviors [78]. This therapeutic intervention includes the child and the caregiver and aims at helping parents to understand the multiple impacts of trauma on the child, to recognize signs and symptoms of trauma, to respond in a supporting way to the child, thus avoiding re-traumatizing. Findings from participating adopted children and their adoptive parents show improvements, such as enhanced positive parenting approaches, decreased parenting stress, and less externalizing and internalizing behaviors of their children [79].

The evaluation of another parenting therapeutic intervention (The Incredible Years parenting program), for adoptive parents and their children, reports that parents feel significantly less stressed and more competent, and their children's behavioral difficulties decrease [80].

Various studies of psychological interventions with adoptive parents were reviewed with regard to the psychic well-being, behavioral functioning, and parent-child relationship of adopted children and adolescents. Interventions using video-feedback help parents reflecting on their interactions with their child, as well as on measures for changing his behavior, thus enhancing adopted children's and adolescents' emotional and behavioral development [81].

References

1. Harms E, Strehlow B. Das Traumkind in der Realität. Göttingen: Vandenhoeck & Ruprecht; 1990.
2. Heinemann C. Neuentscheidungstherapie bei Pflege-, Adoptiv- und Heimkindern mit Scheiterer-Verläufen. Prax Kinderpsychol Kinderpsychiat. 1994;43:130–7.
3. Nickman SL, Rosenfeld AA, Fine P, Macintyre JC, Pilowsky DJ, Howe RA, Derdeyn A, et al. Children in adoptive families: overview and update. J.Amer.Acad. Child. Adolesc Psychiatry. 2005;44(10):987–95.
4. Prew C. Therapy with adoptive families: an innovative approach. Fall: The Prevention Report; 1990. p. 8.
5. Wieder H (1990) Behandlungstechnische Probleme bei der Psychoanalyse adoptierter Kinder.
6. Kernberg P. Child analysis with a disturbed adopted child. Int J Psychoanal Psychother. 1985;11:277–99.
7. Sanzana A, Schmid-Kitsikis E. La présence des absents: les mouvements identificatoires d'un enfant adopté. Psychiatrie de l'enfant XXXVIII. 1995;1:69–107.
8. Wilkinson S, Hough G (1996) Lie as narrative truth in abused adopted adolescents.
9. Steck B. Eltern-Kind-Beziehungsproblematik bei der Adoption. Praxis der Kinderpsychol Kinderpsychiatrie. 1998a;4:240–62.
10. Steck B. Die psychoanalytisch-orientierte Psychodrama-Gruppentherapie bei Kindern und Jugendlichen. Teil 1: Kinderanalyse 6, 278-310. Teil 2. Kinderanalyse. 1998b;6:248–77.
11. Steck B. Die psychoanalytisch-orientierte Psychodrama-Gruppentherapie bei Kindern und Jugendlichen. Teil. 1999;3: Kinderanalyse 7:23–52.
12. Howard JA, Smith SL. Adoption preservation in Illinois: results of a four year study. Normal, IL: Illinois State University; 1995.
13. Brinich PM. Some potential effects of adoption on self and object representations. Psychoanal Study Child. 1980;35:107–33.
14. Lifton BJ. Journey of the adopted self: a quest for wholeness. New York, NY: Basic Books; 1994.
15. Lifton BJ. Ghosts in the adopted family. Psychoanal Inq. 2009;30(1):71–9. https://doi.org/10.1080/07351690903200176.
16. Winnicott DW. Fear of breakdown. No: International Review of Psycho-Analysis; 1974. p. 1.
17. Pinderhughes EE, Matthews JAK, Zhang X, Scott JC. Unpacking complexities in ethnic–racial socialization in transracial adoptive families: a process-oriented transactional system. Dev Psychopathol. 2021;33:493–505. https://doi.org/10.1017/S0954579420001741.
18. Skandrani S, Harf A, El Husseini M. The impact of Children's pre-adoptive traumatic experiences on parents. Front Psych. 2019;10:866. https://doi.org/10.3389/fpsyt.2019.00866.

19. Lamour M, Maury M. Alliance autour du bébé. PUF, Paris: Monographie de la psychiatrie enfant; 2000.
20. Fraiberg S, Adelson E, Shapiro V. Ghosts in the nursery: a Psychoanalyt-ic. Approach to the problems of impaired infant-mother relationship. J. of the American Academy of child. Psychiatry. 1975;14(3):387–421.
21. Kellermann NPF. Geerbtes Trauma'. Die Konzeptualisierung der trans-generationellen Weitergabe von Traumata. Tel Aviver Jahrbuch für deutsche Ge-schichte. 2011;39:137–60.
22. Moré A. Zum psychoanalytischen Verständnis transgenerationaler Übertragungen. Swiss Archives of Neurology, Psychiatry and Psychotherapy. 2018;169(8)
23. Badoni M. (2003): Parents and their child—and the analyst in the middle. Working with a transgenerational mandate. Int. J. Psychoanal. 2002;83, 1111.
24. Maldonado JL. What is your theory of unconscious processes? What are other theories that you would contrast with your conceptualization? Response by Jorge Luis Maldonado. Int J Psychoanal. 2011;92:280–3. https://doi.org/10.1111/j.1745-8315.2011.00425.x.
25. Breuer J, Freud S. Studies on hysteria. 2nd ed. Leipzig: Deuticke; 1895.
26. Anthony RE, Paine AL, Shelton KH. Depression and anxiety symptoms of British adoptive parents: a prospective four-wave longitudinal study. Int J Environ Res Public Health. 2019;16:5153. https://doi.org/10.3390/ijerph16245153.
27. Rushton A, Monck E, Upright H, Davidson M. Enhancing adoptive parenting: devising promising interventions. Child Adolescent Mental Health. 2006;11:25–31. https://doi.org/10.1111/j.1475-3588.2005.00371.x.
28. Juffer F, Bakermans-Kranenburg MJ, Van IJzendoorn MH. The importance of parenting in the development of dis organized attachment: evidence from a preventive intervention study in adoptive families. J Child Psychol Psychiatry. 2005;46:263–74.
29. Juffer F. Bakermans-Kranenburg MJ (2018) working with video-feedback intervention to promote positive parenting and sensitive discipline (VIPP-SD): a case study. J Clin Psychol. 2018;74:1346–57.
30. Harris-Waller J, Granger C, Hussain M. Psychological interventions for adoptive parents: a systematic review. Adoption & Fostering. 2018;42(1):6–21.
31. Robinson F, Luyten P, Midgley N. Child psychotherapy with looked after and adopted children: a UK national survey of the profession. Journal of Child Psychotherapy. 2017;43(2):258–77. https://doi.org/10.1080/0075417X.2017.1324506.
32. Ogden TH. What's true and whose idea was it? Int J Psychoanal. 2003;84:593–606.
33. Mancia M. Implicit memory and early unrepressed unconscious: their role in the therapeutic process (how the neurosciences can contribute to psychoanalysis). Int J Psychoanal. 2006;87(Pt 1):83–103.
34. Buk A. The Mirror neuron system and embodied simulation: clinical implications for art therapists working with trauma survivors. Arts Psychother. 2009;36
35. Bürgin D, Steck B, Schwald A. Verstehen und Deuten im Trauerprozess eines 5¾jährigen traumatisierten Knaben. Kinderanalyse. 2001;4:395–421.
36. Barrois C. Les névroses traumatiques. Paris: Dunod; 1988.
37. Freud S. Beyond the pleasure principle, vol. XVIII. London: Hogarth Press; 1920. p. 7–64.
38. Winnicott DW. Playing and reality. London: Tavistock; 1971a.
39. Cohen D. Life is with others, selected writings on child psychiatry. New Haven: Yale University Press; 2006.
40. Freud A. Normality and pathology in childhood. New York: International University Press; 1965.
41. Bürgin D, Steck B. Indikation psychoanalytischer Psychotherapie bei Kindern und Jugendlichen, Diagnostisch-therapeutisches Vorgehen und Fallbeispiele. Stuttgart: Klett-Cotta; 2013. ISBN 978-3-608-94829-5
42. Bürgin D. Zur Indikation psychoanalytischer Psychotherapie bei Kindern und Jugendlichen. Kinderanalyse. 1992;2(1):22–45.

43. Marion P. Some reflections on the unique time of Nachträglichkeit in theory and clinical practice. Int J Psychoanal. 2012;93(2):317–40. https://doi.org/10.1111/j.1745-8315.2011.00530.x.
44. Bruschweiler-Stern N, Harrison AM, Lyons-Ruth K, Morgan AC, Nahum JP, Sander LW, et al. Explicating the implicit: the local level and the microprocess of change in the analytic situation. Int J Psychoanal. 2002;83(Pt 5):1051–62.
45. Winnicott DW. Therapeutic consultations in child psychiatry. London: Hogarth; 1971b.
46. Quinodoz D. Growing old: a psychoanalyst's point of view. Int J Psychoanal. 2000;90:773–93.
47. Winnicott DW. Home is where we start from: essays by a psychoanalyst. In: Shepherd R, Davis M, editors. Winnicott C. Reading: Addison-Wesley; 1987b.
48. Guyotat J. Mort/naissance et filiation. Etudes de psychopathologie sur le lien de filiation. Paris: Masson; 1980.
49. Nasio JD. Le livre de la douleur et de l'amour. Paris: Editions Payot & Rivages; 1996.
50. Moreno JL. Psychodrama I. New York: Beacon House; 1946.
51. Moreno JL. Psychodrama II. New York: Beacon House; 1959.
52. Anzieu D. Le psychodrame analytique chez l'enfant et l'adolescent. Paris: Presses universitaires de France; 1979.
53. Winnicott DW (1963) Communicating and not communicating leading to a study of certain opposites.
54. Winnicott DW. The maturational processes and the facilitating environment. New York: International Universities Press; 1965.
55. Winnicott DW (1962) Ego integration in child development, in: the maturational processes and the facilitating environment. Pp. 56-63 New York: international universities press, 1965.
56. Bertocci D, Schechter MD. Adopted adults' perception of their need to search: implications for clinical practice. Smith College Studies in Social Work. 1991;61:179–96.
57. Anderson RE. Envy and jealousy. J Coll Stud Psychother. 1987;1:49–81.
58. Stern DN. The interpersonal world of the infant. A view from psychoanalysis and developmental psychology. New York: Basic Books; 1985.
59. Schechter MD, Bertocci D. The meaning of search. In: Brodzinsky DM, Schechter MD, editors. The psychology of adoption. New, Oxford: Oxford University Press; 1990. p. 62–90.
60. Quinodoz D. "J'ai peur de tuer mon enfant" ou "Œdipe abandonné, Œdipe adopté". Rev Franç Psychanal. 1987;51(6):1579–93.
61. Winnicott DW. The use of an object and relating through identifications. In: Winnicott C, Shepherd R, Davis M, editors. Psychoanalytic explorations. Cambridge, MA: Harvard University Press; 1968. p. 218–27.
62. Waber-Thevoz H, Waber JP. Le lien d'adoption à l'épreuve du temps. Neuropsychiatrie de l'Enfance et l'Adolescence. 2000;48:179–98.
63. Brodzinsky D, Livingston Smith S. Commentary: understanding research, policy, and practice issues in adoption instability. Res Soc Work Pract. 2018:1–10.
64. Ozoux-Teffaine O. Enjeux de l'adoption tardive. Nouveaux fondements pour la clinique. La vie de l'enfant Ramonville Saint-Agne: Edition eres; 2004.
65. Barth RP, Miller JM. Building effective post-adoption services: what is the empirical foundation? Familiy relations 49(4), 447-455. Child Dev. 2000;77(3):696–711.
66. Hartinger-Saunders RM, Jones AS, Rittner B. Improving access to trauma-informed adoption services: Applying a Developmental Trauma Framework. Journ Child Adol Trauma. 2019;12:119–30.
67. Harf A, Skandrani S, Radjack R, Sibeoni J, Moro MR, et al. First parent-child meetings in international adoptions: a qualitative study. PLoS One. 2013;8(9):e75300. https://doi.org/10.1371/journal.pone.0075300.
68. Barth RP, Berry M. Preventing adoption disruption. Prev Hum Serv. 1991;9:205–22.
69. Lee BR, Kobulskya JM, Brodzinsky D, Bartha RP. Parent perspectives on adoption preparation: findings from the modern adoptive families project. Child Youth Serv Rev. 2018;85:63–71.
70. Cohen NJ, Coyne J, Duvall J. Adopted and biological children in the clinic: family, parental and child characteristics. J Child Psychol Psychiat. 1993;34(4):545–62.

71. Howard JA, Smith SL. Strenthening adoptive families: a synthesis of post-legal adoption opportunities grants. Normal, IL: Illinois State University; 1997.
72. Prew C, Suter S, Carrington J. Post adoption family therapy: a practice manual. Salem, OR: Children's Services Division; 1990.
73. Groze V, Young J, Corcran-Rumppe K. Post adoption resources for training. Networking and evaluation services (PARTNERS): working with special needs adoptive families in stress. Washington, DC: Prepared with Four Oeaks, Inc., Cedar Rapids, Iowa, for the Department of Health and Human Services, Adoption Opportunities.; 1991.
74. Meakings S, Ottaway H, Coffey A, Palmer C, Doughty J, Shelton K. The support needs and experiences of newly formed adoptive families: findings from the Wales adoption study. Adoption & Fostering. 2018;42(1):58–75. https://doi.org/10.1177/0308575917750824.
75. Conradi L, Agosti J, Tullberg E, Richardson L, Langan H, Ko S, Wilson C. Promising practices and strategies for using trauma-informed child welfare practice to improve foster care placement stability: a breakthrough series collaborative. Child Welfare. 2011;90(6):207–25.
76. Lee BR, Battalen AW, Brodzinsky DM, Goldberg AE. Parent, child, and adoption characteristics associated with post-adoption support needs. Soc Work Res. 2020;44(1)
77. Streeck-Fischer A, van der Kolk B. Down will come baby, cradle and all: diagnostic and therapeutic implications of chronic trauma on child development. Aust N Z J Psychiatry. 2000;34(6):903–18.
78. Sullivan KM, Murray KJ, Ake GS. Trauma-informed care for children in the child welfare system an initial evaluation of a trauma-informed parenting workshop. Child Maltreat. 2015:077559515615961.
79. Allen B, Timmer SG, Urquiza AJ. Parent–child interaction therapy as an attachment-based intervention: theoretical rationale and pilot data with adopted children. Child Youth Serv Rev. 2014;47:334–41.
80. Henderson K, Sargent N. Developing the incredible years. Webster-Stratton parenting skills training program for use with adoptive families. Adopt Foster. 2005;29(4):34–44.
81. Ní Chobhthaigh S, Duffy F. The effectiveness of psychological interventions with adoptive parents on adopted children and adolescents' outcomes: a systematic review. Clin Child Psychol Psychiatry. 2018:1–26. https://doi.org/10.1177/1359104518786339.

Appendix

Each adoptee has his own history, his own difference, which we must learn to live with, without denying it or cultivating it excessively. The construction of a personality consists in recognizing this diversity, accepting, and transcending it.

Marie Brunet (1989, preface)

Epilogue

Adoptees unique life history is marked by three essential perspectives, which represent specific challenges during each developmental period in childhood and adolescence and have life-long influences on the adult adoptee. The main inherent differences of adoptive personal and family life are described.

Psychic Trauma

For the child, adoption always means a relationship breakup with his biological parents and the creation of a new relationship with adoptive parents. This relational dynamic is a lifelong process of the persons involved in this triangle. In transcultural adoptions, the loss of biological parents is compounded by the loss of ethnic, cultural, and linguistic ties. Some children experience this relational loss as a psychic trauma, namely when their grievance, associated with feelings of being rejected, abandoned, or expelled, cannot be overcome, and lead to a desolate self-esteem. Ethnocultural differences are linked to feelings of alienation and exclusion and aggravate self-integration.

A mourning process is required to work through the trauma associated with adoption and to build emotionally sustaining bonds with the adoptive parents. Grieving is complicated by the fact that there is usually uncertainty about the life and death of the biological parents, and the adopted child has no explanation for his

B. Steck, *Adoption as a Lifelong Process*, https://doi.org/10.1007/978-3-031-33038-4

abandonment; in addition, there are no relatives of the biological parents present. A child needs a continuous relationship with a meaningful adult to be able to mourn. If adoptive parents are burdened by own unprocessed losses, e.g., their inability to procreate, they are emotionally unavailable to help their child in his mourning process. Adopted children then try to cope with the adoption event by building up a fantasy world "explaining" what happened to them. In their inner world, real events, received information and own fantasies blend into often confusing and conflicting family romances representations, which may be expressed in a variety of psychic or psychosomatic symptoms.

Revelation of the Adoption Status

The process of informing the child about his adoption takes over years and shapes his developmental history. Every young child deals with the questions of conception and birth. The adopted child wants to know why his adoptive mother did not carry him in her womb and gave him birth. The information must be continuous, adapted to the child's age and ability to understand, and aimed at not harming his self-esteem. Information about origin and adoption are often followed by children's questions about the reasons for their release for adoption. Providing these information calls for enormous empathy and great emotional support from adoptive parents for their child.

The communication process is complicated by adopted children and sometimes by adoptive parents; adopted children can deny their adoption, desiring to forget their past. They may also feel the adoptive parents' anxieties to be disqualified or questioned in favor of idealized biological parents. In addition, adoptive parents often find it difficult to explain the difference between sexual activity and procreative infertility, this to an even greater extent, if they feel insecure in their sexual competence because of their infertility.

Identity Development

The formation of a personal identity includes also genealogical aspects, by which each individual feels connected to previous and future generations, a continuity that adoptees lack in their identity development. In all steps of individuation and separation in childhood and adolescence, adopted children are reminded of their adoption situation and the related relationship breakups. With increasing age and better understanding of adoption, most adoptees are confronted by the necessity to deal with their origins. Their interest may lead to the search for their biological parents. Thereby loyalty conflicts arise because of the dual parental pairs and possibly dual ethno-cultural affiliation. Adopted children may then split the inner images of biological and adoptive parents into good and bad representations. They only identify with the fantasized bad or idealized characteristics of the biological parents, for example, and behave accordingly. This is an attempt to cope with the relationship constellation of dual parenthood (biological and adoptive parents) and to maintain mostly unconscious loyalty ties to the biological parents.

Research and clinical experience show that selection, preparation, and support of adoptive families are of great importance. Whenever difficulties arise in the adoptive family or the adopted child/adolescent presents psychic problems, it is mandatory to adjust therapeutic measures specifically to the individual situation.

Outlook

The challenges for adoptive parents are shaped by a rapidly evolving society, by cultural diversity and by changing family structures (single parenthood, parenthood by sexual and gender minorities) and discontinuous parenting (separation or divorce). The available children for adoption are often older, sometimes disabled, or with personal traumatic experiences of neglect, abuse, or multiple placements.

Adoptive parents are obliged to engage in introspective reflection and psychic processing throughout the entire development of their adopted child. They face the critical task of exercising parental roles and functions and, at the same time, they feel the necessity to reevaluate and try to understand the relational interactions with their adopted child. This process of questioning, self-examination, doubting their parenting ability and personal competence can be accompanied by great distress and sometimes despair. Adoptive parents may feel inept for their task and believe being incapable to fulfill all the requirements. Their convictions—prior to the acceptance of their prospective child—have changed, namely their belief that their unconditional love will repair their child's adverse pre-adoptive experiences. They realize that the adoption experience is associated with much more complex difficulties than they ever imagined. At the same time, adoptive parents know how important it is to reaffirm their right and commitment to their parenthood and their faith and trust in their child. Thanks to their emotional sensitivity and empathy with their child's unique perception and imagination, as well as their acknowledgement of their child's motivations, values, and beliefs, they encourage their child's autonomy aspirations, enabling him to create his own history and individual relationships and to develop his personality. They help their adopted child to overcome his early childhood personal tragic experiences.

When the adopted child's historical and biographical reality and the persons belonging to it remain unknown, he is not able to share these essential elements with his present significant persons. In this sense, the confrontation of adopted children with their fate takes place on an intrapsychic level; their coping with and their meaning attribution to the adoption situation are not confirmed by their historical or biographical reality. The experienced external reality represents forever an uncertainty that adopted children carry with them and which is expressed above all by their sense of vulnerability. To acknowledge the child's unknown historical and biographical reality is essential. Adoptive parents need to recognize the importance of their child's psychic effort to accept his particular filiation. The establishment of stable and reliable relationships with protective and significant attachment figures contributes decisively to the attribution of meaning and psychic elaboration of adopted children's intern world.

The adopted child has the dual character of an abandoned and chosen child. Founders of religions such as Moses and, in the ancient mythologies, founders of civilizations such as Romulus, as well as other heroes or prophets whose births were fabulous or mysterious, were both abandoned and found children. These famous people may be on the forefront of the scene of history because they were driven by a yearning search and passion. Many adopted young people bear witness to their dramatic search, their desire to know their origins and their passion for comprehension through their artistic works.

The History of Oedipus

Laius, king of Thebes, married to Jocasta, consulted for his childlessness the Oracle of Delphi, who predicted that his son would one day kill him and marry his own mother. For fear of the oracle, Laius pierced his son's feet after his birth, tied them together and ordered a shepherd to expose the infant on Mount Cithaeron. But the shepherd entrusted the child to a Corinthian shepherd who brought it to King Polybus of Corinth, whose marriage to Merope had remained childless. The boy was called Oedipus because of his swollen feet and was raised by the royal couple as their own son.

Adult, Oedipus was offended by a peer's statement about his origins: "Some man at a banquet who had drunk too much shouted out that I am not my father's son." Since he received no answer to the question of his origin from Merope and Polybus— what he believed to be his birth parents—he in turn consulted the oracle of Delphi and was informed that he would kill his father and marry his mother. To avoid the fulfillment of this prophecy, Oedipus did not return to Corinth. He went from Delphi to Thebes, and in a narrow pass at a fork of three paths was asked by the driver of a chariot to clear the way. In the following fight, Oedipus killed the charioteer and his passenger, Laius, his birth father.

Laius was on his way for consulting the oracle how he could free Thebes from the Sphinx, recognizable by her female head, her lion's body, her eagle's wings, and her serpent's tail. Hera, the wife of Zeus, had sent the Sphinx to punish Thebes for a crime, committed by Laius who had kidnapped the boy Chrysippus[1]. The Sphinx posed the following riddle to anyone passing by: "What creature with only one voice walks on four legs in the morning, on two legs at noon and on three legs in the evening?" She devoured anyone who could not solve the riddle.

Oedipus, arriving at the gates of Thebes, guessed the answer: it is man who crawls on all fours as an infant, stands on two legs in manhood and leans on a stick

---

[1] Chrysippus, son of king Pelops, was kidnapped by the Theban prince Laius, his tutor.

in old age. The Sphinx then threw itself from Mount Phikion and crashed in the valley. Out of gratitude, Oedipus was given the royal throne by Creon, brother of Jocasta. After Laius' death, Oedipus ruled Thebes and married Iocasta, the widow of Laius, without knowing that she was his birth mother.

From this marriage two sons (Eteocles and Polyneices) and two daughters (Antigone and Ismene) were born. Thebes was now ravaged by the plague. The oracle of Delphi, again consulted, proclaimed that Thebes would only be freed from the plague when the murderer of Laius was expelled from the city. Finally, the blind seer Tiresias revealed to Oedipus the events which had taken place. The Shepherd—who should have abandoned Oedipus—and the revelation of Oedipus' adoption by Merope, after the death of Polybus, confirmed the events. Jocasta hanged herself and Oedipus blinded himself.

Accompanied by his daughter Antigone, Oedipus—after long years of wandering—moved to Colonus in Attica, where he died. Eteocles and Polyneices fought each other for the control of Thebes after their father Oedipus abdicated and died. Creon, successor to Oedipus as king of Thebes, declared Polyneices who had fought against his own country as a traitor and ordered to let him decompose in public. Antigone returned to Thebes, where she disregarded Creon's order and buried her brother out of devotion and loyalty to the Gods and her family. Creon, enraged by her disobedience, wanted to lock her up alive in the family tomb as punishment. But Antigone and Haimon, Creon's son and the fiancé of Antigone, had already committed suicide.

In his Oedipus works, Sophocles portrayed the curse, which was passed from generation to generation in the Labdakid dynasty at the royal house in Thebes.

Back Cover

Adoption represents an event of intense and unpredictable experiences. Each adoption is a testimony of manifold human resources and of a unique personal commitment.

Adoption does not end with the acceptation of a child, but shapes the entire lives of adoptive parents, adopted children and biological parents.

Adoptive parents and adopted children are confronted with specific challenges on their shared life path. Many parents of adopted children experience stressful situations that are associated with great psychic strain for them and their children.

The adoption situation represents a complex reality for all members of the family and requires personal engagement and confrontation of each individual and the whole family. The adopted child is expected to accept his biological roots and his growing up as an adopted child. Individual members of an adoptive family cope with the adoption situation in varying ways and with different levels of processing ability. Integrating this highly significant event into the individual biography and family history is an exceptionally demanding task and an extraordinary achievement.

This book provides insights into the specific challenges adoptive families and adopted children face. It is aimed at adoptive families and professionals who are confronted with the adoption situation: Physicians, psychiatrists, child and youth psychiatrists, psychologists, psychotherapists, social workers, pedagogues, teachers, lawyers, as well as placement agencies, guardianship and child and youth protection authorities.

Index

© The Editor(s) (if applicable) and The Author(s), under exclusive license to
Springer Nature Switzerland AG 2023
B. Steck, *Adoption as a Lifelong Process*,
https://doi.org/10.1007/978-3-031-33038-4